Natural Products Chemistry: Advances in Synthetic, Analytical and Bioactivity Studies, Volume II

Natural Products Chemistry: Advances in Synthetic, Analytical and Bioactivity Studies, Volume II

Guest Editor

Giovanni Ribaudo

MDPI

Basel • Beijing • Wuhan • Barcelona • Belgrade • Novi Sad • Cluj • Manchester

Guest Editor
Giovanni Ribaudo
Department of Molecular and
Translational Medicine
University of Brescia
Brescia
Italy

Editorial Office
MDPI AG
Grosspeteranlage 5
4052 Basel, Switzerland

This is a reprint of the Special Issue, published open access by the journal *Molecules* (ISSN 1420-3049), freely accessible at: https://www.mdpi.com/journal/molecules/special_issues/ED4NLND979.

For citation purposes, cite each article independently as indicated on the article page online and as indicated below:

Lastname, A.A.; Lastname, B.B. Article Title. *Journal Name* **Year**, *Volume Number*, Page Range.

ISBN 978-3-7258-7018-9 (Hbk)
ISBN 978-3-7258-7019-6 (PDF)
https://doi.org/10.3390/books978-3-7258-7019-6

Cover image courtesy of Giovanni Ribaudo

Contents

About the Editor

Giovanni Ribaudo

Giovanni Ribaudo, PhD, received his Master's degree *cum laude* in Medicinal Chemistry and Technology at the University of Padova (Italy) in 2011 and his PhD in 2015 at the same Institution, after carrying out part of his research at the State University of New York, Albany (NY, USA). Between 2015 and 2019, Dr. Ribaudo worked as a post-doctoral researcher at the University of Padova collaborating with a private company in the field of natural-compound chemistry. In 2019, Dr. Ribaudo joined the Department of Molecular and Translational Medicine of the University of Brescia, where he is currently a lecturer in Medicinal Chemistry and in Drug Analysis for Pharmacy and Biotechnology. His research activity employs a combination of synthetic, analytical (HPLC, NMR, mass spectrometry) and computational medicinal chemistry tools, and his main research interests are the design and screening of small molecules interacting with peculiar DNA arrangements and nature-inspired drug-like bioactive compounds.

Dr. Ribaudo has co-authored more than 130 scientific papers, all published in recognized international journals, and 2 book chapters, and he is the inventor of 2 patents. In 2024, he was listed among the World's Top 2% Scientists in the field of Medicinal Chemistry.

molecules

MDPI

Editorial

Natural Products Chemistry: Advances in Synthetic, Analytical and Bioactivity Studies, Volume II

Giovanni Ribaudo

Department of Molecular and Translational Medicine, University of Brescia, Viale Europa 11, 25123 Brescia, Italy; giovanni.ribaudo@unibs.it

The idea of collecting novel contributions relating to the chemistry of natural compounds in this Special Issue stemmed from the success of the first edition of the collection entitled "Natural Products Chemistry: Advances in Synthetic, Analytical and Bioactivity Studies", which was published in *Molecules* in 2023 [1].

The field of chemical sciences, and of medicinal chemistry in particular, has always been strongly related to the world of natural products. Small organic compounds of natural origin are chemically diverse molecules, and they are characterized by a variety of scaffolds and functional groups. Moreover, chirality represents an additional feature [2].

The study of natural compounds is intriguing because of their potential applications, but it also carries several challenges from the point of view of their extraction and analytical characterization. At the same time, organic chemists put their best effort in the efficient synthesis and derivatization and optimization of natural compounds to produce optimized analogs, thus unleashing the potential of the semi-synthetic derivatives [3]. Flavonoids, alkaloids and terpenes are only some of the chemical classes that attract the interest of the medicinal chemist for the identification and development of novel therapeutic options [4,5]. Eventually, it must be considered that currently used theoretical drug discovery tools allow us to rationalize and translate into modern medicinal chemistry the traditional uses of nature-inspired molecules [6–8]. Indeed, medicinal chemistry is one of the fields of chemical sciences in which natural compounds traditionally find wide application. Such molecules are investigated for their anticancer roles through peculiar mechanisms [9], as antibacterial agents [10] and with the aim of developing novel tools against neurodegeneration [11,12]. Nevertheless, natural compounds are the focus of many other fields [13]. In this connection, food chemistry [14], engineering and material sciences represent only few examples [15,16].

This Special Issue aimed at collecting research papers and review articles related to the different aspects of the chemistry of natural compounds, including extraction, structural elucidation, synthesis and biological evaluation of natural, semi-synthetic derivatives and nature-inspired molecules. Particular attention was also dedicated to compounds of pharmaceutical interest. As a result, between 2024 and 2025, eight articles were published in this Special Issue, testifying the strong interest of the scientific community towards the chemistry of natural compounds under different perspectives. In particular, the Special Issue collected four research articles and four reviews. Moreover, it must be noted that this volume showed an international reach, as authors across the globe submitted their contributions. Indeed, corresponding authors from China, Ecuador, Italy, Japan, Poland, Saudi Arabia, South Africa, and USA, along with their collaborators from many other countries such as Egypt, Palestine, and Ukraine participated to this Special Issue with their research.

Molecules **2026**, *31*, 374 https://doi.org/10.3390/molecules31020374

In further detail, the research papers are concerned with the following: Dushna and colleagues synthesized N-oxide derivatives of alkaloids and characterized them through electrochemical studies. In the context of organic synthesis, Webber and Russu described trimethylenemethane cyclopentyl-annulations as a strategy to obtain a functionalized angular triquinane skeleton. Ayoup and colleagues reported the synthesis, characterization and antiproliferative activity of fluorinated isoflavones. Hu and colleagues analyzed the constituents, of medicinal interest, of *Andrographis paniculata* (Burm. f.).

Concerning review articles, Khwaza and Aderibigbe focused their contribution on the pharmacological properties of derivatives of ursolic acid. Adriana Monserrath Orellana-Paucar reviewed the therapeutic properties of turmeric essential oil components. In their contribution, Kato-Noguchi and Kato reviewed the defense molecules of the invasive plant species *Ageratum conyzoides*, while Antonio Evidente provided an overview of α-pyrones as phytotoxins produced by plant pathogen fungi.

The contributions collected in the Special Issue are listed below, following the order presented above.

- Dushna, O.; Dubenska, L.; Gawor, A.; Karasińki, J.; Barabash, O.; Ostapiuk, Y.; Blazheyevskiy, M.; Bulska, E. Structural Characterization and Electrochemical Studies of Selected Alkaloid N-Oxides. *Molecules* **2024**, *29*, 2721. https://doi.org/10.3390/molecules29122721.
- Webber, S.M.; Russu, W.A. Investigation of Trimethylenemethane Cyclopentyl-Annulations as a Strategy to Obtain a Functionalized Angular Triquinane Skeleton. *Molecules* **2024**, *29*, 5358. https://doi.org/10.3390/molecules29225358.
- Ayoup, M.S.; Daqa, M.; Salama, Y.; Hazzam, R.; Hawsawi, M.B.; Soliman, S.M.; Al-Maharik, N. Efficient Consecutive Synthesis of Fluorinated Isoflavone Analogs, X-Ray Structures, Hirshfeld Analysis, and Anticancer Activity Assessment. *Molecules* **2025**, *30*, 795. https://doi.org/10.3390/molecules30040795.
- Hu, E.; Cheng, R.; Liu, A.; Wang, Y.; Long, H.; Hou, J.; Wang, D.; Wu, W.; Wu, X. Metabolomic Profiles and Differential Constituents of Andrographis paniculata (Burm. f.) in Different Growth Stages and Parts. *Molecules* **2025**, *30*, 1490. https://doi.org/10.3390/molecules30071490.
- Khwaza, V.; Aderibigbe, B.A. Potential Pharmacological Properties of Triterpene Derivatives of Ursolic Acid. *Molecules* **2024**, *29*, 3884. https://doi.org/10.3390/molecules29163884.
- Orellana-Paucar, A. Turmeric Essential Oil Constituents as Potential Drug Candidates: A Comprehensive Overview of Their Individual Bioactivities. *Molecules* **2024**, *29*, 4210; https://doi.org/10.3390/molecules29174210.
- Kato-Noguchi, H.; Kato, M. Defense Molecules of the Invasive Plant Species Ageratum conyzoides. *Molecules* **2024**, *29*, 4673. https://doi.org/10.3390/molecules29194673.
- Evidente, A. An Overview of α-Pyrones as Phytotoxins Produced by Plant Pathogen Fungi. *Molecules* **2025**, *30*, 2813. https://doi.org/10.3390/molecules30132813.

In conclusion, the success of this Special Issue once again testifies the interest of the scientific community on the field of natural compounds, and prompts further research in the field.

Acknowledgments: G.R. acknowledges J.T. and G.E.R. for the support.

Conflicts of Interest: The author declares no conflicts of interest.

References

1. Ribaudo, G. Natural Products Chemistry: Advances in Synthetic, Analytical and Bioactivity Studies. *Molecules* **2023**, *28*, 5577. [CrossRef] [PubMed]

https://doi.org/10.3390/molecules31020374

2. Hong, J. Role of Natural Product Diversity in Chemical Biology. *Curr. Opin. Chem. Biol.* **2011**, *15*, 350–354. [CrossRef] [PubMed]
3. Hu, L.-J.; Duan, Z.-Z.; Wang, Y.; Ye, W.-C.; Che, C.-T. Strategies and Advances in the Biomimetic Synthesis of Natural Products. *Engineering* **2025**, *44*, 30–36. [CrossRef]
4. Nath, R.; Manna, S.; Panda, S.; Maity, A.; Bandyopadhyay, K.; Das, A.; Khan, S.A.; Debnath, B.; Akhtar, M.J. Flavonoid Based Development of Synthetic Drugs: Chemistry and Biological Activities. *Chem. Biodivers.* **2025**, *22*, e202401899. [CrossRef] [PubMed]
5. Amirkia, V.; Heinrich, M. Alkaloids as Drug Leads—A Predictive Structural and Biodiversity-Based Analysis. *Phytochem. Lett.* **2014**, *10*, xlviii–liii. [CrossRef]
6. Singla, R.K.; Sharma, P.; Dubey, A.K.; Gundamaraju, R.; Kumar, D.; Kumar, S.; Madaan, R.; Shri, R.; Tsagkaris, C.; Parisi, S.; et al. Natural Product-Based Studies for the Management of Castration-Resistant Prostate Cancer: Computational to Clinical Studies. *Front. Pharmacol.* **2021**, *12*, 732266. [CrossRef] [PubMed]
7. Ding, B.; Yu, Y.; Geng, S.; Liu, B.; Hao, Y.; Liang, G. Computational Methods for the Interaction between Cyclodextrins and Natural Compounds: Technology, Benefits, Limitations, and Trends. *J. Agric. Food Chem.* **2022**, *70*, 2466–2482. [CrossRef] [PubMed]
8. Ribaudo, G.; Coghi, P.; Yang, L.J.; Ng, J.P.L.; Mastinu, A.; Memo, M.; Wong, V.K.W.; Gianoncelli, A. Computational and Experimental Insights on the Interaction of Artemisinin, Dihydroartemisinin and Chloroquine with SARS-CoV-2 Spike Protein Receptor-Binding Domain (RBD). *Nat. Prod. Res.* **2022**, *36*, 5358–5363. [CrossRef] [PubMed]
9. Chen, J.-W.; Chen, S.; Chen, G.-Q. Recent Advances in Natural Compounds Inducing Non-Apoptotic Cell Death for Anticancer Drug Resistance. *Cancer Drug Resist.* **2023**, *6*, 709–727. [CrossRef] [PubMed]
10. Lewis, K.; Lee, R.E.; Brötz-Oesterhelt, H.; Hiller, S.; Rodnina, M.V.; Schneider, T.; Weingarth, M.; Wohlgemuth, I. Sophisticated Natural Products as Antibiotics. *Nature* **2024**, *632*, 39–49. [CrossRef] [PubMed]
11. Chen, X.; Drew, J.; Berney, W.; Lei, W. Neuroprotective Natural Products for Alzheimer's Disease. *Cells* **2021**, *10*, 1309. [CrossRef] [PubMed]
12. Moeini, R.; Memariani, Z.; Asadi, F.; Bozorgi, M.; Gorji, N. Pistacia Genus as a Potential Source of Neuroprotective Natural Products. *Planta Med.* **2019**, *85*, 1326–1350. [CrossRef] [PubMed]
13. Parthasarathy, A.; Mantravadi, P.K.; Kalesh, K. Detectives and Helpers: Natural Products as Resources for Chemical Probes and Compound Libraries. *Pharmacol. Ther.* **2020**, *216*, 107688. [CrossRef] [PubMed]
14. De Araújo, F.F.; De Paulo Farias, D.; Neri-Numa, I.A.; Pastore, G.M. Polyphenols and Their Applications: An Approach in Food Chemistry and Innovation Potential. *Food Chem.* **2021**, *338*, 127535. [CrossRef] [PubMed]
15. O'Neill, E.C.; Kelly, S. Engineering Biosynthesis of High-Value Compounds in Photosynthetic Organisms. *Crit. Rev. Biotechnol.* **2017**, *37*, 779–802. [CrossRef] [PubMed]
16. Benli, H. Bio Mordants: A Review. *Environ. Sci. Pollut. Res.* **2024**, *31*, 20714–20771. [CrossRef] [PubMed]

https://doi.org/10.3390/molecules31020374

molecules

MDPI

Article

Structural Characterization and Electrochemical Studies of Selected Alkaloid N-Oxides

Olha Dushna [1,2], Liliya Dubenska [2], Andrzej Gawor [1], Jakub Karasiński [1], Oksana Barabash [2], Yurii Ostapiuk [2], Mykola Blazheyevskiy [3] and Ewa Bulska [1,*]

1 Biological and Chemical Research Centre, Faculty of Chemistry, University of Warsaw, Żwirki i Wigury 101, 02-093 Warsaw, Poland; o.dushna@cnbc.uw.edu.pl (O.D.); agawor@chem.uw.edu.pl (A.G.); jkarasinski@chem.uw.edu.pl (J.K.)

2 Faculty of Chemistry, Ivan Franko National University of Lviv, Kyryla i Mefodiya 6, 79-005 Lviv, Ukraine; liliya.dubenska@lnu.edu.ua (L.D.); oksana.barabash@lnu.edu.ua (O.B.); yurii.ostapiuk@lnu.edu.ua (Y.O.)

3 Department of General Chemistry, National University of Pharmacy, Valentynivska 4, 61-168 Kharkiv, Ukraine; blazejowski@ukr.net

* Correspondence: ebulska@chem.uw.edu.pl

Abstract: In this work, we synthesized and confirmed the structure of several alkaloid N-oxides using mass spectrometry and Fourier-transform infrared spectroscopy. We also investigated their reduction mechanisms using voltammetry. For the first time, we obtained alkaloid N-oxides using an oxidation reaction with potassium peroxymonosulfate as an oxidant. The structure was established based on the obtained fragmentation mass spectra recorded by LC-Q-ToF-MS. In the FT-IR spectra of the alkaloid N-oxides, characteristic signals of N-O group vibrations were recorded (bands in the range of 928 cm^{-1} to 971 cm^{-1}), confirming the presence of this functional group. Electrochemical reduction studies demonstrated the reduction of alkaloid N-oxides at mercury-based electrodes back to the original form of the alkaloid. For the first time, the products of the electrochemical reduction of alkaloid N-oxides were detected by mass spectrometry. The findings provide insights into the structural characteristics and reduction behaviors of alkaloid N-oxides, offering implications for pharmacological and biochemical applications. This research contributes to a better understanding of alkaloid metabolism and degradation processes, with potential implications for drug development and environmental science.

Keywords: alkaloids; N-oxide alkaloids; synthesis; mass spectrometry; FT-IR spectroscopy

1. Introduction

Alkaloids (ALs) constitute a large group of substances of plant and synthetic origin that are extensively utilized by humans [1]. Alkaloids have a variety of biological activities and are widely used in medicine [2–4]. The ALs are utilized in the formulation of anti-inflammatory, analgesic, stimulating, antimicrobial, anticancer, antifungal, antispasmodic, neuropharmacological, and other drugs [5–7]. Recent studies [8,9] have also shown the potential usefulness of some ALs in the fight against SARS-CoV-2, specifically berberine, an alkaloid found in the fruits of barberry and turmeric, and quinine, an alkaloid from the quinoline series. These ALs have been demonstrated to have the ability to inhibit viral replication, suggesting potential applications in the treatment of SARS-CoV-2 [8,9].

In addition, plants containing ALs are a common component of the human diet, present in both food and beverages [10]. Some well-known examples of ALs found in the human diet include caffeine from coffee seeds, theobromine from cocoa seeds, theophylline from tea leaves, tomatine from tomatoes, and solanine from potatoes [2].

Some of the ALs, including those widely used in pharmacy, have a toxic effect on humans and animals. The misuse of ALs such as morphine, cocaine, caffeine, and nicotine can have fatal consequences [11].

Consuming food products that contain alkaloids can also cause disease [12]. Several pyrrolizidine and tropane ALs, widely distributed in plants and plant products, have been identified as hepatotoxic and carcinogenic, representing one of the most dangerous classes of phytotoxins affecting the peripheral and central nervous systems, especially the organs involved in digestion and metabolism [13–15]. In accordance with European recommendations (Commission Regulation (EU) 2021/1399 [16], Commission Regulation (EU) 2020/2040 [17], Commission Regulation (EU) 2016/239 [18]), control limits for tropane alkaloids (atropine, scopolamine) are set at 1 μg/kg in plant-origin products, while pyrrolizidine alkaloids range from 1 μg/kg to 750 μg/kg, depending on the matrix. For example, in tea, the AL content should not exceed 1 μg/kg, and in herbal infusions of lemon balm and peppermint, the limit is set at 400 μg/kg. Therefore, the careful control of food products and the regulation of AL use in medicine are important current tasks.

ALs undergo various biochemical transformations in living organisms. Major metabolic pathways, facilitated by hepatic enzymes, encompass hydrolysis, conjugation, and oxidation [19]. AL N-oxides are typical intermediates of AL metabolism and are often excreted from the body in this form. However, oxides can also exhibit bioactivity; in particular, N-oxides of the pyrrolizidine alkaloids, the formed oxidation products, can readily react with proteins, create DNA adducts, and induce tumors via a genotoxic mechanism [20,21]. On the other hand, some alkaloid N-oxides formed during the N-oxidation reaction are considered safe markers with no harmful effects on the human body and are easily excreted through urine [22]. For instance, the primary metabolites of the nicotine alkaloid are cotinine and nicotine N-oxide. An average smoker, consuming 10 cigarettes daily, excretes approximately 0.56 mg of nicotine N-oxide unchanged in the urine within 24 h [23–25]. This indicates that alkaloid N-oxides formed during the metabolic process could potentially function as markers for monitoring alkaloids in biological fluids, especially concerning the consumption of alkaloid-based medications and food items containing alkaloids.

Moreover, alkaloid N-oxides represent a common form of existence for many alkaloids in plants [26]. Therefore, it is crucial to monitor the content of food products and plant materials such as tea and honey, emphasizing not only the alkaloids themselves but also their N-oxides. For the identification and determination of the alkaloid N-oxides in various objects, there is a need for their standard solutions. Therefore, a standardized methodology for the synthesis of alkaloid N-oxides is required.

This investigation aimed to establish an environmentally sustainable and economically viable methodology for the synthesis of alkaloid N-oxides while validating their structural integrity. This endeavor involved the utilization of mass spectrometry and infrared spectroscopy. In contemporary laboratory settings, the integration of high-performance chromatography with mass spectrometry detection (MS or MS/MS) is prevalent for the analysis of various substances, including food products and herbal medicinal raw materials. Therefore, augmenting the existing database and discerning the disparities between the mass spectra of alkaloids and their N-oxide counterparts are imperative tasks. The study of infrared spectra of alkaloid N-oxides opens the possibility of rapid and cheap determination of such compounds.

The subsequent phase of our research focused on elucidating the mechanism underlying the reduction process involved in synthesizing alkaloid N-oxides, which may mimic metabolic or degradation reactions occurring in vivo. This investigation holds particular significance given the potential physiological relevance of such reactions. In recent years, a combined approach leveraging electrochemical (EC) methods alongside mass spectrometry (MS) has emerged as a powerful tool for addressing this challenge [27,28]. By coupling EC methods with MS detection, this approach not only complements existing biochemical studies techniques but also offers advantages in terms of efficiency and cost-effectiveness. Moreover, it facilitates the identification of electrochemical reaction products, shedding light on their potential roles as metabolic or degradation by-products. This integrated methodology represents a cornerstone in the fields of metabolomics and bioanalytical chemistry, providing valuable insights into complex biological processes and chemical transformations [28–32].

This study focused on five alkaloids that belong to different chemical groups and serve different purposes. These include both natural and synthetic compounds, as depicted in Figure 1. Specifically, the alkaloids selected are atropine (a tropane), quinine (a quinuclidine), platyphylline (a pyrrolizidine), nicotine (a pyridine), and nefopam (a synthetic benzoxazocine). This selection is strategically diverse, enabling a comprehensive examination of various classes of alkaloids, each renowned for its unique pharmacological activities and widespread utility in medical applications. It should be added that alkaloid N-oxides are formed regardless of the type of alkaloid skeleton. The process typically involves the oxidation of a nitrogen atom in the alkaloid structure to form an N-oxide functional group. This transformation can occur during an oxidation reaction. The presence of N-oxide groups can affect the pharmacological properties of the alkaloid, including its bioavailability, metabolic stability, and interaction with biological targets. Thus, investigating the potential formation of alkaloid N-oxides with different skeletal types can be a valuable aspect of research, providing insight into their metabolic pathways.

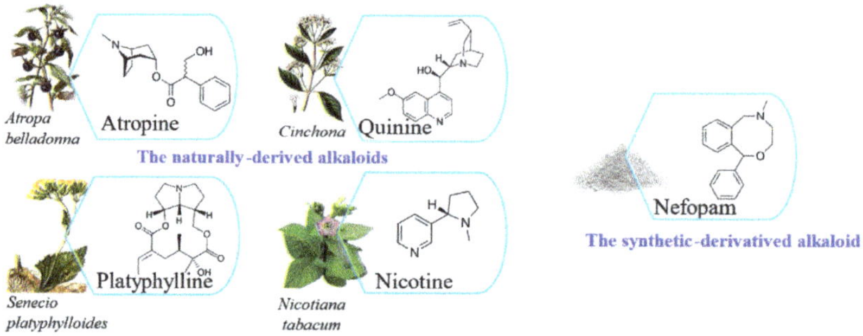

Figure 1. The alkaloids employed in this study were utilized for the synthesis of alkaloid N-oxides.

2. Results and Discussion

2.1. Synthesis of Alkaloid N-Oxides

Alkaloid N-oxides can be easily synthesized in the laboratory [33]. Hydrogen peroxide and organic peroxyacids are commonly employed as oxidants [34–38]. The commercial reagent potassium peroxymonosulfate (KPMS) was used as an oxidant, enabling the synthesis of the main metabolites of alkaloids in just 15 min [39–42]. The oxidation of alkaloids is rapid at room temperature, except for nicotine. The formation of nicotine N-oxide at 20–25 °C takes 40 min, and slight heating of the solution accelerates the reaction. A 5-fold excess of KPMS should also be used.

The main factor affecting the completeness of the oxidation of an alkaloid to its N-oxide is pH. Alkaloids are oxidized to their N-oxides in an alkaline environment. The optimum pH for oxidation is close to the pKa of the alkaloid. Table 1 shows the optimal conditions for obtaining the studied alkaloid N-oxides. Previously, we reported the preparation of nefopam N-oxide [39], nicotine N-oxide [42], platyphylline N-oxide [40], and atropine N-oxide [41]. In this study, we present, for the first time, the synthesis of quinine N-oxide via this specific method and oxidation reaction (Table 1). Thus, we have standardized the methodology for the synthesis of alkaloid N-oxides.

Table 1. Optimal conditions for obtaining alkaloids N-oxides.

Optimal Conditions \ Alkaloids	Nefopam N-Oxide [39]	Nicotine N-Oxide [42]	Platyphylline N-Oxide [40]	Atropine N-Oxide [41]	Quinine N-Oxide
$pH_{oxidation}$ (provided by BRB)	8.0	9.3	8.4	10.2	9.5
Oxidation temperature, °C	20–25	40	20–25	20–25	20–25

The oxidation reaction of atropine with peroxymonosulfate to atropine N-oxide is depicted in Scheme 1. This second-order reaction has a rate constant of 0.193 $L{\cdot}mol^{-1}{\cdot}min^{-1}$, and its kinetics adhere to the principles of specific acid-base catalysis [41].

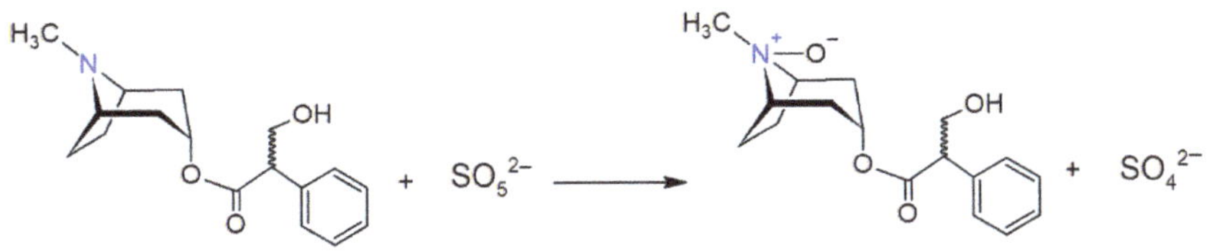

Scheme 1. The reaction of obtaining atropine N-oxide using the oxidant peroxymonosulfate.

2.2. *Studies on Structure of Alkaloid N-Oxides by Mass Spectrometry*

Identification and characterization of alkaloid N-oxides were achieved by liquid chromatography coupled with high-resolution mass spectrometry (LC-Q-ToF-MS). Mass spectra were recorded for both the alkaloids and the synthetically obtained alkaloid N-oxides to identify the obtained N-oxides and confirm the presence of an additional oxygen atom in the structure. Table 2 presents the measured and theoretically calculated values of $[M + H]^+$ for all the studied compounds. Moreover, the mass accuracy was calculated to confirm the chemical formula of the investigated compounds. The mass accuracy for compounds was computed by calculating the absolute difference between the theoretical and experimentally observed mass-to-charge ratios (m/z), dividing this difference by the theoretical m/z, and expressing the result in parts per million (ppm). The obtained values of mass accuracy did not exceed the permissible threshold of 5 ppm, which is deemed acceptable for high-resolution mass spectrometry [43,44] and reliably confirms that N-oxides ALs were obtained.

Table 2. Characteristics of the mass spectra of the studied compounds.

Compound	Chemical Formula	Theoretical $[M + H]^+$	Measured $[M + H]^+$	Mass Accuracy, ppm
Nefopam	$C_{17}H_{19}NO$	254.1539	254.1542	1.18
Nefopam N-oxide	$C_{17}H_{19}NO_2$	270.1488	270.1491	1.11
Atropine	$C_{17}H_{23}NO_3$	290.1750	290.1756	2.07
Atropine N-oxide	$C_{17}H_{23}NO_4$	306.1699	306.1700	0.33
Quinine	$C_{20}H_{24}N_2O_2$	325.1910	325.1918	2.46
Quinine N-oxide	$C_{20}H_{24}N_2O_3$	341.1859	341.1859	0
Platyphylline	$C_{18}H_{27}NO_5$	338.1969	338.1964	−1.48
Platyphylline N-oxide	$C_{18}H_{27}NO_6$	354.1918	354.1927	2.54
Nicotine	$C_{10}H_{14}N_2$	163.1229	163.1229	0
Nicotine N-oxide	$C_{10}H_{14}N_2O$	179.1179	179.1176	−1.67

An essential prerequisite for the structure elucidation of alkaloid N-oxides was a comprehensive understanding of the fragmentation process of these compounds. Below is a detailed interpretation of the mass spectra of selected alkaloid N-oxides acquired in MS^2. The following pairs of compounds were studied as research compounds: quinine and its

N-oxide, atropine and its N-oxide, nefopam and its N-oxide, and nicotine and its N-oxide. Figures 2–5 illustrate the fragmentation mass spectra of study compounds where the m/z values correspond to the exact mass values on the mass spectrum. The obtained m/z values of the fragmented ions were compared with the theoretical values. Figures 2–5 show theoretical values for the proposed schemes. Figure 3C and Figures S1–S3 (Supplementary Materials) show the detailed fragmentation scheme of alkaloids and alkaloid N-oxides.

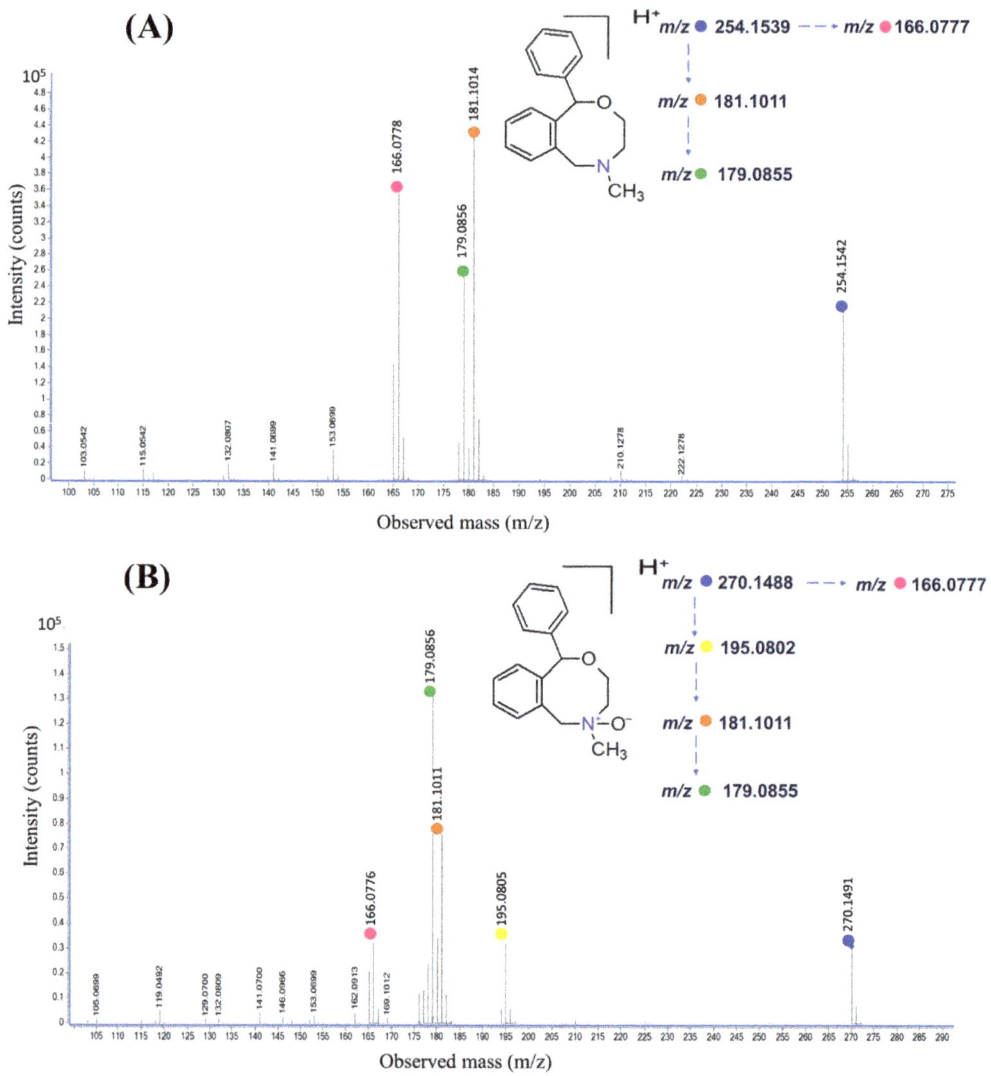

Figure 2. Elucidation of fragmentation patterns of nefopam (**A**) and nefopam N-oxide (**B**).

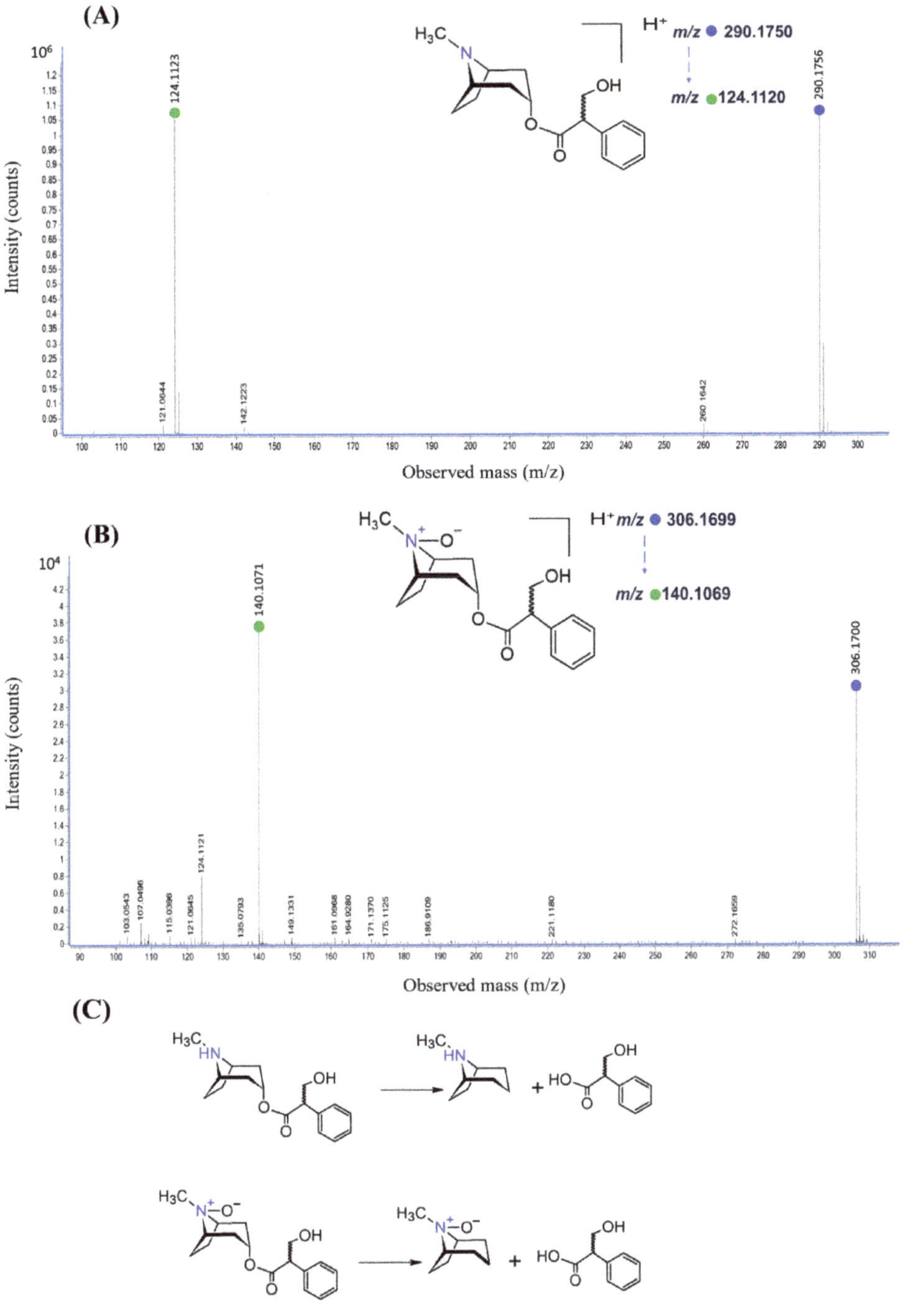

Figure 3. Elucidation of fragmentation patterns of atropine (**A**) and atropine N-oxide (**B**) and proposed fragmentation pattern of atropine and atropine N-oxide (**C**).

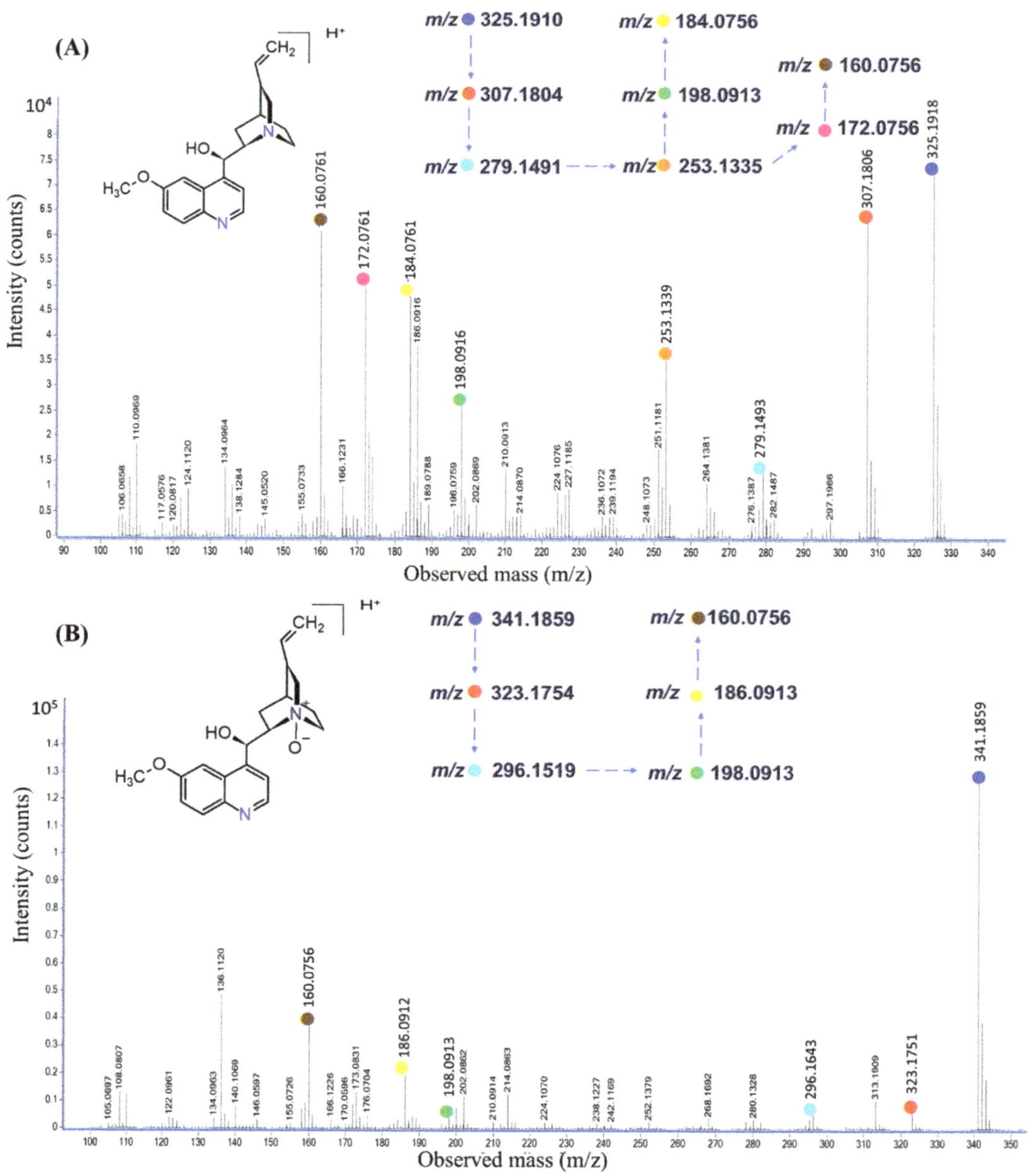

Figure 4. Elucidation of fragmentation patterns of quinine (**A**) and quinine N-oxide (**B**).

2.2.1. Nefopam and Nefopam N-Oxide

In the fragmentation mass spectrum of the protonated molecular ion of nefopam at m/z 254, product ions at m/z 181, 179, and 166 were observed, as obtained in Figure 2A. The major fission fragment product ion at m/z 181 resulted from a loss of C_3H_7NO moiety from the benzoxazocine ring. Further detachment of two hydrogen atoms from an ion at m/z 181 will lead to the formation of an ion at m/z 179. Accurate mass measurement of these ions confirmed their chemical formulas. The fragmentation pathways are given in

Figure S3 (Supplementary Materials). The obtained mass spectrum is fully consistent with previous research provided by Yu et al. [45].

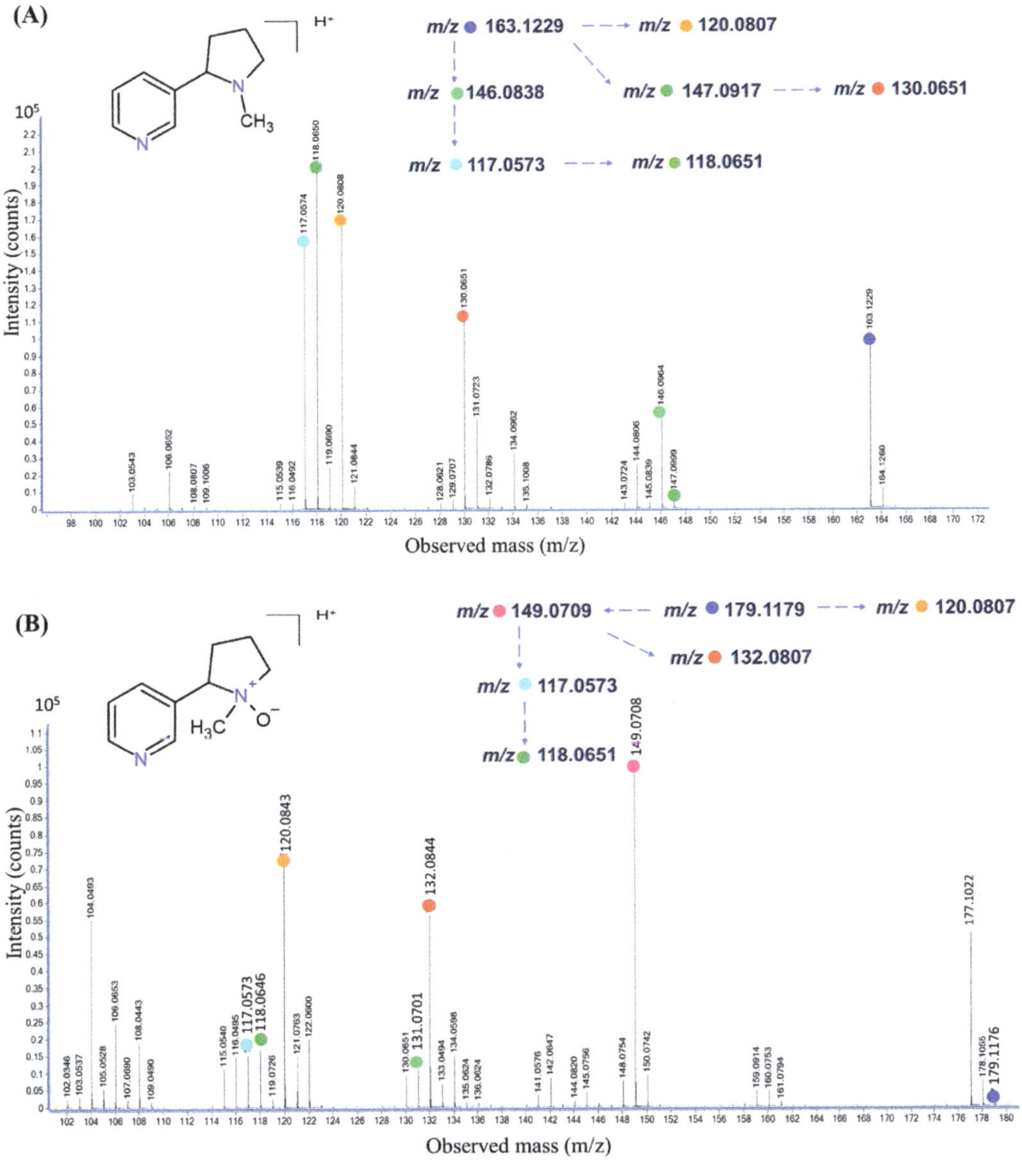

Figure 5. Elucidation of fragmentation patterns of nicotine (**A**) and nicotine N-oxide (**B**).

In the fragmentation mass spectrum of nefopam N-oxide, a pattern like that of the fragmentation mass spectrum of nefopam was observed. However, a small fraction of nefopam N-oxide underwent fragmentation, resulting in the formation of an ion at m/z 195. This suggests the cleavage of the C_3H_9NO fragment from the protonated molecular ion of nefopam N-oxide (m/z 270) (Figure 2B). These results align with those described by Yu et al. [45].

2.2.2. Atropine and Atropine N-Oxide

The fragmentation of the protonated molecular ion of atropine results in the main product ion at m/z 124 ($C_8H_{13}N$) and of atropine N-oxide at m/z 140 ($C_8H_{13}NO$) (Figure 3). Additionally, a signal at m/z 142 was detected on the fragmentation mass spectrum for atropine, serving as a secondary product of atropine fragmentation. These results align with those described by Chen et al. and Luo et al. [46,47].

2.2.3. Quinine and Quinine N-Oxide

On the fragmentation mass spectrum of the protonated molecular ion of quinine at m/z 325, product ions at m/z 307, 279, 253, 198, 186, 184, 172, and 160 were observed (Figure 4A). Also, we registered for the protonated molecular ion of quinine N-oxide at m/z 341 and product ions at m/z 323, 296, 198, 186, and 160 (Figure 4B). The obtained fragmentation mass spectrum of quinine is in complete agreement with prior studies [48,49]. Furthermore, we compared the two obtained mass spectra of quinine and quinine N-oxide among ourselves. The signals at m/z 186 and 160 correspond to the fragmentation of the quinoline ring, and these signals are present in both mass spectra. The difference between the signals at m/z 307 for quinine and m/z 323 for quinine N-oxide is 16, indicating that the oxidation of quinine occurs at the tertiary nitrogen atom in the quinuclidine fragment.

2.2.4. Nicotine and Nicotine N-Oxide

The fragmentation mass spectrum of the protonated molecular ion of nicotine at m/z 163 observed product ions at m/z 146, 147, 130, 120, 118, and 117 (Figure 5A). Similarly, for the protonated molecular ion of nicotine N-oxide at m/z 179, we registered product ions at m/z 179, 149, 132, 120, 118, and 117 (Figure 5B). We also compared the two mass spectra of nicotine and nicotine N-oxide. The signals present in both mass spectra at m/z 120, 118, and 117 correspond to protonated fragments of pyridine derivatives. This is indicative of the formation of nicotine N-oxide by the piperidine fragment. These results agree with Liang et al., Smyth et al., and Tsugawa et al., as described by [50–53]. However, we believe that the fragmentation of nicotine and nicotine N-oxide is more likely to occur, as depicted in Figure S2 (Supplementary Materials).

2.3. *Studies on Structure of N-Oxide Alkaloids by FT-IR Spectrometry*

The IR spectra of alkaloids and their alkaloid N-oxides, presented in Figure 6, indicate specific characteristics of the molecular structure of the investigated compounds. Table 3 provides vibration signals for all groups present in the structures of alkaloids and their N-oxides. From the IR spectra data, a notable distinction between the spectra of alkaloids and their N-oxides is the presence of N-O group vibrations (bands in the range of 928 cm^{-1} to 971 cm^{-1}). These bands, characteristic of the N-O stretch, are crucial for identifying N-oxides but are relatively weak and fall into the fingerprint region, making them less prominent. The N-O group vibration signal is highlighted in Figure 6.

The region from 2500 cm^{-1} to 3660 cm^{-1} is represented by broad peaks corresponding to the stretching of O–H and C–H bonds, indicating the presence of active hydrogen bonds in the molecules of alkaloid N-oxides.

Additionally, these peaks also suggest the presence of hydroxyl and methyl groups. Peaks in the range of 1403 cm^{-1} to 1608 cm^{-1} reflect vibrations of aromatic systems (C=C and C–C), indicating the existence of aromatic ring systems in the molecules of alkaloids, particularly in nicotine, quinine, and atropine. Furthermore, in the case of platyphylline and atropine N-oxides, absorption bands in the range of 1451 cm^{-1} to 1637 cm^{-1} were identified, corresponding to the vibrations of C=O in the alkaloid molecules, suggesting the presence of carbonyl group in the structure of these molecules. In general, the rest of the IR spectroscopic data of investigated alkaloid N-oxides agree with those reported in the literature [49,54–56].

The N–O group vibration signal is highlighted in a black circle.

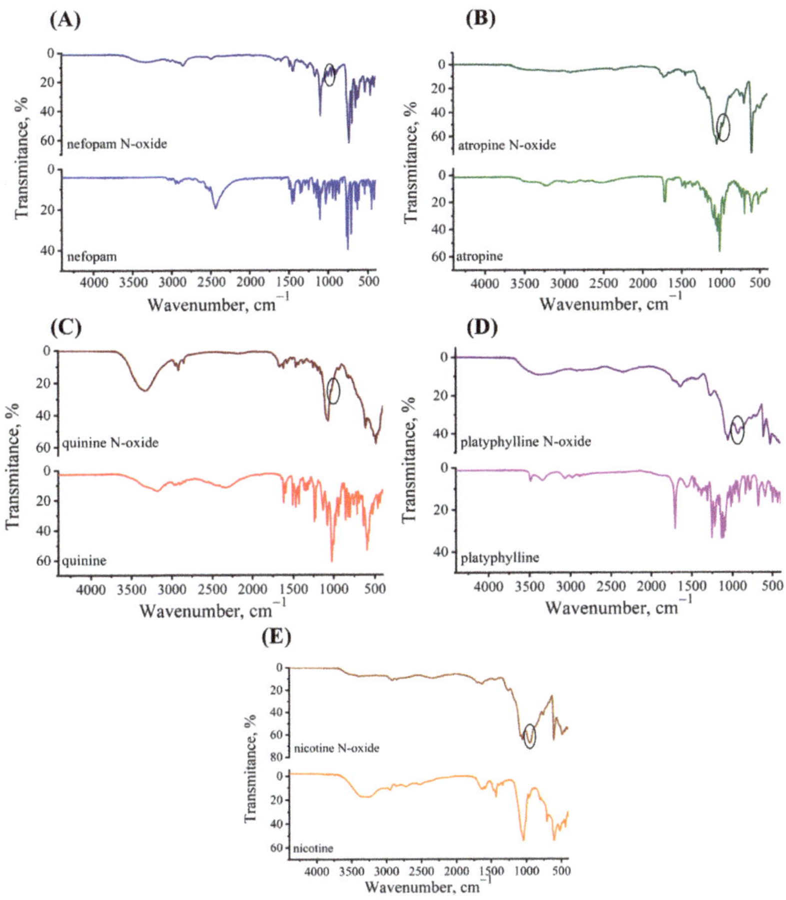

Figure 6. The FT-IR spectra of alkaloid N-oxides and alkaloids: (**A**) nefopam N-oxide and nefopam; (**B**) atropine N-oxide and atropine; (**C**) quinine N-oxide and quinine; (**D**) platyphylline N-oxide and platyphylline; (**E**) nicotine N-oxide and nicotine. The N-O group vibration signal is highlighted in circles.

Table 3. Selected assigned IR vibrations of alkaloids and their N-oxides.

Alkaloids	Experimental Wavenumbers, cm^{-1} (Signal Intensity) [a]		Type of Vibration and Bond	Functional Group
	Alkaloids	**Alkaloids N-Oxide**		
Atropine	3500–3223 w	3660–2500 w	ν [b] (O–H)	Hydroxy
	3080 w	3066 w	ν (C–H)	Phenyl
	1721 m	1724 m	ν (C=O)	Carboxylic
	1494 w	1403–1500 w	ν (C=C)	Phenyl
	1200 m		ν (C–N)	Tropane
	–	1229 m		
	–	971 s	ν (N–O)	N-oxide group

Table 3. *Cont.*

Alkaloids	Experimental Wavenumbers, cm^{-1} (Signal Intensity) [a]		Type of Vibration and Bond	Functional Group
Nefopam	3044 w	3063 w	ν (C–H)	Phenyl
	1600 w	1600 w	ν (C–C)	Phenyl
	1497–1437 m	1446–1493 m	ν (C=C)	Phenyl
	1240 m	1267 m	ν (C–N)	Benzoxazocine
	–	952 m	ν (N–O)	N-oxide
Quinine	3550–3053 m	3600–3000 m	ν (O–H)	Hydroxy
	2943 w	2955 w	ν (C–H)	Quinoline
	1618 m	1617 m	ν (C–C)	Quinoline
	1647–1594 m	1668–1571 w	ν (C=N)	Quinoline
	1473–1431 m	1467–1431 m	ν (C=C)	Quinoline
	1235 w	1253 m	ν (C–N)	Quinuclidine
	1025 s	1066 s	ν (C–O)	6-Methoxyquinoline
	–	928 s	ν (N–O)	N-oxide group
Platyffiline	3488–3210 w	3488–3200 w	ν (O–H)	Hydroxy
	3067 w	2937 w	ν (C–H)	12-Hydroxysenecionan
	2977 w	2919 w	ν (C–H)	12-Hydroxysenecionan
	1707 m	1705 w	ν (C=O)	12-Hydroxysenecionan-11,16-dione
	1554 w	1552 w	ν (C–C)	12-Hydroxysenecionan-11,16-dione
	1437 w	1437 w	ν (C–O)	12-Hydroxysenecionan-11,16-dione
	1241 m	1270 m	ν (C–N)	Pyrrolizidine
	–	931 s	ν (N–O)	N-oxide
Nicotine	3360–3079 m	3250–3000 m	ν (C–H)	Pyridine
	2950 w	2952 w	ν (C–H)	1-Methylpyrrolidin
	1628 m	1628 m	ν (C–C)	Pyridine
	1643–1530 w	1650–1579 m	ν (C=N)	Pyridine
	1473–1433 m	1467–1431 m	ν (C=C)	Pyridine
	1220 w	1253 m	ν (C–N)	Pyrrolidine
	–	948 s	ν (N–O)	N-oxide

[a] Intensity: s = strong; m = medium; w = weak. [b] Symbol ν means stretching deformation.

2.4. Study of Alkaloid N-Oxide Reduction with the Electrochemical Approach

The electrochemical (EC) approach was employed to gain deeper insights into the metabolism and degradation mechanisms of alkaloid N-oxides in biological systems. Nowak et al. extensively reviewed the simulation of drug metabolism through various methods, including EC [57]. From a pharmaceutical perspective, the EC approach offers several advantages, such as being cost-effective, easy to use, and avoiding ethical concerns associated with using human or animal materials. This makes it a highly appealing option for drug metabolism research [58]. This approach was also used in this work.

Alkaloid N-oxides are easily reduced on the surface of mercury-based electrodes over a wide pH range, resulting in the formation of either one or two peaks (depending on the alkaloid N-oxides and the pH of the solution). Figure 7A shows the polarograms of the reduction of alkaloid N-oxides obtained in optimal conditions [39–42]. The arrow in Figure 7A indicates that polarograms of reduced alkaloid N-oxides were shifted up towards axis *Y* for a better view. Previously, we selected optimal conditions for the reduction of alkaloid N-oxides, including the pH of reduction and the scan rates. In this work, for the first time, we investigated the electrochemical behavior of quinine N-oxide; namely, the optimal conditions for its reduction on the surface of a dropping mercury electrode were established. On the dropping mercury electrode (DME), quinine N-oxide is reduced in the form of a single peak at a potential of −1.15 V (Figure 7A). It should be noted that the first peak on the polarogram of quinine N-oxide (E = −1.03 V—Figure 7A) corresponds to the reduction of quinine itself, according to [59].

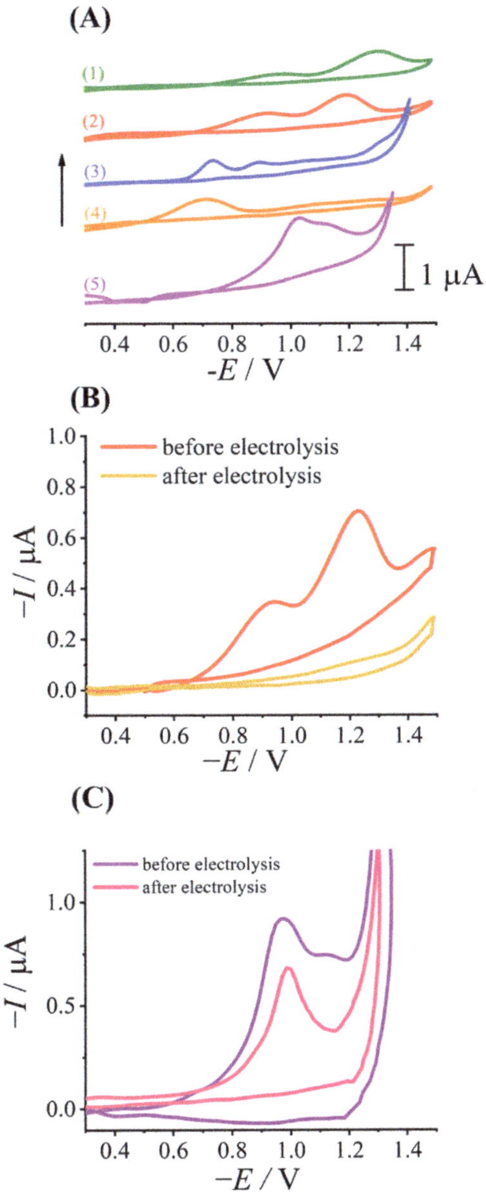

Figure 7. (**A**) Cyclic polarograms of atropine N-oxide (1), nefopam N-oxide (2), nicotine N-oxide (3), platyphylline N-oxide (4), and quinine N-oxide (5) under optimal conditions. The concentration of alkaloid N-oxides was 40 μmol/L. Scan rate—0.5 V/s. (**B**) Cyclic polarograms of nefopam N-oxide before and after electrolysis. The concentration of nefopam N-oxide was 20 μmol/L. Scan rate—0.5 V/s. (**C**) Cyclic polarograms of quinine N-oxide before and after electrolysis. The concentration of quinine N-oxide was 20 μmol/L. Scan rate—0.5 V/s.

It was determined that the reduction current of all research alkaloid N-oxides exhibits a diffusion–adsorption nature. The optimal environment for the reduction of alkaloid

N-oxides is within the pH range of 3 to 7, which is provided by the Britton–Robinson buffer (BRB).

Also, we investigated and described the mechanism of alkaloid N-oxide reduction on the surface of mercury electrodes [39–42]. When we obtained the two peaks of the reduction of the N-oxides of the alkaloids, this process corresponds to two single-electron transfer processes. The first single-electron transfer to the N-oxide yields an amine radical cation together with a hydroxide ion, and the second reduction yields the original structure of the alkaloid. This process is reflected in the appearance of two peaks on the voltammogram, as observed in the reduction of atropine N-oxide and nefopam N-oxide [39,41]. In the case of the polarogram of alkaloid N-oxides showing a single cathodic peak, it indicates the one-stage reduction of the alkaloid N-oxide, involving one electron and one proton. In this context, the reduction of the alkaloid N-oxide yields a hydroxylamine derivative. Subsequently, this hydroxylamine derivative can revert to the original alkaloid through a protonation reaction in a mildly acidic environment. However, this process cannot be registered under voltammetry conditions. This one-step reduction process of alkaloid N-oxides has been observed for nicotine N-oxide and platyphylline N-oxide [40,42]. It is important to note that both proposed mechanisms of reduction of alkaloid N-oxides are agreed on by data in the literature [60,61].

To confirm the hypothesis regarding the mechanism of alkaloid N-oxide reduction on the electrode surface, identification and structural determination were carried out using mass spectrometry (MS). Initially, prolonged electrolysis of solutions of alkaloid N-oxides was performed using a macro electrode of mercury as the working electrode (to increase the surface area and accelerate the process). Electrolysis was conducted for two compounds at a concentration of 20 μM for 6 h: the nefopam N-oxide at the potential of the first peak ($E = -1.00$ V) and the quinine N-oxide at the potential of the peak ($E = -1.15$ V). By maintaining such experimental conditions, we aimed to ensure that the reduction reaction selectively targeted the alkaloid N-oxide compound in accordance with the specified potential. The primary objective of the prolonged electrolysis duration was to facilitate the generation of the principal reduction product of the alkaloid N-oxide on the surface of the mercury electrodes. Throughout this process, we meticulously tracked and observed the emergence of only one product, aligning precisely with the compound described within the theoretical framework of the reduction mechanism. The polarograms of the reduction nefopam N-oxide and quinine N-oxide before and after electrolysis are shown in Figure 7B,C. Other research shows that alkaloids do not reduce at the DME.

During electrolysis, the signals of reduction alkaloid N-oxides decreased, and after 6 h, they completely disappeared. This indicates the complete reduction of alkaloid N-oxides. The same pattern was observed in the chromatograms obtained by the LC-Q-ToF-MS method. The reduction peak at $E = -1.03$ V (Figure 7C) was registered on the polarogram of quinine after 6 h of electrolysis, which corresponds to the reduction of quinine itself and not its N-oxide (see above).

The mass spectra for nefopam N-oxide and its electrolysis product were received. We have established that the nefopam N-oxide ($[M + H]^+ = 270.1480$) is reduced to the nefopam ($[M + H]^+ = 254.5434$). Similarly, the quinine N-oxide is reduced to the protonated anionnitroxide radical derivative ($[M + H]^+ = 342.1929$), which, in turn, transforms back to the quinine ($[M + H]^+ = 325.1864$) due to protonation.

Thus, we have confirmed the reduction of alkaloid N-oxides on the electrode surface to the original alkaloids. This detailed mass spectrometric analysis provides clear evidence for the reduction mechanisms proposed. Furthermore, the identification of intermediate products and final reduction compounds through MS offers a deeper understanding of the electrochemical reduction pathways and confirms the stepwise reduction processes.

This electrochemical approach offers advantages in terms of ease of handling, practicality, and environmental friendliness, presenting a viable alternative to conventional oxidation or reduction reactions commonly employed in organic biomolecule synthesis. Given the benefits of electrochemical synthesis in producing target molecules, it holds promising prospects for surpassing limitations associated with traditional synthesis methods. Moreover, the ability to simulate metabolic pathways and degradation processes in a controlled and ethical manner enhances the relevance of this approach in pharmaceutical and biochemical research, providing novel insights into the behavior of alkaloid N-oxides and their potential applications in drug development and analysis.

3. Materials and Methods

3.1. Chemical and Reagents

Following alkaloid substances were used in this work: nefopam hydrochloride, atropine sulfate, nicotine sulfate, platyphylline hydrotartrate, and quinine hydrochloride. Detailed characteristics of alkaloid substances are given in Table 4. Potassium peroxymonosulfate (KPMS) (CAS No. 70693-62-8) was used as an oxidizing agent. The Britton–Robinson buffer (BRB) was used as a background electrolyte. To prepare the BRB, 20.2 g of $Na_2B_4O_7{\cdot}10H_2O$, 28.7 mL of CH_3COOH, and 17.6 mL of H_3PO_4 were dissolved in the volumetric flask [39–42]. Analytical reagent-grade chemicals were purchased from Sigma-Aldrich (Darmstadt, Germany), EMD Millipore (Darmstadt, Germany), and Baker (Deventer, The Netherlands). Samples were diluted with deionized water obtained by the Milli-Q System (resistivity 18.2 MΩ cm; EMD Millipore, Darmstadt, Germany). Formic acid (~98%) used for liquid chromatographic purposes was purchased from Honeywell Chemicals (Bracknell, UK).

Table 4. Characteristics of alkaloid substances.

Compound	CAS No.	Molecular Mass	pKa	Purity, %
Nefopam	23327-57-3	253.34	8.98	≥99.0
Nicotine	54-11-5	162.23	8.02	99.0
Atropine	5908-99-6	289.36	9.84	99.7
Platyphylline	480-78-4	337.41	8.1	98.5
Quinine	6119-47-7	324.18	8.0	≥99.0

3.2. Instrumentation

3.2.1. Mass Spectrometry

An Agilent 1290 Infinity system (Agilent Technologies, Wood Dale, IL, USA) coupled with an Agilent 6450 UHD Accurate-Mass Q-TOF mass spectrometer (Agilent Technologies, Wood Dale, IL, USA) was used to obtain high-resolution mass spectra. Electrospray ionization (ESI) in positive ion mode was applied. ESI conditions were as follows: nebulizing gas temperature, 300 °C; nebulizing gas flow, 7 L/min; sheath gas temperature, 350 °C; and sheath gas flow, 11 L/min. Nitrogen was used as a nebulizer and sheath gas. The collision energy was 20 eV. Full-scan spectrums and fragmentation mass spectrums were acquired in the (100–1000) m/z range.

The chromatographic separation of the compounds was carried out using a Synergi 2.5 μm Polar-RP 100 Å, 100 mm × 2 mm column, and gradient elution. Phase A (0.1% formic acid in water) and phase B (0.1% formic acid in acetonitrile) were used as mobile phases. The injection volume was 2 μL. Mass spectra were obtained for the studied compounds at a concentration of approximately 5 μmol/L in a solution of 1:1 methanol/water.

3.2.2. FT-IR Spectroscopy

The samples of alkaloids and alkaloid N-oxides in dry form were analyzed with a Fourier-transform infrared spectrophotometer IRSpirit FTIR (Shimadzu, Japan), equipped with a diamond-tipped ATR accessory. The data were collected in absorbance mode, and the wavelength ranged from 4400 cm^{-1} to 400 cm^{-1}. A spectral resolution of 4 cm^{-1} was used. Software LabSolutions IR 2.13 (Shimadzu, Japan) was used for spectrum collection and spectrum processing.

To transfer to a dry form, we extracted the alkaloid N-oxides in dry form. Specifically, alkaloid N-oxides were extracted from the aqueous solution using 10 mL of chloroform in three separate extractions. Subsequently, the extracts containing alkaloid N-oxides in chloroform were dried at room temperature until dry crystals formed.

3.2.3. Electrochemistry

We used the digital device MTech OVA-410 (MTech Lab, Lviv, Ukraine) with three-electrode cell (working dropping mercury electrode (DME), a saturated calomel reference electrode, and platinum wire auxiliary electrode) [62]. The applied DME had τ = 12 s in 0.1 mol/L NH_4Cl with an open circuit. The current was measured at a fixed time (10 s) in the life of the drop.

Cyclic voltammetry and linear sweep voltammetry with a scan rate of 0.5 V/s were used to study the mechanism of reduction of alkaloid N-oxides. The prepared solutions for measurement were transferred to an electrochemical cell, and dissolved oxygen was removed with purified argon for 10 min. Polarograms were recorded in the potential range from 0 V to −1.5 V with a scan rate of 0.5 V/s (and back for cyclic voltammetry).

To establish the detailed structure of the products of the electrochemical reaction of the reduction of alkaloid N-oxides, a long electrolysis was carried out for 6 h using mercury macroelectrode as a working electrode.

4. Conclusions

In this work, for the first time, we comprehensively investigated some synthesized alkaloid N-oxides using KPMS as an oxidant. The standardized methodology developed here for the synthesis of alkaloid N-oxides is promising for pharmaceutical research, facilitating their production for further study and offering avenues for new drug development.

Mass spectrometry and Fourier-transform infrared spectroscopy were used to establish and confirm the structure. Using electrochemical methods, in particular voltammetry, the mechanism of reduction of alkaloid N-oxides on the surface of mercury electrodes was confirmed. For the first time, we have isolated the products of electrochemical reduction of alkaloid N-oxides and determined their structures using high-resolution mass spectrometry. It turned out that most alkaloid N-oxides are restored to the original form of the alkaloid itself. Such elucidation of reduction mechanisms using electrochemical methods in combination with mass spectrometry is a significant step forward in revealing alkaloid metabolism and degradation pathways. Understanding the electrochemical behavior of alkaloid N-oxides on electrode surfaces sheds light on potential reactions in living organisms. This research is critical to understanding the fate and effects of alkaloids and has implications for drug metabolism and toxicity studies.

In addition, the obtained results improve our ability to monitor the content of alkaloids and their N-oxides in food products, thereby improving food safety practices. Overall, this comprehensive study represents a significant advance in alkaloid N-oxide research spanning pharmacology, toxicology, and food science. Further research in this area holds great potential for harnessing the benefits of alkaloids and their derivatives in biomedical and agricultural contexts.

Supplementary Materials: The following supporting information can be downloaded at https://www.mdpi.com/article/10.3390/molecules29122721/s1. Figure S1. Proposed fragmentation pattern of quinine (A) and quinine N-oxide (B). Figure S2. Proposed fragmentation pattern of nicotine (A) and nicotine N-oxide (B). Figure S3. Proposed fragmentation pattern of nefopam (A) and nefopam N-oxide (B).

Author Contributions: O.D., L.D., M.B. and E.B.: conceptualization; O.D., M.B., A.G., J.K., E.B. and L.D.: methodology; O.D., O.B., J.K. and Y.O.: analytical investigations; O.D., A.G. and E.B.: data curation; O.D., A.G., E.B. and L.D.: writing—original draft; O.D., A.G., L.D., Y.O. and E.B.: writing—review and editing. All authors have read and agreed to the published version of the manuscript.

Funding: This work was financed by the Ministry of Education and Science of Ukraine (Grant Number 0116U001541) and was partly supported by the Simons Foundation (Award Number: 1290588). This research was co-funded by the University of Warsaw as part of the "Excellence Initiative—Research University (2020–2026)" under the program of the Ministry of Science and Higher Education of Poland.

Institutional Review Board Statement: Not applicable.

Informed Consent Statement: Not applicable.

Data Availability Statement: Data are contained within the article and Supplementary Materials.

Acknowledgments: This study was carried out at the Biological and Chemical Research Centre, the University of Warsaw, which was established within the project co-financed by the European Union from the European Regional Development Fund under the Operational Programme Innovative Economy 2007–2013. This study was carried out in laboratories of the University of Warsaw, accredited in accordance with ISO/IEC 17025:2017 "General requirements for the competence of testing and calibration laboratories" (accreditation number: AB 1525) by the Polish Centre for Accreditation, and in laboratories of the Faculty of Chemistry, Ivan Franko National University of Lviv.

Conflicts of Interest: The authors declare no conflicts of interest.

References

1. Manna, K.; Somraj Singh, W.; Goswami, S.; Ashif Ikbal, A.M.; Rajkhowa, A.; Debnath, B. Metabolites Study of Experimental Plant Derived Alkaloids: A Review. *Nat. Prod. J.* **2023**, *13*, 64–78. [CrossRef]
2. Kurek, J. Introductory Chapter: Alkaloids—Their Importance in Nature and for Human Life. In *Alkaloids—Their Importance in Nature and Human Life*; IntechOpen: London, UK, 2019.
3. Rajput, A.; Sharma, R.; Bharti, R. Pharmacological Activities and Toxicities of Alkaloids on Human Health. *Mater. Today Proc.* **2022**, *48*, 1407–1415. [CrossRef]
4. Faisal, S.; Badshah, S.L.; Kubra, B.; Emwas, A.-H.; Jaremko, M. Alkaloids as Potential Antivirals. A Comprehensive Review. *Nat. Prod. Bioprospect.* **2023**, *13*, 4. [CrossRef]
5. Russo, M.; Moccia, S.; Spagnuolo, C.; Tedesco, I.; Russo, G.L. Roles of Flavonoids against Coronavirus Infection. *Chem. Biol. Interact.* **2020**, *328*, 109211. [CrossRef]
6. Aryal, B.; Raut, B.K.; Bhattarai, S.; Bhandari, S.; Tandan, P.; Gyawali, K.; Sharma, K.; Ranabhat, D.; Thapa, R.; Aryal, D.; et al. Potential Therapeutic Applications of Plant-Derived Alkaloids against Inflammatory and Neurodegenerative Diseases. *Evid.-Based Complement. Altern. Med.* **2022**, *2022*, 1–18. [CrossRef]
7. Tuzimski, T.; Petruczynik, A. New Trends in the Practical Use of Isoquinoline Alkaloids as Potential Drugs Applicated in Infectious and Non-Infectious Diseases. *Biomed. Pharmacother.* **2023**, *168*, 115704. [CrossRef]
8. M Mostafa, E.; Gamal, M.; M Ghoneim, M.; Hussein, S.; H El-Ghorab, A.; A Abdelgawad, M.; Musa, A. Repurposing of FDA Approved Alkaloids as COVID 19 Inhibitors; in Silico Studies. *Pharmacogn. J.* **2021**, *13*, 110–123. [CrossRef]
9. Wink, M. Potential of DNA Intercalating Alkaloids and Other Plant Secondary Metabolites against SARS-CoV-2 Causing COVID-19. *Diversity* **2020**, *12*, 175. [CrossRef]
10. Akinboye, A.J.; Kim, K.; Choi, S.; Yang, I.; Lee, J.-G. Alkaloids in Food: A Review of Toxicity, Analytical Methods, Occurrence and Risk Assessments. *Food Sci. Biotechnol.* **2023**, *32*, 1133–1158. [CrossRef]
11. Beyer, J.; Drummer, O.H.; Maurer, H.H. Analysis of Toxic Alkaloids in Body Samples. *Forensic Sci. Int.* **2009**, *185*, 1–9. [CrossRef]
12. Koleva, I.I.; van Beek, T.A.; Soffers, A.E.M.F.; Dusemund, B.; Rietjens, I.M.C.M. Alkaloids in the Human Food Chain—Natural Occurrence and Possible Adverse Effects. *Mol. Nutr. Food Res.* **2012**, *56*, 30–52. [CrossRef]
13. Schrenk, D.; Gao, L.; Lin, G.; Mahony, C.; Mulder, P.P.J.; Peijnenburg, A.; Pfuhler, S.; Rietjens, I.M.C.M.; Rutz, L.; Steinhoff, B.; et al. Pyrrolizidine Alkaloids in Food and Phytomedicine: Occurrence, Exposure, Toxicity, Mechanisms, and Risk Assessment—A Review. *Food Chem. Toxicol.* **2020**, *136*, 111107. [CrossRef]
14. de Nijs, M.; Crews, C.; Dorgelo, F.; MacDonald, S.; Mulder, P.P.J. Emerging Issues on Tropane Alkaloid Contamination of Food in Europe. *Toxins* **2023**, *15*, 98. [CrossRef]
15. Gumus, Z.P. Assessment of Toxic Pyrrolizidine and Tropane Alkaloids in Herbal Teas and Culinary Herbs Using LC-Q-ToF/MS. *Foods* **2023**, *12*, 3572. [CrossRef]
16. The European Commission. *Commission Regulation (EU) 2021/1399 of 24 August 2021 Amending Regulation (EC) No 1881/2006 as Regards Maximum Levels of Ergot Sclerotia and Ergot Alkaloids in Certain Foodstuffs*; The European Commission: Brussels, Belgium, 2021.
17. The European Commission. *Commission Regulation (EU) 2020/2040 of 11 December 2020 Amending Regulation (EC) No 1881/2006 as Regards Maximum Levels of Pyrrolizidine Alkaloids in Certain Foodstuffs*; The European Commission: Brussels, Belgium, 2020.

18. The European Commission. *Commission Regulation (EU) 2016/239 of 19 February 2016 Amending Regulation (EC) No 1881/2006 as Regards Maximum Levels of Tropane Alkaloids in Certain Cereal-Based Foods for Infants and Young Children*; The European Commission: Brussels, Belgium, 2016.
19. Robinson, T. The Metabolism and Biochemical Actions of Alkaloids in Animals. *Stud. Nat. Prod. Chem.* **2000**, *22*, 3–54.
20. Dusemund, B.; Nowak, N.; Sommerfeld, C.; Lindtner, O.; Schäfer, B.; Lampen, A. Risk Assessment of Pyrrolizidine Alkaloids in Food of Plant and Animal Origin. *Food Chem. Toxicol.* **2018**, *115*, 63–72. [CrossRef]
21. Fu, P.P.; Chou, M.W.; Xia, Q.; Yang, Y.-C.; Yan, J.; Doerge, D.R.; Chan, P.C. Genotoxic Pyrrolizidine Alkaloids and Pyrrolizidine Alkaloid *N*-Oxides—Mechanisms Leading to DNA Adduct Formation and Tumorigenicity. *J. Environ. Sci. Health Part C* **2001**, *19*, 353–385. [CrossRef]
22. He, Y.; Zhu, L.; Ma, J.; Lin, G. Metabolism-Mediated Cytotoxicity and Genotoxicity of Pyrrolizidine Alkaloids. *Arch. Toxicol.* **2021**, *95*, 1917–1942. [CrossRef]
23. Hukkanen, J.; Jacob, P.; Benowitz, N.L. Metabolism and Disposition Kinetics of Nicotine. *Pharmacol. Rev.* **2005**, *57*, 79–115. [CrossRef]
24. Park, S.B.; Jacob, P.; Benowitz, N.L.; Cashman, J.R. Stereoselective Metabolism of (S)-(-)-Nicotine in Humans: Formation of Trans-(S)-(-)-Nicotine N-1′-Oxide. *Chem. Res. Toxicol.* **1993**, *6*, 880–888. [CrossRef]
25. Benowitz, N.L.; Griffin, C.; Tyndale, R. Deficient C-Oxidation of Nicotine Continued. *Clin. Pharmacol. Ther.* **2001**, *70*, a120252. [CrossRef]
26. Widjaja, F.; Zheng, L.; Wesseling, S.; Rietjens, I.M.C.M. Physiologically Based Kinetic Modeling of Senecionine N-Oxide in Rats as a New Approach Methodology to Define the Effects of Dose and Endpoint Used on Relative Potency Values of Pyrrolizidine Alkaloid N-Oxides. *Front. Pharmacol.* **2023**, *14*, 1125146. [CrossRef]
27. Potęga, A.; Göldner, V.; Niehaves, E.; Paluszkiewicz, E.; Karst, U. Electrochemistry/Mass Spectrometry (EC/MS) for Fast Generation and Identification of Novel Reactive Metabolites of Two Unsymmetrical Bisacridines with Anticancer Activity. *J. Pharm. Biomed. Anal.* **2023**, *235*, 115607. [CrossRef]
28. Li, Z.; Shen, F.; Mishra, R.K.; Wang, Z.; Zhao, X.; Zhu, Z. Advances of Drugs Electroanalysis Based on Direct Electrochemical Redox on Electrodes: A Review. *Crit. Rev. Anal. Chem.* **2024**, *54*, 269–314. [CrossRef]
29. Rogowska, A.; Pomastowski, P.; Szultka-Młyńska, M.; Walczak-Skierska, J.; Rafińska, K.; Rafiński, Z.; Buszewski, B. Investigation of the Mechanism of Zearalenone Metabolization in Different Systems: Electrochemical and Theoretical Approaches. *Toxicon* **2022**, *210*, 19–24. [CrossRef]
30. Grint, I.; Crea, F.; Vasiliadou, R. The Combination of Electrochemistry and Microfluidic Technology in Drug Metabolism Studies. *ChemistryOpen* **2022**, *11*, e202200100. [CrossRef]
31. Herl, T.; Matysik, F. Recent Developments in Electrochemistry–Mass Spectrometry. *ChemElectroChem* **2020**, *7*, 2498–2512. [CrossRef]
32. Rodrigues, M.O.; Eberlin, M.N.; Neto, B.A.D. How and Why to Investigate Multicomponent Reactions Mechanisms? A Critical Review. *Chem. Rec.* **2021**, *21*, 2762–2781. [CrossRef]
33. Blazheyevskiy, M. *Application of Derivatization by Means of Peroxy Acid Oxidation and Perhydrolysis Reactions in Pharmaceutical Analysis*; Ivan Franko National University of Lviv: Lviv, Ukraine, 2017.
34. Aisyah, A.; Tamaela, N.B.; Santoso, J.; Syah, Y.M.; Mujahidin, D. Synthesis of Quinine N-Oxide and an NMR Tutorial in Its Structure Determination. *J. Sains Teh Dan Kina* **2016**, *17*, 11–20. [CrossRef]
35. Fawzy, A. Oxidative Degradation of Atropine Drug by Permanganate Ion in Perchloric and Sulfuric Acid Solutions: A Comparative Kinetic Study. *Adv. Biochem.* **2016**, *4*, 58. [CrossRef]
36. Ogawa, T.; Niwa, H.; Yamada, K. An Efficient Enantioselective Synthesis of Indicine N-Oxide, an Antitumor Pyrrolizidine Alkaloid. *Tetrahedron* **1993**, *49*, 1571–1578. [CrossRef]
37. Vaz, N.; Manjunatha, A.S. Mechanistic Insight into the Oxidation of Atropine Sulfate Monohydrate with Aqueous Acidic Chloramine-T: Design of Kinetic Modeling. *Bulg. Chem. Commun.* **2016**, *48*, 671–677.
38. Meti, M.D.; Nandibewoor, S.T.; Chimatadar, S.A. Spectroscopic Investigation and Reactivities of Ruthenium(III) Catalyzed Oxidation of Anticholinergic Drug Atropine Sulfate Monohydrate by Hexacyanoferrate(III) in Aqueous Alkaline Media: A Mechanistic Approach. *Synth. React. Inorg. Met. Nano-Met. Chem.* **2014**, *44*, 263–272. [CrossRef]
39. Dubenska, L.; Dushna, O.; Pysarevska, S.; Blazheyevskiy, M. A New Approach for Voltammetric Determination of Nefopam and Its Metabolite. *Electroanalysis* **2020**, *32*, 626–634. [CrossRef]
40. Dubenska, L.O.; Dushna, O.M.; Plyska, M.V.; Blazheyevskiy, M.Y. Method of Polarographic Determination Of Platyphylline In A Form Of N-Oxide And Its Validation In Solution For Injection. *Methods Objects Chem. Anal.* **2020**, *15*, 83–92. [CrossRef]
41. Dubenska, L.; Dushna, O.; Blazheyevskiy, M.; Pysarevska, S.; Klymiuk, I. Kinetic and Polarographic Study on Atropine N-Oxide: Its Obtaining and Polarographic Reduction. *Chem. Pap.* **2021**, *75*, 4147–4155. [CrossRef]
42. Dushna, O.; Dubenska, L.; Plotycya, S.; Rydchuk, M.; Blazheyevskiy, M. The Alternative Voltammetric Method for the Determination of Nicotine and Its Metabolite Nicotine N-Oxide. *J. Electrochem. Soc.* **2022**, *169*, 016513. [CrossRef]
43. Gawor, A.; Bulska, E. A Standardized Protocol for Assuring the Validity of Proteomics Results from Liquid Chromatography–High-Resolution Mass Spectrometry. *Int. J. Mol. Sci.* **2023**, *24*, 6129. [CrossRef]
44. Köfeler, H.C.; Gross, M.L. Correction of Accurate Mass Measurement for Target Compound Verification by Quadrupole Time-of-Flight Mass Spectrometry. *J. Am. Soc. Mass. Spectrom.* **2005**, *16*, 406–408. [CrossRef]

45. Yu, J.; Solon, E.; Shen, H.; Modi, N.B.; Mittur, A. Pharmacokinetics, Distribution, Metabolism, and Excretion of the Dual Reuptake Inhibitor [^{14}C]-Nefopam in Rats. *Xenobiotica* **2016**, *46*, 1026–1048. [CrossRef]
46. Chen, H.; Chen, Y.; Du, P.; Han, F.; Wang, H.; Zhang, H. Sensitive and Specific Liquid Chromatographic–Tandem Mass Spectrometric Assay for Atropine and Its Eleven Metabolites in Rat Urine. *J. Pharm. Biomed. Anal.* **2006**, *40*, 142–150. [CrossRef]
47. Luo, R.Y.; Comstock, K.; Ding, C.; Wu, A.H.B.; Lynch, K.L. Comparison of Liquid Chromatography-High-Resolution Tandem Mass Spectrometry (MS2) and Multi-Stage Mass Spectrometry (MS3) for Screening Toxic Natural Products. *J. Mass. Spectrom. Adv. Clin. Lab.* **2023**, *30*, 38–44. [CrossRef]
48. Marcsisin, S.R.; Jin, X.; Bettger, T.; McCulley, N.; Sousa, J.C.; Shanks, G.D.; Tekwani, B.L.; Sahu, R.; Reichard, G.A.; Sciotti, R.J.; et al. CYP450 Phenotyping and Metabolite Identification of Quinine by Accurate Mass UPLC-MS Analysis: A Possible Metabolic Link to Blackwater Fever. *Malar. J.* **2013**, *12*, 214. [CrossRef]
49. Iurchenko, I.; Blazheyevskiy, M.; Koretnik, O.; Shlusar, O. Iodometric Determination of Quinine Sulfate in Tablets Using N-Oxidation with Diperoxysebacic Acid. *Int. J. Sch. Res. Chem. Pharm.* **2023**, *3*, 001–012. [CrossRef]
50. Liang, S.-S.; Shiue, Y.-L.; Kuo, C.-J.; Guo, S.-E.; Liao, W.-T.; Tsai, E.-M. Online Monitoring Oxidative Products and Metabolites of Nicotine by Free Radicals Generation with Fenton Reaction in Tandem Mass Spectrometry. *Sci. World J.* **2013**, *2013*, 1–8. [CrossRef]
51. Smyth, T.J.; Ramachandran, V.N.; McGuigan, A.; Hopps, J.; Smyth, W.F. Characterisation of Nicotine and Related Compounds Using Electrospray Ionisation with Ion Trap Mass Spectrometry and with Quadrupole Time-of-flight Mass Spectrometry and Their Detection by Liquid Chromatography/Electrospray Ionisation Mass Spectrometry. *Rapid Commun. Mass. Spectrom.* **2007**, *21*, 557–566. [CrossRef]
52. Tsugawa, H.; Nakabayashi, R.; Mori, T.; Yamada, Y.; Takahashi, M.; Rai, A.; Sugiyama, R.; Yamamoto, H.; Nakaya, T.; Yamazaki, M.; et al. A Cheminformatics Approach to Characterize Metabolomes in Stable-Isotope-Labeled Organisms. *Nat. Methods* **2019**, *16*, 295–298. [CrossRef]
53. Famele, M.; Mancinelli, R.; Ferranti, C.; Zoratto, F. Proof of Nicotine Transfer to Rat Pups through Maternal Breast Feeding to Evaluate the Neurobehavioral Consequences of Nicotine Exposure. *Ann. Dell'Istituto Super. Sanità* **2018**, *54*, 176–184. [CrossRef]
54. Panek, J.J.; Błaziak, K.; Jezierska, A. Hydrogen Bonds in Quinoline N-Oxide Derivatives: First-Principle Molecular Dynamics and Metadynamics Ground State Study. *Struct. Chem.* **2016**, *27*, 65–75. [CrossRef]
55. Lin, L.; Bao, H.; Wang, A.; Tang, C.; Dien, P.-H.; Ye, Y. Two New N-Oxide Alkaloids from Stemona Cochinchinensis. *Molecules* **2014**, *19*, 20257–20265. [CrossRef]
56. Brandes, B.; Halz, J.H.; Merzweiler, K.; Deigner, H.-P.; Csuk, R. Synthesis and Structure of Azelastine-N-Oxides. *J. Mol. Struct.* **2022**, *1251*, 132033. [CrossRef]
57. Nowak, P.; Woźniakiewicz, M.; Kościelniak, P. Simulation of Drug Metabolism. *TrAC Trends Anal. Chem.* **2014**, *59*, 42–49. [CrossRef]
58. Jurva, U.; Weidolf, L. Electrochemical Generation of Drug Metabolites with Applications in Drug Discovery and Development. *TrAC Trends Anal. Chem.* **2015**, *70*, 92–99. [CrossRef]
59. Dar, R.A.; Brahman, P.K.; Tiwari, S.; Pitre, K.S. Electrochemical Studies of Quinine in Surfactant Media Using Hanging Mercury Drop Electrode: A Cyclic Voltammetric Study. *Colloids Surf. B Biointerfaces* **2012**, *98*, 72–79. [CrossRef]
60. Reybier, K.; Nguyen, T.H.Y.; Ibrahim, H.; Perio, P.; Montrose, A.; Fabre, P.-L.; Nepveu, F. Electrochemical Behavior of Indolone-N-Oxides: Relationship to Structure and Antiplasmodial Activity. *Bioelectrochemistry* **2012**, *88*, 57–64. [CrossRef]
61. Moreno, E.; Pérez-Silanes, S.; Gouravaram, S.; Macharam, A.; Ancizu, S.; Torres, E.; Aldana, I.; Monge, A.; Crawford, P.W. 1,4-Di-N-Oxide Quinoxaline-2-Carboxamide: Cyclic Voltammetry and Relationship between Electrochemical Behavior, Structure and Anti-Tuberculosis Activity. *Electrochim. Acta* **2011**, *56*, 3270–3275. [CrossRef]
62. MTech Lab. Available online: http://chem.lnu.edu.ua/mtech/devices.htm (accessed on 4 June 2024).

molecules

MDPI

Review

Potential Pharmacological Properties of Triterpene Derivatives of Ursolic Acid

Vuyolwethu Khwaza * and Blessing A. Aderibigbe *

Department of Chemistry, University of Fort Hare, Alice Campus, Alice 5700, Eastern Cape, South Africa
* Correspondence: vkhwaza@ufh.ac.za (V.K.); baderibigbe@ufh.ac.za (B.A.A.); Tel.: +27-40-602-2266 (B.A.A.)

Abstract: Ursolic acid (UA) and its derivatives have garnered significant attention due to their extensive pharmacological activity. UA is a pentacyclic triterpenoid found in a variety of plants, such as apples, rosemary, thyme, etc., and it possesses a range of pharmacological properties. Researchers have synthesized various derivatives of UA through structural modifications to enhance its potential pharmacological properties. Various in vitro and in vivo studies have indicated that UA and its derivatives possess diverse biological activities, such as anticancer, antifungal, antidiabetic, antioxidant, antibacterial, anti-inflammatory and antiviral properties. This review article provides a review of the biological activities of UA and its derivatives to show their valuable therapeutic properties useful in the treatment of different diseases, mainly focusing on the relevant structure-activity relationships (SARs), the underlying molecular targets/pathways, and modes of action.

Keywords: ursolic acid; natural product; triterpenoids; pharmacological activities; derivatives

1. Introduction

Natural products are chemical compounds extracted or isolated from living organisms. The molecular structural diversity of natural products and their unique pharmacological activities have attracted the attention of medicinal chemists. Natural products and their bioactive molecules act as valuable resources for drug discovery in medicinal chemistry [1]. In recent decades, drugs derived from or inspired by natural products have significantly contributed to disease treatment [2]. Between 1981 and 2019, 1881 drugs were approved, with 71 (3.8%) being natural products and 356 (18.9%) resulting from semisynthetic modification of natural products [3]. The discovery of artemisinin stands out as a significant achievement in the development of natural products [4].

Triterpenoids, the largest group of natural bioactive molecules, have been widely explored due to their pharmacological properties [5–7]. The IUPAC name of UA (**1**) is 3-(β-hydroxy-urs-12-en-28-oic acid) and its chemical structure is shown in Figure 1. It is a pentacyclic triterpenoid of the ursane type, derived from various plant species. Historically, UA was first identified in the extract of apple epicuticular waxes during the 1920s [8,9]. Since then, numerous reports have detailed the isolation of UA from different plant species and the evaluation of its biological activities. Additionally, several studies have introduced new methods for developing novel formulations of UA and modifying its chemical structure to enhance its therapeutic effects in both in vivo and in vitro studies by improving its poor water solubility and bioavailability. In terms of biological activities, UA, with a basic chemical structure containing five 6-membered rings (A, B, C, D and E), has a remarkable variety of biological properties such as anticancer [10,11], antiviral [12–14], anti-inflammatory [15–18], anti-oxidant [19,20], antifungal [21–25], antibacterial [26,27], antidiabetic effects [28–32], etc. (as depicted in Figure 1).

In this review, we present an update on the structural modifications and therapeutic effects of UA and its derivatives on various infectious and non-infectious diseases. Additionally, we summarize the proposed mechanisms of action and molecular targets of UA and its derivatives.

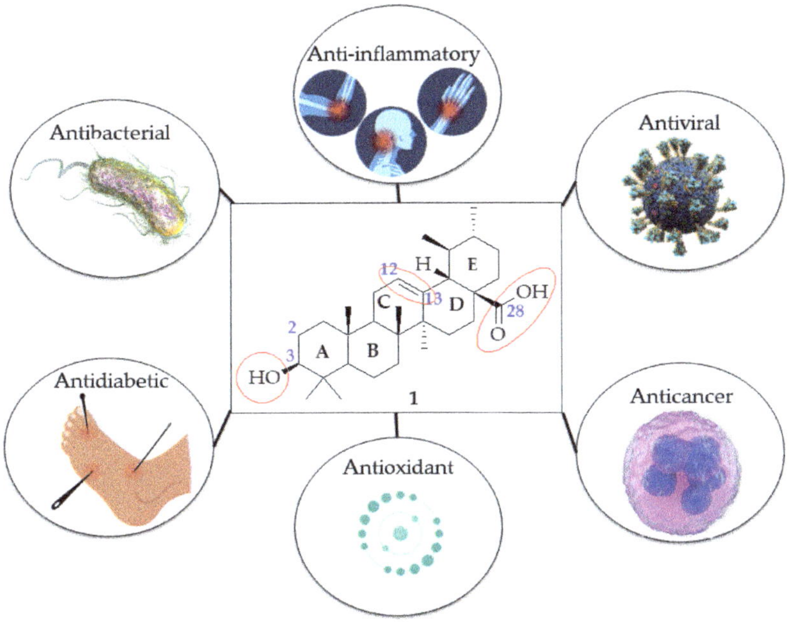

Figure 1. The chemical structure of UA with highlighted major active sites and its biological properties.

2. UA Derivatization

The chemical structure of UA features three primary active sites for structural modification as highlighted in Figure 1. These sites include the carboxylic group at C-28, the β-hydroxy group at C-3, and an alkene between C-12 and C-13. These sites have been extensively explored for their potential pharmacological activities, with anticancer derivatives being among the most studied [33]. Modification of the C-28 carboxylic acid or C-3 hydroxyl group not only significantly enhances its biological activity but also decreases its toxicity [34,35]. In addition to the important role played by the C-28 amide and C-3 ester groups in inhibiting NF-κB, Jiang et al. reported the antitumor efficacy of long-chain diamine derivatives of UA through potential NF-κB inhibition. Derivatives with longer chain diamine side chains (n = 6) had better activity than those with shorter chains (n = 4 and 5). The presence of an O-acetyl substitution at C-28 proved to give more activity than the presence of a hydroxyl group at the same position [36]. Modifications have been employed in trying to change the oxidation state and /or the lipophilicity at C-3 [33]. Some studies have revealed that the configuration at C-3 plays a vital role in the antiproliferative activity of UA, and, at the same time, a free hydroxyl group at the same position decreases its anticancer efficacy [37]. Modifications such as the retention of the carbonyl at C-28 and the incorporation of several substituted aromatic rings at C-3 improved the anticancer activity of UA [38]. The introduction of a tetrazole moiety at the C-28 position of UA increases HIF-1α inhibitory activity while a bulky group at the C-3 position decreases the activity [39]. Wang et al. reported that compounds containing ester groups showed stronger antitumor activity towards MCF-7, HeLa and HepG2 cells than compounds with acylhydrazine, amide and carbonyl moieties. Though the introduction of N,N-dialkylamide decreased cytotoxicity activity, the compounds containing dimethylamino groups on the amide side chain displayed the strongest antitumor activity of all the derivatives indicating the role played by the groups on the amino side chain in enhancing cytotoxicity [40].

In summary, UA derivatization typically involves modifying specific functional groups on the UA structure. Common UA modifications include:

Esterification: introducing ester groups can improve lipophilicity and membrane permeability [41,42].
Amidation: converting carboxyl groups to amides can enhance stability and bioactivity [43–45].
Glycosylation: adding sugar moieties can improve solubility and bioavailability [46].
Oxidation/Reduction: modifying hydroxyl or carbonyl groups to influence activity and selectivity [47].
Acylation: adding acyl groups to enhance lipophilicity and cellular uptake [37].

3. Pharmacokinetic Studies

Although UA is recognized for its ability to inhibit the proliferation of various cancer cell lines, its pharmacokinetics are constrained by its low aqueous solubility. The effectiveness of cancer treatment relies on the drug's ability to reach the tumor at therapeutic concentrations [48]. Preclinical trials have shown that UA is poorly absorbed through the intestines and rapidly eliminated by liver metabolism when orally administered. Intravenous administration of UA resulted in its diffusion throughout the body with non-specific distribution [49]. Since the oral route is considered better than the intravenous, efforts have been made to enhance the bioavailability of phytochemical antitumor agents following oral administration. The slow release of UA from UA-loaded nanoparticles resulted in lower cytotoxicity than the free UA [48]. Frolova et al. employed fluorescently labelled UA to track the penetration and distribution dynamics of UA in vitro. The confocal images after 12 h of incubation inferred the location of UA on the inner membranes (endosomes, Golgi apparatus and endoplasmic reticulum). After 18h, the labelled UA was bound to the mitochondrial receptors while the signal could be identified within the nucleus after 24 h [35].

Khan et al. determined that UA nano lipid vesicles (UALVs) and UA-loaded lipid vesicle gel (UALVG) exhibited distinct pharmacokinetic profiles following intranasal administration. UALVs showed a peak plasma concentration (C_{max}) at 30 min (142.9 $\pm$ 5.49 ng/mL) with a T_{max} of 30 min, whereas in the brain, the T_{max} was 2 h (C_{max} 325.2 $\pm$ 20.86 ng/g). On the other hand, UALVG had a T_{max} of 2 h (C_{max} 184.73 ng/g) in plasma and 6 h (C_{max} 398.9 ng/g) in brain tissue. Penetration enhancement effects of the lipids and vesicular size meant that the T_{max} and C_{max} values would differ between the UALV and UALVG. The nanoformulation was non-toxic both to the nasal mucosa and the brain [50].

4. Biological Activities

UA is known for its diverse biological effects, such as its ability to combat cancer, diabetes, viruses, etc. (see Figure 1). Reviewing various reported studies, the sections below briefly introduce the pharmacological activities of UA and its derivatives.

4.1. Anti-Inflammatory Activity

Inflammation is the body's natural response to a variety of stimuli, including pathogens, chemicals, and autoimmune triggers. It is essential for tissue repair and defense against these stimuli and is marked by symptoms like redness, pain and swelling [51]. Inflammation is an intricate process linked to the development of several diseases, such as cardiovascular conditions, cancer, neurodegenerative disorders, etc. [52].

UA's mechanism of action involves an increase in proteins crucial for the terminal differentiation of keratinocytes, such as filaggrin, loricrin, and involucrin [53]. UA boosts intercellular lipids, especially ceramide, aiding in the restoration of the epidermal barrier [53,54]. Additionally, UA can reduce intracellular reactive oxygen species (ROS) production and mitigate the oxidative effects of UVB radiation by preventing lipid peroxidation [55,56]. The anti-inflammatory properties of UA are attributed to the suppression of NF- and the genes it regulates, including pro-inflammatory cytokines, Cyclooxygenase-2 (COX-2), and lipoxygenase [57].

Pentacyclic triterpenes are a highly potent class of natural products due to their diverse biological properties and structural variety [43]. UA, a plant-derived medicinal compound, targets different extracellular and intracellular mechanisms related to inflammation, angiogenesis, metastasis, and apoptosis. Moreover, UA synthetic derivatives have demonstrated good potential in disease prevention [52]. The anti-inflammatory activities of UA and its derivatives are attributed to their ability to inhibit histamine release from mast cells and suppress the activities of cyclooxygenase and lipoxygenase enzymes [53]. Additionally, they inhibit inducible nitric oxide synthase (iNOS) and elastase, reduce the inflammatory cytokine-induced expression of E-selectin on endothelial cells by preventing NF-kappa B (NF-κB) activation, and decrease the production of intracellular reactive oxygen species [58]. However, despite these benefits, UA faces some technological challenges, including low water solubility (~5.6 μg/mL), poor absorption, and low bioavailability, which limit its clinical potential [59].

Wei et al. [43] developed UA derivatives incorporating piperazine, triazolone, and oxadiazole groups to develop effective anti-inflammatory agents. Many of these molecules demonstrated significant anti-inflammatory effects at a dosage of 100 mg/kg. Notably, compound **2** (Figure 2) demonstrated a potent inhibitory effect on ear inflammation among all the synthesized molecules, with an inhibition of 69.76%, surpassing that of ibuprofen (25.17%) and indomethacin (26.83%) at a dosage of 100 mg/kg (i.p.), making it 2- and 3-fold more potent than these standard drugs used as control. The cytotoxicity of the derivatives was evaluated using the MTT assay, and none exhibited significant cytotoxic activity, unlike UA. Additionally, molecular docking results revealed that the UA derivatives showed a high affinity for the COX-2 active site, suggesting their anti-inflammatory effects are likely due to COX-2 inhibition. These findings suggest that compound **2** is a promising anti-inflammatory therapeutic.

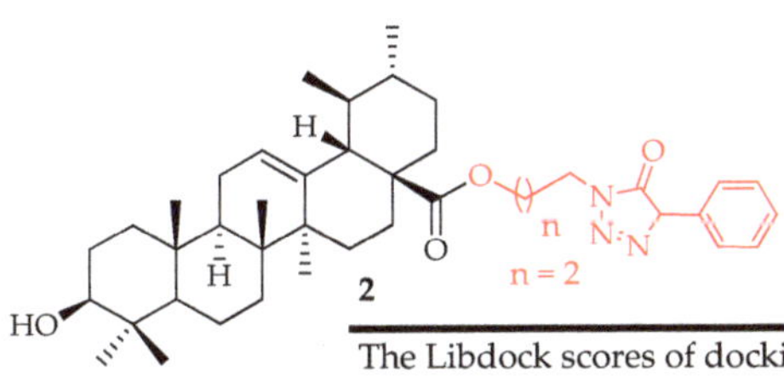

The Libdock scores of docking (compounds **2** and UA) with COX-2		
Compound	Inhibition rate (%)	LibDock score(kcal/mol)
2	69.76	151.72
UA	57.67	126.69

Figure 2. UA derivative 2 and its anti-inflammatory outcomes compared to UA.

Zhang et al. [60] designed and synthesized three compounds by attaching 1,2,3-triazole groups to UA to explore new anti-inflammatory agents. These compounds were evaluated for anti-inflammatory effects employing an ear edema model. The most potent compound was subjected to in vitro assays for COX-2/ COX-1 inhibition. Overall, the derivatives demonstrated significant anti-inflammatory activity. Notably, compound **3** (Figure 3) showed the highest activity, with an 82.81% inhibition rate following intraperitoneal administration, surpassing celecoxib used as a positive control. Molecular docking revealed the interaction mechanism between the COX-2 enzyme and compound **3**. Further studies indicated that compound **3** had strong COX-2 inhibitory activity, with an IC_{50} value of 1.16 μM and a selectivity index (SI) of 64.66, comparable to celecoxib with an IC_{50} value of 0.93 μM and SI of 65.47. These findings show that this chemotype holds promise for developing new anti-inflammatory agents targeting COX-2. It was observed that the position and the physical and chemical properties of different substituents on the phenyl ring had little effect on the anti-inflammatory activities of these compounds. This suggests that the electronic effect of the group attached to the benzene ring was insignificant.

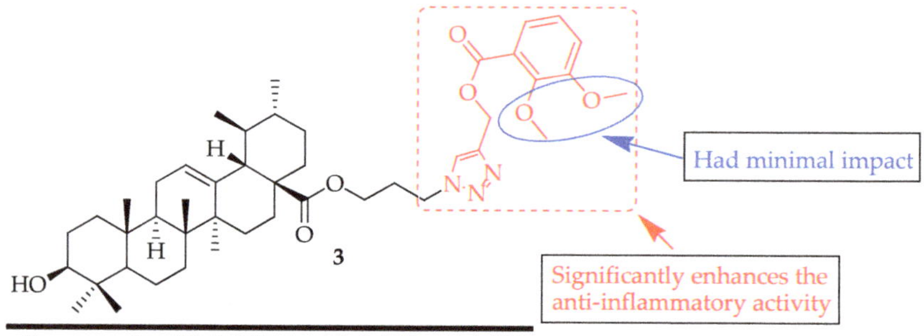

Compound	IC_{50}(μM)	Inhibition rate(%)
3	1.38 ± 0.65	82.81
UA	4.80 ± 0.58	55.34
Celecoxib	2.80 ± 0.65	65.00

Figure 3. UA derivative **3** and its anti-inflammatory outcomes compared to UA and reference drug.

The same authors [61] synthesized and screened two series of novel UA-based 1,2,4-triazolo [1,5-a]pyrimidine derivatives for their anti-inflammatory properties. They evaluated the compounds by examining how these compounds inhibit the inflammatory response induced by LPS in RAW 264.7 macrophages in vitro. The researchers examined how varying concentrations of the compounds affected the release of nitric oxide (NO) and inflammatory cytokines (i.e., TNF-α and IL-6). They also assessed the compounds' in vitro toxicity. The findings showed that compound **4** (Figure 4) could significantly decrease the production of the inflammatory factors. A docking analysis was performed to explore how compound **4,** UA, and Celecoxib interact with the active site of the COX-2 receptor. The enzyme study conducted in vitro indicated that compound **4** achieves its anti-inflammatory effects by inhibiting COX-2. This research illustrated that incorporating a 1,2,4-triazolo[1,5-a]pyrimidine group into UA unexpectedly increased the anti-inflammatory potency of its derivatives. Previous research [20] showed a significant enhancement in the anti-inflammatory effect of UA by not modifying the carboxylic acid group (C-28). This study similarly found that certain compounds demonstrated more potent inhibition of IL-6 compared to compounds with an ethyl group added at the C-28 position.

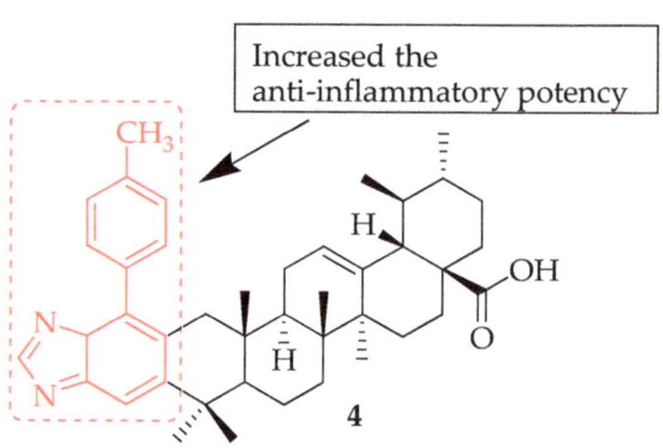

Figure 4. UA derivative **4** with the incorporated 1,2,4-triazolo[1,5-a]pyrimidine moiety and its corresponding effects.

Wu and colleagues [62] designed, synthesized, and evaluated three sets of UA derivatives that incorporated an aminoguanidine moiety for their antibacterial and anti-inflammatory properties. The anti-inflammatory tests revealed that a majority of the compounds demonstrated strong activity. Notably, compound **5** (Figure 5) showed the highest potency, achieving 81.61% inhibition following intraperitoneal administration. This was more effective than UA and the standard reference drugs ibuprofen and indomethacin. SAR analysis demonstrated that the aminoguanidine group was crucial for anti-inflammatory properties. These findings suggested that keeping the carboxylic group (C-28) was advantageous for maintaining this activity.

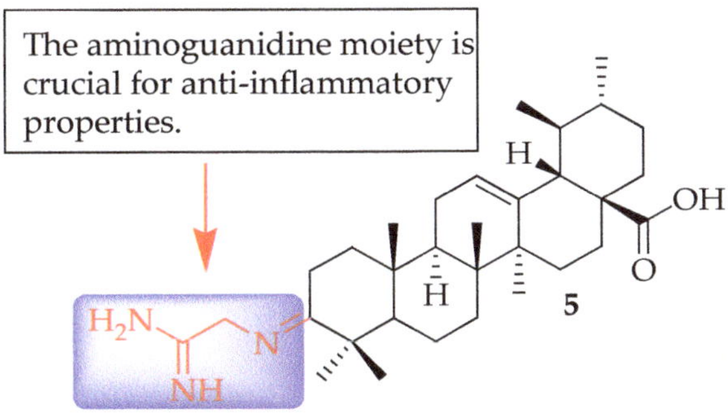

Compound	IC_{50}(μM)	Inhibition rate(%)
5	1.14 ± 0.3	81.61
UA	2.76 ± 0.41	55.35
Indometacin	3.56 ± 0.89	42.42
Ibuprfen	3.35 ± 0.55	45.86

Figure 5. UA derivative **5** and their anti-inflammatory outcomes compared to UA and reference drugs.

Qi et al. [63] conducted a study in which they synthesized 16 new hybrids of UA. These hybrids were linked through 1,2,3-triazole to modified gallate moieties, employing CuAAC 1,3-cycloaddition reactions. In the in vitro tests, it was shown that all these derivatives were successful in reducing oxidative stress and inflammation. Significantly, compound **6** (Figure 6) effectively reduced the expression of pro-inflammatory cytokines in lipopolysaccharide (LPS)-induced RAW264.7 cells in a dose-dependent manner, notably suppressing mRNA levels of iNOS ($p < 0.05$) and COX-2 ($p < 0.01$). Compound **6**'s ability to inhibit pro-inflammatory cytokines was associated with its suppression of the LPS-induced PI3K/Akt signalling pathway. Additionally, in vivo studies using zebrafish demonstrated that compound **6** effectively reduced inflammation in the gastrointestinal tract and exhibited favourable safety profiles in cytotoxicity assessments. According to their analysis of SARS, they noted that the potent anti-inflammatory effects of these new compounds could be explained by several factors: (1) the incorporation of triazole and gallate groups as polar components along with a nonpolar triterpene structure create hybrid compounds, possessing amphiphilic properties. This improves the solubility and availability of the hybrid derivatives; (2) the strong anti-inflammatory potency of hybrid triterpene derivatives containing a triazole linker is linked to the existence of two adjacent polar substituents in the aromatic position, consistent with the research findings of Zhang et al. [62]; (3) incorporating a gallate component into the hybrid compound led to remarkable antioxidant properties, potentially accountable for the inhibition of ROS; and (4) the incorporation of shielded gallates featuring a methoxy-methylenedioxy component enhanced the antioxidant and anti-inflammatory activities. Compounds containing this methoxymethylenedioxy segment could be seen as a latent form, combining polyphenol and aldehyde attributes. Reports suggest that integrating 1,3-benzodioxole components can enhance a compound's antioxidant, hypolipidemic effect, and anti-inflammatory (i.e., COX-2 inhibition) [64,65] properties. Hence, hybrids featuring 1,3-dioxo-lane protection may outperform derivatives with unbound phenolic OH groups in terms of antioxidant activity. The amide or ester linkage between the C-28 position of UA and the linker, along with the ether connection between the linker and the gallate element, exhibits resistance to hydrolysis, ensuring the stability of hybrid derivatives. This study offered a new reference for developing molecules for health issues related to antioxidation and anti-inflammation properties.

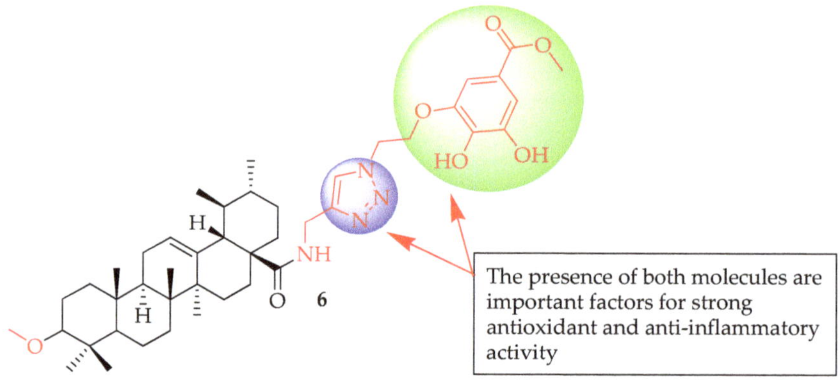

Figure 6. UA derivative **6** and the corresponding effect of the incorporated moieties.

Li et al. [66] synthesized derivatives of UA and assessed their ability to inhibit HIF-1α and their anti-inflammatory properties. Compound **7** (Figure 7) demonstrated stronger inhibition of HIF-1α compared to the standard UA. In vivo tests showed that compound **7** reduced inflammation similarly to celecoxib at the same dose. Additionally, compound **7** moderately inhibited COX-2, akin to celecoxib. Overall, among the newly developed derivatives, compound **7** shows potential as a starting point for further optimization in the search for new HIF-1α inhibitors and anti-inflammatory drugs.

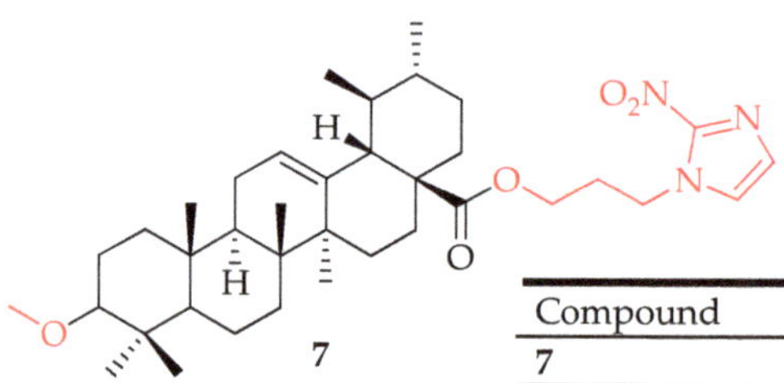

Compound	IC_{50}(μM)	Inhibition rate(%)
7	0.80 ± 0.01	68.13
UA	4.80 ± 0.58	55.34
Celecoxib	2.80 ± 0.65	65.00

Figure 7. UA derivative **7** and its anti-inflammatory outcomes compared to UA and Celecoxib.

Overall, the reported UA derivatives exhibit notable anti-inflammatory activity by inhibiting key inflammatory mediators and pathways. These derivatives can suppress the production of pro-inflammatory cytokines and downregulate the expression of COX-2 and inducible iNOS. Additionally, some UA derivatives may enhance the activity of antioxidant enzymes, reducing oxidative stress associated with inflammation. The combined effects of these mechanisms highlight their potential application for treating inflammatory diseases or conditions, making them valuable candidates for further research and development in anti-inflammatory therapies. Below (Table 1) is a summary of the anti-inflammatory activities of UA derivatives including the method of modification, the tested Models/Assays used, and the observed effects.

Table 1. The anti-inflammatory activity of various UA derivatives (**2–7**), including the method of modification, the tested cancer cell lines, and the observed effects.

Compounds	Modification Method	Tested Models/Assays	Observed Effects	Ref.
2	Incorporated piperazine, triazolone, and oxadiazole groups at the C-3 position	Ear edema model	Decreased ear swelling, reduced COX-2 expression	[43]
3	attached 1,2,3-triazole groups at the C-28 position	Para-xylene-induced mice ear-swelling	Reduced inflammation, reduced COX-2 expression	[61]
4	Incorporated a 1,2,4-triazolo[1,5-a]pyrimidine group at C-28 position.	xylene-induced ear edema model	Decreased the production of the inflammatory factors, inhibited COX-2	[61]
5	Incorporated an aminoguanidine moiety	xylene-induced ear edema	Reduced inflammation	[62]
6	Linked UA with modified gallate moieties through 1,2,3-triazole employing CuAAC 1,3-cycloaddition reactions	RAW 264.7 macrophages	Inhibited pro-inflammatory cytokines by suppressing the LPS-induced PI3K/Akt signalling pathway, suppressed mRNA levels of iNOS ($p < 0.05$) and COX-2) ($p < 0.01$).	[63]
7	introduced a 1,2,3-triazoles moiety, 1,2,4-triazoles moiety or a nitroimidazoles ring to the C-28 of UA nucleus	xylene-induced ear edema	Inhibited HIF-1α, and COX-2.	[66]

4.2. Anticancer Activity

Currently, cancer poses a significant threat to human health in developing countries. Therefore, there is an urgent demand for new strategies and approaches to develop effective anticancer agents for cancer treatment. Currently, various studies in cancer research are focused on UA because of its efficacy throughout different stages of cancer progression and its minimal toxicity. Even though the exact mechanisms behind its effects are not well understood, many studies have demonstrated that UA can produce significant anticancer properties by regulating related factors such as apoptosis, proliferation, metastasis, and angiogenesis [67–69]. Indeed, UA has strong antitumor activities and its interesting molecular structure with three major active pharmacophores, such as β-hydroxy (C-3), carboxylic moiety (C-28), and alkene (C-12–C-13), makes it a distinctive compound for appropriate structural modifications to develop more innovative anticancer agents [37,59].

Structural modification of a molecule affects its receptor binding and biological activity and alters its pharmacokinetic profile and physiochemical properties [70]. To determine the significant pharmacophores of a molecular drug, a thorough understanding of its synthetic and natural analogues is required. UA has significant anticancer properties on different cancer cells without impacting healthy cells. Although the precise molecular mechanisms of UA are still unclear, scientists have demonstrated that UA exerts its anticancer effects through various pathways, including the induction of autophagy and apoptosis [35], inhibition of angiogenesis and metastasis [71], inhibition of cell invasion, arresting the cell cycle [72], and reversing drug resistance of chemotherapy [73,74].

UA appears to induce apoptosis of many cancer cell lines through various mechanisms. Apoptosis, also referred to as programmed cell death I, is a conserved intrinsic cellular mechanism playing a significant role in pathological and physiological conditions [75,76]. Cell death occurs through two distinct mechanisms: the intrinsic pathway (i.e., mitochondrial pathway) and the extrinsic pathway (i.e., receptor pathway) [77]. Chuang et al. treated hepatocellular carcinoma cells (SK-Hep-1) with different concentrations of UA (0, 10, 20, 30, 40, 50, and 60 μM) for 24, 48, or 72 h. The results showed a reduction in cell viability in a time- and dose-dependent manner, along with nuclear chromatin shrinkage, indicating that UA may induce apoptosis by inhibiting the p38MAPK- and PI3K/AKT-signaling pathways [78].

In another study by Luo et al., UA was found to trigger apoptosis in hepatoma cells (HepG2) by activating AMP-activated protein kinase (AMPK) and promoting glycogen synthase kinase 3β (GSK 3β) phosphorylation [79]. In gallbladder carcinoma cells (SGC-996 and GBC-SD), UA inhibits cell proliferation and induces S-phase cell cycle arrest and apoptosis by modulating the expression of relevant molecules. Moreover, UA administration via intraperitoneal injection reduced xenograft gallbladder tumor growth in nude mice by activating caspase-3 and caspase-9 [80].

Fan et al. synthesized twelve novel UA-based hybrid compounds and evaluated them against glioma cell lines. Among the synthesized compounds, compound **8** (Figure 8) exhibited stronger inhibition of U251 cell proliferation compared to UA. Compound **8** suppressed the growth of glioma cells, triggered apoptosis, and halted cell cycle progression by down-regulating metabolic pathways [81]. Mendes et al. [82] prepared a collection of novel ring-A cleaved UA derivatives and evaluated their impact on inhibiting proliferation in non-small cell lung cancer (NSCLC) cells using both 3D and 2D culture models. The most effective compound was found to be compound **9** (Figure 8) with a secondary amine at position C-3 of a cleaved ring-A. Among the amide derivatives, those with secondary amides and bulkier side chains exhibited a significant reduction in cytotoxic activity. In contrast, secondary amides with smaller alkyl side chains resulted in the most potent compounds, with compound **9** demonstrating five times greater potency than the parent compound UA across all tested cell lines. The molecular mechanism investigation of this compound indicated the promotion of apoptosis via the activation of caspase-7/-8, along with the suppression of Bcl-2. Compound **9** also induced autophagy with elevated levels of Beclin-1 or LC3A/B-II and reduced levels of mTOR and p62.

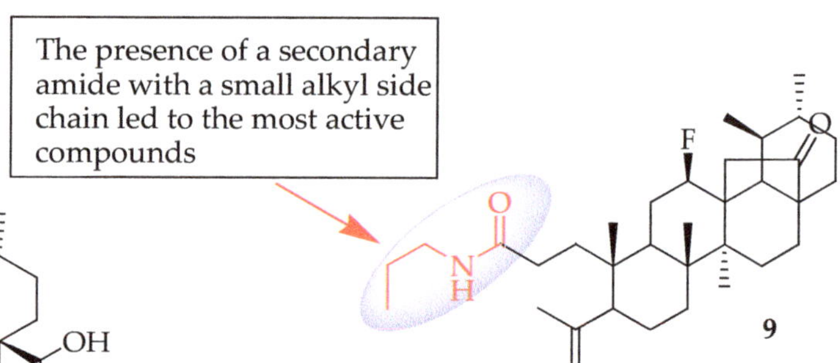

9

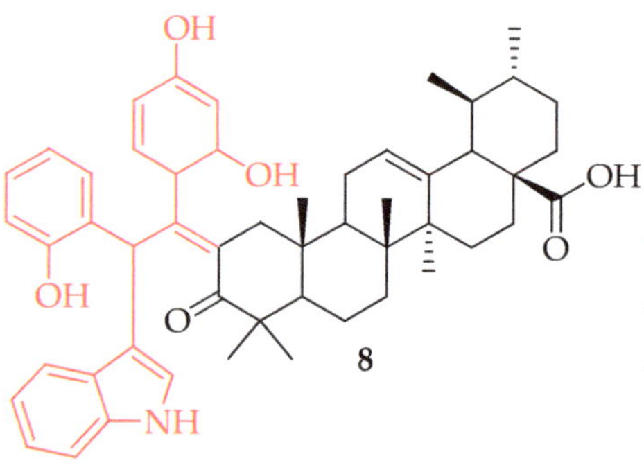

8

	IC$_{50}$ (μM)		
Compound	H460	H322	H460
UA	14.8 ± 0.6	15.3 ± 2.8	21.1 ± 1.6
9	2.6 ± 0.9	3.3 ± 0.9	4.4 ± 0.6

Figure 8. UA derivatives (**8**, **9**) and their anticancer outcomes compared to UA.

Derivative **10** (Figure 9) showed higher cytotoxicity than the parent UA in MCF-7 and TET21N cell lines with IC$_{50}$ values of 1.59 ± 0.11 and 0.81 ± 0.08 μM, respectively. It was also significantly more effective in inducing mitochondria-dependent apoptosis, evidenced by the release of cytochrome c, activation of caspase-3, and poly(ADP-ribose)polymerase cleavage, a known caspase-3 target [83].

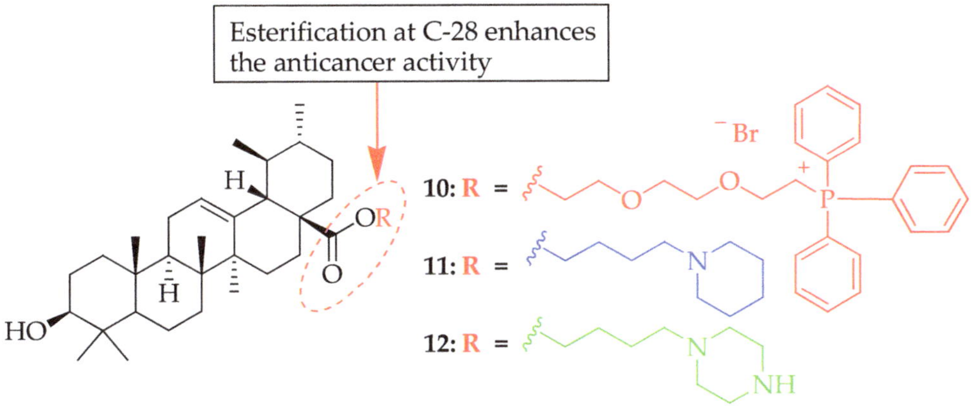

Compound	IC_{50} (μM)	
UA	>20(MCF-7)	>10(TET21N)
10	1.59 ± 0.911(MCF-7)	0.81 ± 0.8(TET21N)
UA	26.51 ± 1.1(MGC-803)	31.39 ± 0.85(Bcap-37)
11	4.99 ± 0.40(MGC-803)	8.56 ± 0.44 (Bcap-37)
UA	28.9 ± 1.3(H460)	26.8 ± 2.3(A549)
12	3.9 ± 0.2(H460)	3.4 ± 0.5(A549)

Figure 9. UA derivatives (**10–12**) and their anticancer outcomes compared to UA.

Liu et al. assessed the in vitro anticancer effects of compound **11** (Figure 9) on human breast cancer cells (Bcap-37) and gastric cancer cells (MGC-803) using an MTT assay. Compound **11** demonstrated a more potent inhibitory effect than UA. The mechanism of compound **11** was studied by Hoechst 33258 staining, acridine orange/ethidium bromide staining, terminal deoxynucleotidyl transferase biotin-dUTP nick-end labelling assay, and flow cytometry, which indicated that compound **11** can initiate apoptosis in MGC-803 cells, achieving an apoptosis rate of 34.59% after 36 h of treatment with 10 μM concentration [84]. The results indicate that: (1) Substituting the C28-COOH group of UA with a fatty alkyl group significantly reduced its effectiveness. (2) A notable improvement in cell growth inhibition was observed when an amino group was introduced at the C28 position. (3) Esterification of the C3-OH and C28-COOH groups with succinic anhydride and benzyl bromide, respectively, significantly enhanced the biological activity. However, introducing aromatic amines at the C-3 position resulted in a loss of activity, highlighting the importance of maintaining a polar group at the C-3 position for cytotoxic activity.

In a recent study conducted by Gou et al., a novel UA derivative compound **12** (Figure 9) exhibited a potent anticancer effect against lung cancer cells (A549 and H460 cells) than parent UA. It also revealed a stronger antiproliferation effect by inducing cell apoptosis and G0/G1 phase arrest, which is linked to the ER stress pathway, particularly the activation of the PERK/eIF2a/CHOP axis [85].

Meng et al. designed and synthesized eighteen UA derivatives and evaluated their cytotoxicity in vitro against two cancer cell lines, namely BEL7402 and SGC7901, by MTT assay. Four compounds (i.e., **13**, **14**, **15** and **16** (Figure 10)) showed a significantly higher inhibitory rate than the parent UA on both cell lines, and the interactions between the four compounds and NF-κB were also studied by docking simulations [86].

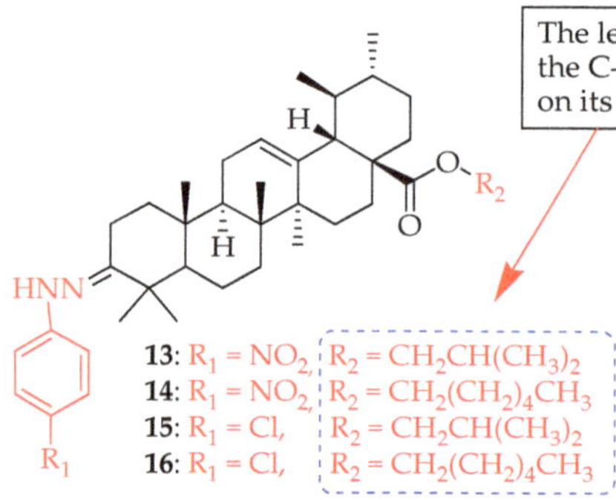

	IC_{50} (μM)	
Compound	BEL-7402	SGC-7901
UA	>50	>50
13	7.08	15.62
14	8.57	6.30
15	5.63	8.73
16	4.49	7.01

Figure 10. UA derivatives (**13–16**) and their anticancer outcomes compared to UA.

Wu et al. reported that UA derivative **17** (Figure 11) bearing an aminoguanidine moiety possesses the ability to inhibit HIF-1α transcriptional activity in low-oxygen conditions with an IC_{50} value of 4.0 μM. Compound **17** decreased HIF-1α protein expression by inhibiting its synthesis, lowered vascular endothelial growth factor production, and impeded cancer cell proliferation [38]. Compound **18** (Figure 11) synthesized by Jin et al. exhibited the most potent activity against three cancer cells (SMMC-7721, HeLa, and MDA-MB-231) and induced the apoptosis of cervical cancer cells (HeLa cells), halted cell cycle progression at the G0/G1 phase, decreased mitochondrial membrane potential, and elevated intracellular reactive oxygen species levels. Moreover, it suppressed MEK1 kinase activity and disrupted the Ras/Raf/MEK/ERK-signaling pathways [87].

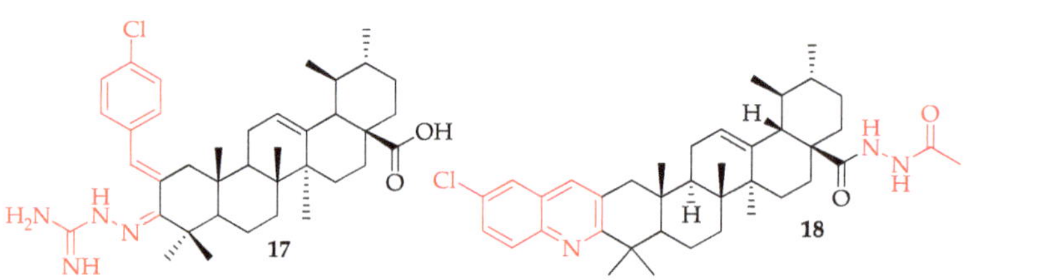

IC_{50}(μM)	
Compound	HRE
UA	>100
17	4.0

	IC_{50}(μM)			
Compound	MDA-MB-231	HeLa	SMMC-7721	QSG7701
UA	>50	>50	>50	
18	0.12 ± 0.01	0.08 ± 0.01	0.34 ± 0.03 1	0.76 ± 0.72

Figure 11. UA derivatives (**17**, **18**) and their anticancer outcomes compared to UA.

Gu et al. synthesized compounds **20–23** (Figure 12), which exhibited significant antitumor activities against three different human cancer cell lines (HeLa, SMMC-7721, MDA-MB-231), demonstrating greater potency than the positive control, etoposide. Compounds **20–23** were synthesized by dissolving UA in acetone and oxidizing it with Jones reagent, resulting in a 75% yield of 3-oxo-ursolic acid (**19**). Compound **19** was then treated with the respective o-amino benzaldehyde under a nitrogen atmosphere to produce compounds **20–23**, with yields ranging from 62% to 68%. Compound **21** induced apoptosis in MDA-MB-231 cell lines in a dose-dependent manner. Additionally, cell cycle analysis showed that compound **21** promoted G0/G1 phase arrest in MDA-MB-231 cell lines [88].

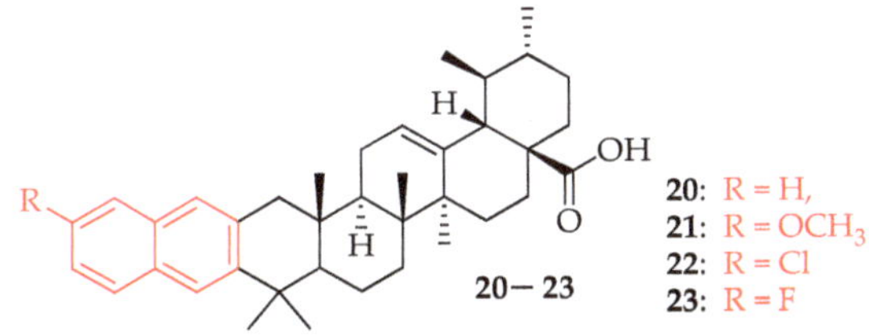

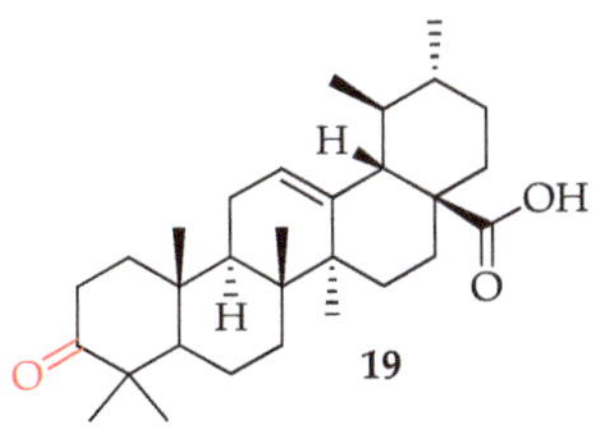

Compound	IC$_{50}$ (μM) SMMC-7721	HeLa	MDA-MB-231
UA	>40	>40	>40
Etoposide	21.03 ± 0.17	7.21 ± 0.79	16.27 ± 0.45
20	13.40 ± 0.08	0.37 ± 0.04	0.75 ± 0.05
21	12.49 ± 0.08	0.36 ± 0.05	0.61 ± 0.07
22	14.62 ± 0.05	1.22 ± 0.08	1.36 ± 0.03
23	13.34 ± 0.13	1.87 ± 0.03	0.90 ± 0.10

Figure 12. UA derivatives (**20–23**) and their anticancer outcomes compared to UA/model drug.

Meng et al. synthesized eleven novel derivatives by altering positions C-2, C-3, and C-28 of UA. These derivatives were evaluated for their cytotoxicity against human cancer cells (BGC-823, HeLa and HepG2) via MTT assay. The results revealed that all the synthesized compounds had strong antiproliferative activity against HepG2, BGC-823, and HeLa cells, and the compounds that indicated the most potent activity higher than gefitinib (positive control) were derivatives **24** and **25 (Figure 13**). Converting UA into an amide group at the C-28 position enhanced the antitumor activity, as observed in compounds **24** and **25**. Additionally, alkyl side chains at the C-3 position, like alkanoyloxy imino chains, play a crucial role in inhibiting tumor cell growth [89].

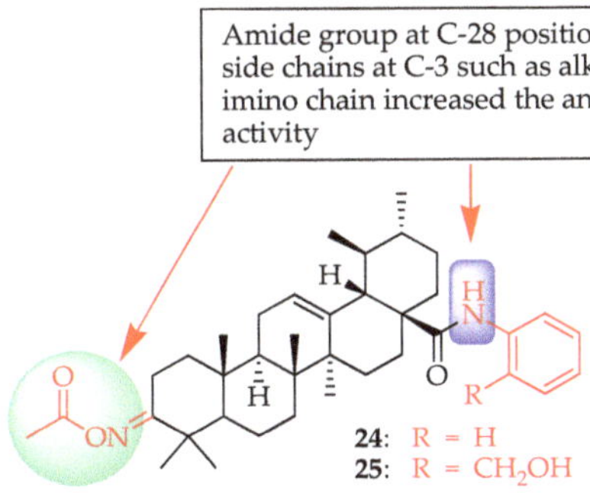

Compound	IC$_{50}$ (μM) HeLa	HepG2	BGC-823
UA	>50	>50	>50
Gefitinib	17.1	20.7	19.3
24	9.25	21.2	8.06
25	13.8	23.7	9.15

Figure 13. UA derivatives (**24**, **25**) and their anticancer outcomes compared to UA or a model drug.

Wang et al. [40] synthesized indolequinone derivatives of UA **26–28** (Figure 14) which inhibited cell migration, triggered apoptosis, and induced their cell cycle arrest of MCF-7 cells at the S phase in a concentration-dependent manner. When tested against MCF-7, HeLa, and HepG2 cells, compound **28** exhibited the best activity with IC$_{50}$ values of 1.66, 3.16, and 10.35 μM, respectively with very low cytotoxicity against gastric mucosal cell lines (Ges-1, IC$_{50}$ = 20.74 μM). Treating the cells with different concentrations of compound **28** raised ROS levels from 3.99% (control) to 43.23% (4 μM), suggesting that apoptosis induced by **28** was attributed to the production of ROS. The fact that **28** decreased the expression levels of p-AKT and p-mTOR indicated its ability to inhibit the P13K/AKT/mTOR-signaling pathway, an intracellular pathway important in cell cycle regulation and directly related to cell proliferation and cancer. The SAR analysis demonstrated that compounds with dimethylamino groups on the amide side chain displayed much stronger cytotoxic activities than all of the other derivatives, indicating that such moieties on the amide side chain were beneficial to their cytotoxic activity.

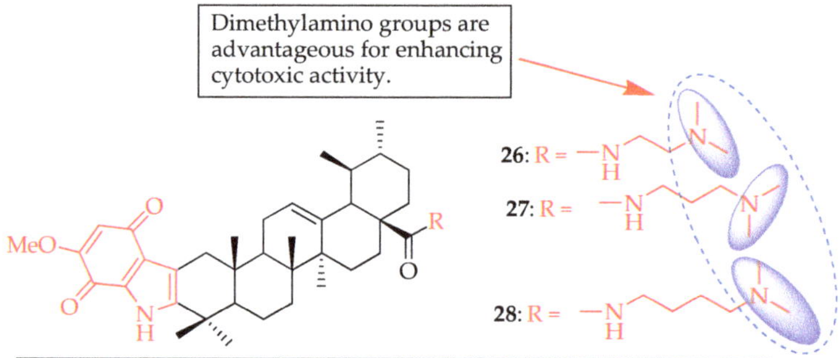

Compound	IC_{50} (μM)			
	MCF-7	HeLa	HepG2	Ges-1
26	2.52 ± 0.07	3.47 ± 0.16	21.27 ± 2.01	21.63 ± 0.27
27	2.23 ± 0.19	3.38 ± 0.60	14.90 ± 1.79	20.89 ± 0.45
28	1.66 ± 0.21	3.16 ± 0.24	10.35 ± 1.63	20.74 ± 0.61
Etoposide	5.14 ± 0.32	5.74 ± 0.42	8.73 ± 1.21	20.71 ± 0.49

Figure 14. UA derivatives (**26–28**) and their anticancer outcomes compared to UA/reference drug.

Zhang et al. developed a series of new UA containing tetrazole derivatives and assessed their inhibitory activity on the hypoxia-inducible factor 1α (HIF-1α), migration, angiogenesis, and proliferation. The most potent compounds were **29** (IC_{50} = 0.8 μM), **30** (IC_{50} = 1.4 μM), **31** (IC_{50} = 1.6 μM), **32** (IC_{50} = 2.2 μM), and **33** (IC_{50} = 4.7 μM) (Figure 15). Of the compounds tested, compound **33** showed the most promising HIF-1α inhibitory activity and did not show any significant cytotoxicity at a concentration of 30 μM against a Hep3B cell line. Analysis of the SARs of the compounds showed an increase in the HIF-1α inhibitory effect upon introducing a tetrazole moiety at C-28 of UA while bulky groups at C-3 proved to decrease the HIF-1α inhibitory activity [39].

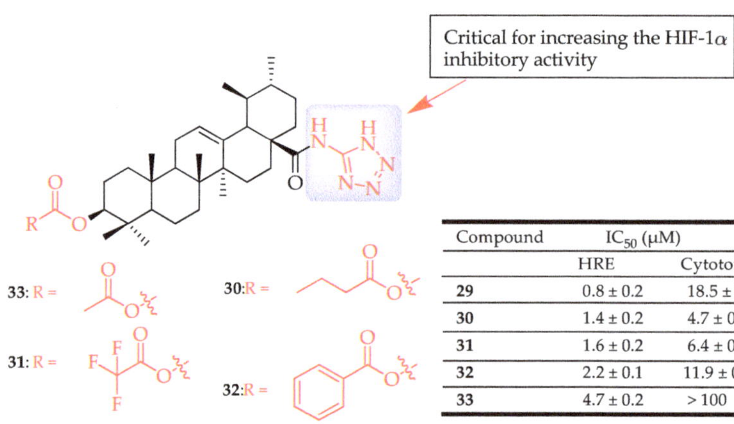

Compound	IC_{50} (μM)	
	HRE	Cytotoxicity
29	0.8 ± 0.2	18.5 ± 0.2
30	1.4 ± 0.2	4.7 ± 0.2
31	1.6 ± 0.2	6.4 ± 0.2
32	2.2 ± 0.1	11.9 ± 0.2
33	4.7 ± 0.2	> 100

Figure 15. UA derivatives (**29–33**) and their anticancer outcomes.

Popov et al. synthesized novel UA derivatives with a combination of two different azole types (1,3,4-oxadiazole and 1,2,3-triazole or 1,2,5-oxadiazole and 1,2,3-triazole) at different positions of UA. These hybrid compounds were evaluated for their cytotoxicity against immortalized human fibroblasts, A549, U-87 MG, HepG2, and MCF-7 cell lines. Compounds **34** and **35** (Figure 16) showed cytotoxicity comparable to that of UA on MCF-7 cells. Compound **35** had a 3-O-acetyl group which is known to have the potential of enhancing cytotoxicity [90]. Though **35** was less active than UA against the three cell lines, it exhibited excellent cytotoxicity against MCF-7 cells with IC_{50} = 1.55 μM, even better than doxorubicin (IC_{50} = 4.51 μM). Linking heterocyclic fragments of 1,2,3-triazole and 3-(methyl)-4-methyl-1,2,5-oxadiazole-2-oxide to the C-28 position of UA creates a favorable condition for the cytotoxic activity of these hybrid derivatives [91].

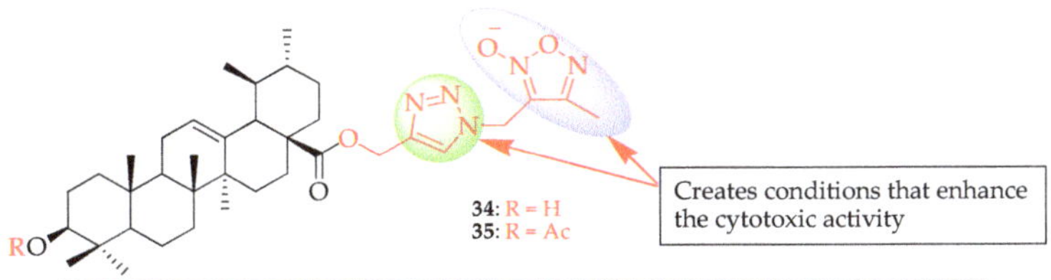

Compound	IC_{50}				
	Immortalized human fibroblasts	MCF-7	U-87 MG	A549	HepG2
Doxorubicin	3.33 ± 0.67	4.51 ± 1.12	2.05 ± 0.22	6.17 ± 1.17	10.02 ± 1.67
UA	90.89 ± 5.5	25.05 ± 3.17	43.82 ± 3.88	41.02 ± 3.77	37.28 ± 5.02
34	25.85 ± 3.04	22.9 ± 10.02	29.71 ± 6.52	> 100	12.89 ± 2.63
35	10.41 ± 1.2	1.55 ± 0.08	>100	> 100	> 100

Figure 16. UA derivatives (**34**, **35**) and their anticancer outcomes compared to UA or a model drug.

Zhang et al. synthesized a series of NO-donating UA-benzylidine derivatives and evaluated their in vitro antitumor activity against four human cancer cell lines (HepG-2, MCF-7, HT-29, and A549). The different constituents of the benzylidene at C-2 resulted in different inhibitory activity. Compound **36** (Figure 17) was found to be the most promising candidate with IC_{50} values of 65.8, 4.28, and 78.39 μM on HepG2, HT-29, and A549 cells, respectively. The cytotoxicity of **36** against these different cancer cell lines was attributed to replacing the 4-H atom at benzylidene with chlorine, introducing nitrooxyethyl at C-28, and the oxidation of C-3. Compound **36** induced apoptosis via arrest of the cycle at the G1 phase and mitochondria-mediated pathway. The very low IC_{50} (4.28 μM) of compound **36** against HT-29 showed its potential application for the treatment of colon cancer [92].

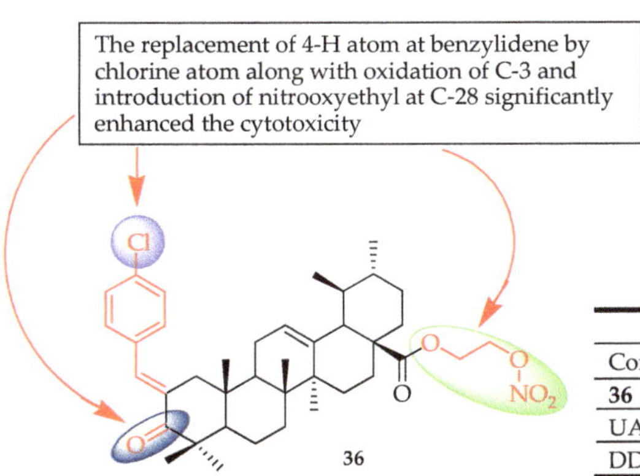

	IC_{50} (μM)			
Compound	HepG2	MCF-7	HT-29	A549
36	65.8 ± 6.3	>100	4.28 ± 3.5	78.39 ± 5.6
UA	44.35 ± 4.9	>100	41.86 ± 1.3	48.13 ± 2.2
DDP	22.21 ± 2.1	22.97 ± 3.4	12.23 ± 1.2	21.48 ± 3.7

Figure 17. UA derivative **36** and its anticancer outcomes compared to UA or model drug.

Compound **37** (Figure 18), one of the most active compounds synthesized by Wang and colleagues, lowered the ratio of the apoptosis regulators BCL2/BAX, resulting in disrupted mitochondrial potential and triggering apoptosis. Additionally, this compound effectively suppressed the growth of Hela xenografts in nude mice. Furthermore, a SAR analysis showed that several factors significantly influenced the cytotoxicity. These factors include the acetylation of the C-3 group, the type of nitrogen heterocycle, the length of linkers between the C-28 (COOH) and nitrogen heterocycles, and various substituents on the piperazine ring [93].

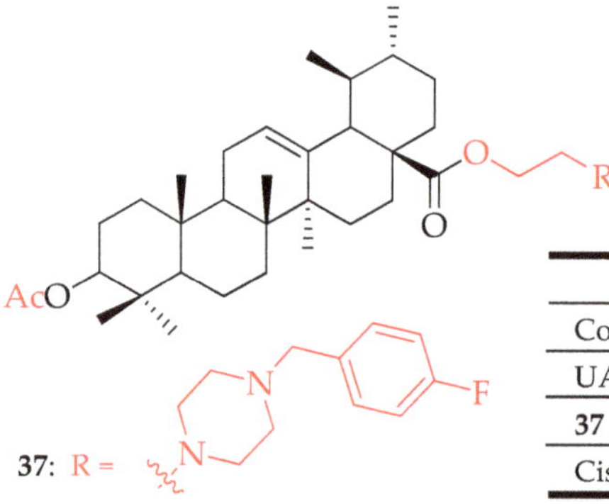

	Inhibition rates (%)		IC_{50} (μM)	
Compound	HeLa	MKN45	HeLa	MKN45
UA	13	18	15.1 ± 2.7	16.7 ± 1.4
37	89	84	2.6 ± 1.1	2.1 ± 0.3
Cisplatin	77	62	15.1 ± 0.9	2.8 ± 0.1

Figure 18. UA derivative (**37**) and its anticancer outcomes compared to UA Cisplatin.

Spivak et al. evaluated the anticancer properties of their novel C-28 guanidine-functionalized UA-based derivatives. Compounds **38** and **39** (Figure 19) exhibited better anticancer activity than UA when tested against HeLa, Jurkat, Hek293, K562, and U937 cell lines. Although compound **39** showed a weaker apoptotic effect, especially on the Jurkat cell line, it showed comparable results in decreasing the number of vital Jurkat cells (6.8, 14.3, and 20.7% of early and late apoptotic cells and necrotic cells, respectively). Based on the biological evaluation, compound **39** is assumed to trigger programmed cell death, which includes apoptotic mechanisms and arresting of the cell cycle in the S-phase [94].

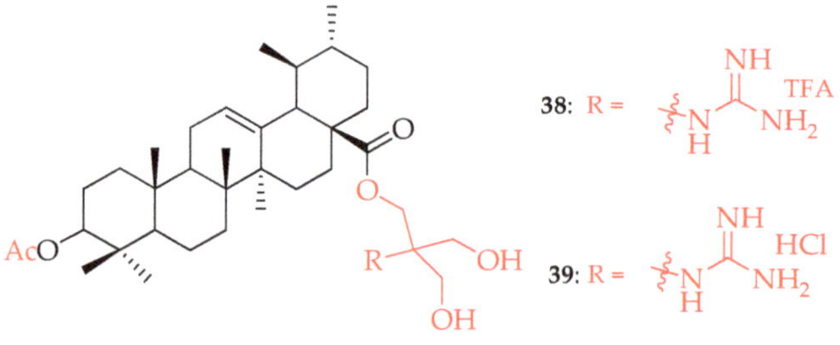

Compound	IC_{50} (μmol/L)					
	Jurkat	K562	U937	HEK293	HeLa	Fibroblasts
UA	23 ± 0.34	68 ± 0.11	17 ± 0.12	96 ± 0.22	88 ± 0.35	324 ± 0.16
38	6.8 ± 0.32	40 ± 0.29	2.1 ± 0.41	13 ± 0.19	11 ± 0.27	47 ± 0.15
39	3.8 ± 0.23	11 ± 0.18	5.3 ± 0.29	14 ± 0.34	12 ± 0.29	51 ± 0.26

Figure 19. UA derivatives (**38**, **39**) and their anticancer outcomes compared to UA.

Li et al. developed a novel UA derivative, having a nitrogen heterocyclic scaffold, which suppressed cell proliferation and triggered apoptosis in breast cancer cell lines. IC_{50} values for suppression of SUM149PT and HCC1937 cell viability by compound **40**

(Figure 20) were 4–6 μM compared to 8-10 μM by UA on the same cell lines. Compound **40** arrested the G_0/G_1 cell cycle, thereby inducing suppression of cancer cell viability. Treatment of SUM149PT and HCC1937 cells with 5 μM of **40** and UA revealed that the ability of **40** to induce apoptosis was higher than that of UA. The results showed that the incorporation of piperazine and thiourea at the C-28 and C-3 positions of UA significantly inhibits breast cancer cell viability [95].

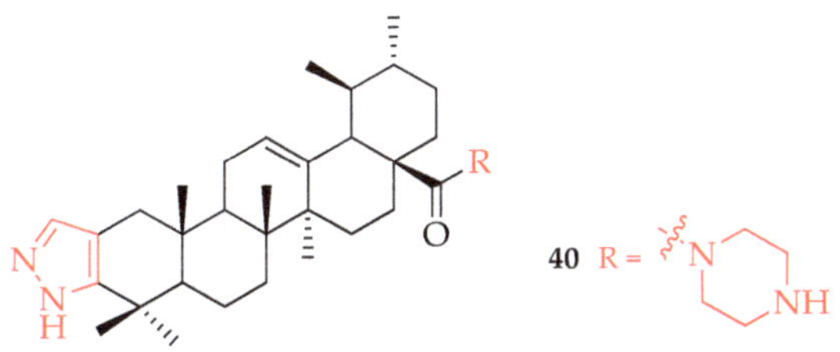

Figure 20. UA derivative **40** incorporated with nitrogen heterocyclic scaffolds.

Jiang et al. synthesized a series of UA derivatives having long-chain diamine gallic acid moieties as potential NF-κB inhibitors. Compound **41** (Figure 21) had the best activity against the four cell lines. The C-3 carbonyl moiety on compound **41** interacted with key residues on NF-κB through hydrogen bonding, thereby inhibiting its activity. Compound **41** inhibited the binding of NF-κB to DNA, suppressed NF-κB activation, inhibited A549 cell migration in vitro, and arrested A549 cell line at the G1 phase. The results showed the potential of the UA derivatives in inhibiting the NF-κB pathway, thus being able to suppress migration and reverse MDR in A549 lung cancer cells [36]. The SAR study reveals that diamide linkers at the C-28 position play an important role in the biological activity of the compound. Comparing the inhibitory concentrations of the pairs (with similar substitution and variation in n) indicated that the longer diamide side chain (n = 6) showed relatively enhanced activity than the shorter diamide side chain (n = 4 and 5).

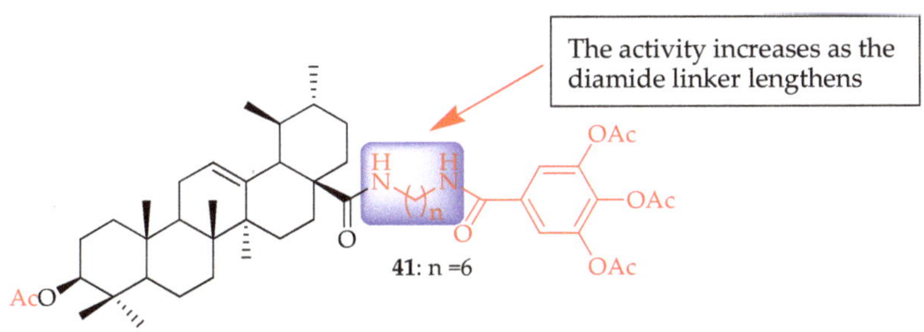

Compound	IC_{50} (μM)				
	T24	A549	HepG2	SKOV3	HL-7702
41	6.01 ± 0.87	5.22 ± 0.65	6.82 ± 1.07	8.95 ± 1.26	> 50
UA	37.88 ± 1.12	40.91 ± 0.92	42.37 ± 0.87	45.53 ± 1.21	> 50
HCPT	11.69 ± 0.75	2.73 ± 1.02	3.19 ± 0.56	6.01 ± 0.67	14.83 ± 1.01

Figure 21. UA derivatives and their anticancer outcomes compared to UA or model drug.

Fontana et al. evaluated the involvement of NF-κB in the cytotoxicity of UA derivatives towards the cell lines HepG2, Hep3B, and HA22T/VGH of hepatocellular carcinoma. Methylation of the carboxylic acid moiety did not improve the activity of the compounds while oxidation of C-3 resulted in the loss of activity. Compound **42** (Figure 22) showed inhibitory effects on NF-κB comparable to the ones of UA against the selected cell lines, showing its potent cytotoxicity towards hepatocellular carcinoma [33].

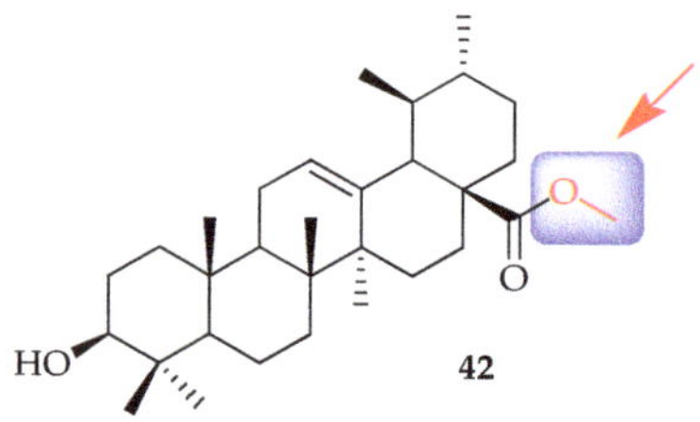

42

Methylation of the carboxylic acid moiety did not improve the activity

Compound	IC_{50} (μM)		
	HA22T/VGH	HepG2	Hep3B
UA	23.1 ± 8.7	40.8 ± 11.9	52.0 ± 1.0
42	38.0 ± 4.0	45.0 ± 5.0	38.0 ± 2.0

Figure 22. UA derivative **42** and their anticancer outcomes compared to UA.

UA derivatives have shown significant anticancer activity through various mechanisms, including induction of apoptosis, inhibition of tumor cell proliferation, and modulation of signaling pathways, such as NF-κB, which is associated with cancer progression. These derivatives can disrupt the cell cycle, promote the generation of ROS, and enhance the expression of pro-apoptotic proteins while downregulating anti-apoptotic factors. Additionally, these derivatives have demonstrated the capability to inhibit angiogenesis by affecting tumor microenvironment interactions and inflammatory responses. Overall, the structural modification of UA has led to the development of derivatives with superior anticancer properties, making them promising candidates for further preclinical and clinical development in cancer therapy. Table 2 summarizes the anticancer activities of the reported UA derivatives, including the method of modification, the tested cancer cell lines, and the observed effects. Subsequent research is still needed to explore the in-depth structure-activity relationships and the antitumor mechanism of these derivatives.

Table 2. The anticancer activity of various UA derivatives, including the method of modification, the tested cancer cell lines, and the observed effects.

Compounds	Modification Method	Tested Cancer Cell Lines	Observed Effects	Ref.
8	Used Jones reagent to deliver the C-3 oxidized UA derivative then incorporated benzaldehyde and indole.	U251 (Glioblastoma)	Suppressed the growth of glioma cells, triggered apoptosis, and halted cell cycle progression by down-regulating metabolic pathways	[81]
9	Introduced a secondary amine at position C-3 of a cleaved ring-A	NSCLC (Lung cancer)	Induced apoptosis and autophagy	[82]
10	Linked the triphenylphosphonium group to a UA at the C-28 position through the hydrophobic n-butyl or hydrophilic triethylene glycol spacer	MCF-7 (Breast adenocarcinoma) and TET21N (Neuroblastoma)	Induced mitochondria-dependent apoptosis	[83]
11	Reacted UA with 1,2-dibro-moethane, 1,3-dibromopropane, 1,4-dibromobutane or butyl bromide in DMF in the presence of K_2CO_3, and then reacted with corresponding amines to yield the targeted compounds.	Bcap-37 (Breast cancer) and MGC-803 (Gastric cancer)	Induced apoptosis on MGC-803 cells,	[84]
12	UA was coupled with 1,4-dibromo-butane in the presence of K_2CO_3 and KI in DMF. The resulting intermediate was subsequently reacted with piperazine.	A549 and H460 (Lung cancer)	Inhibited cell proliferation, induced apoptosis, Increased cell cycle arrest in the G0/G1 phase	[85]

Table 2. *Cont.*

Compounds	Modification Method	Tested Cancer Cell Lines	Observed Effects	Ref.
13–16	They oxidized the UA via John reagent (PCC), introduced various bromo-alkanes at the C-28 position, and then added 1-(4-nitrophenyl)hydrazine at the C-3 position.	BEL7402 (liver cancer) and SGC7901 (Gastric cancer)	Reduced tumor growth, enhanced cytotoxicity, and inhibited the NF-*k*B pathway of tumor cells.	[86]
17	Fused aminoguanidine moiety at the UA skeleton.	HCT116 (Colon cancer), A549: (Lung cancer), Hep3B (Liver cancer), HeLa (Cervical cancer)	reduced HIF-1α protein levels inhibited hypoxia-induced expression of VEGF at both the mRNA and protein levels and inhibited the proliferation of cancer cells in vitro.	[38]
18	Incorporated hydrazide, and oxadiazole moieties into UA structure.	SMMC-7721 (Liver cancer), HeLa (Cervical cancer), MDA-MB-231 (Breast cancer)	Enhanced cytotoxicity, Induced apoptosis of HeLa cells, arrested cell cycle at the G0/G1 phase, elevated intracellular reactive oxygen species level, decreased mitochondrial membrane potential, inhibited MEK1 kinase activity, and impeded Ras/Raf/MEK/ERK transduction pathway	[87]
21	Incorporated hydrazide derivatives into UA structure.	SMMC-7721 (Liver cancer), HeLa (Cervical cancer), MDA-MB-231 (Breast cancer)	Induced apoptosis in MDA-MB-231 cell lines in a dose-dependent manner. Additionally, promoted G0/G1 phase arrest in MDA-MB-231 cell lines.	[88]
24, 25	They oxidized UA using Jone's reagent, followed by treatment with NH_2-OH·HCl. The resulting intermediate was then reacted with Ac_2O. This intermediate was subsequently condensed with suitable amino and phenol compounds in the presence of triethylamine.	HeLa (Cervical cancer), HepG2 (Liver cancer), BGC-823(Gastric cancer)	Inhibited cell proliferation, Enhanced cytotoxicity	[89]
26–28	Designed novel indolequinone derivatives of UA-bearing ester, hydrazide, or amide moieties	MCF-7 (Breast cancer), HeLa (Cervical cancer), HepG2 (Liver cancer)	Enhanced cytotoxicity, suppresses the migration of MCF-7 cells, elevates intracellular reactive oxygen species (ROS) levels, and decreases mitochondrial membrane potential. upregulated Bax, cleaved caspase-3/9, cleaved PARP levels and downregulated Bcl-2 level of MCF-7 cells, inhibited cell proliferation	[40]
29–33	UA was modified by introducing a tetrazole moiety, with the tetrazole group directly attached to the nitrogen atom of the amide group at the C-28 position. The C-3 hydroxy group was either left unmodified, oxidized, esterified, or converted to hydrazine	Hep3B cells (Liver cancer)	Inhibited the HIF-1α	[39]
34, 35	Combined UA with two different azole types (1,3,4- oxadiazole and 1,2,3-triazole or 1,2,5- oxadiazole and 1,2,3-triazole) at different positions of UA.	MCF-7 (Breast cancer), HepG2 (Liver cancer), A549 (Lung cancer), **U-87MG** (Glioblastoma)	Enhanced cytotoxicity	[90]
36	Incorporated different constituents of the benzylidene at C-2	HepG2 (Liver cancer), HT-29 (Colon cancer), A549 (Lung cancer)	Induced apoptosis via arrest of the cycle at the G1 phase and mitochondria-mediated pathway. Enhanced cytotoxicity	[92]
37	Acetylation of the hydroxyl group at the C-3 position. Introduction of 2-chloroethanol at the C-28 position. Addition of methanesulfonyl chloride (MsCl) in pyridine. Reaction with piperazine. Oxidation with PCC. Introduction of 4-fluorobenzyl bromide at the piperazine moiety	MKN45 (Gastric cancer)	Decreased the apoptosis regulator (BCL2/BAX) ratio, disrupted mitochondrial potential, induced apoptosis, and suppressed the growth of Hela xenografts in nude mice.	[93]

Table 2. *Cont.*

Compounds	Modification Method	Tested Cancer Cell Lines	Observed Effects	Ref.
38, 39	Converted the UA into C-28-amino-functionalized derivatives	HeLa, Jurkat, Hek293, K562, and U937	Inducted the cell cycle arrest at the S-phase and apoptosis.	[94]
40	UA was treated with acetic anhydride in dry pyridine under the 4-dimethylamino pyridine. The 3-acetyl UA was treated with oxalyl chloride to produce an intermediary 28-acyl chloride. This compound was then mixed with piperazine to produce the targeted compound.	SUM149PT (Breast cancer), HCC1937(Breast cancer),	Suppressed cell proliferation and triggered apoptosis in both cell lines	[95]
41	Acylated the C-3(OH) position. Converted the carboxylic group at the C-8 position oxalyl chloride ($(CO)_2C_{12}$). The intermediated was reacted with hexamethylenediamine ($H_2N(CH_2)_6NH_2$). Then reacted with 3,4,5-triacetoxybenzoic acid to form the amide bond.	A549 (Lung cancer), HepG2 (Liver cancer) KOV3 (Ovarian cance) T24 (Bladder cancer)	Inhibited the binding of NF-κB to DNA, suppressed NF-κB activation, inhibited A549 cell migration in vitro, and arrested A549 cell line at the G1 phase.	[36]
42	Methylated the C-28 carboxylic group of UA using diazomethane to produce the methyl ester	HepG2, Hep3B and HA22T/VGH (Liver cancer)	Inhibited cell growth and induced an inhibition of NF-κB activation in hepatocellular carcinoma cell lines	[33]

4.3. Antimicrobial

The extensive use and misuse of antibiotics give rise to microbial drug resistance, which is a serious challenge. Currently, several therapeutic compounds are being developed, however, the issue of drug resistance is increasing. Drug resistance is one of the world's most serious health issues [96]. Bacterial infections caused by drug-resistant pathogens are much worse compared to antibiotic-susceptible ones [97]. The only way to combat these bacterial infections is to develop novel antibiotics or combinations of two or more antibiotics with different modes of action. Previous research suggests that UA and its analogues may inhibit bacterial growth by disrupting metabolic pathways [9]. Other research has found that lipophilic molecules like pentacyclic triterpenoids can disrupt membrane stability and halt cell growth [98]. Triterpenoids are thought to inhibit bacterial efflux pumps, DNA synthesis, and macromolecular synthesis in Gram-positive bacteria [98–100]. Due to the lack of data, the exact antibacterial mechanism for triterpenoids is not yet known, but it was demonstrated that the lack of β-hydroxyl group in position C-3 of betulinic acid derivatives did not exert antibacterial activities against *Staphylococcus aureus* and *Escherichia coli* [101]. Triterpenoids' biological activity is enhanced by modifying them at the C-28 COOH position via amination and esterification [102–105]. It has been brought to light that triterpenoids and their derivatives may be useful weapons to solve the issue of multidrug resistance and reduce the side effects of antibiotics [101].

4.3.1. Antibacterial Activity

UA and its derivatives present a multifaceted antibacterial approach, targeting membrane integrity, biofilm formation, enzyme activity, efflux mechanisms, oxidative stress, and metabolic pathways. These diverse mechanisms not only reduce bacterial growth and survival but also enhance the effects of conventional antibiotics, making UA a promising candidate in the fight against bacterial infections, especially those involving resistant strains. Additionally, studies have explored the use of UA in conjunction with antibiotics as a promising alternative for treating bacterial infections. For instance, Wojnicz et al. [106] investigated the combination of UA and ciprofloxacin, which is used to treat recurrent urinary tract infections caused by *E. coli*. Their findings revealed an improved antibiofilm efficacy against *E. coli*, potentially due to the acidic nature of UA.

UA (32 μg/mL) also reportedly synergizes with colistin when used to treat clinical *Klebsiella pneumoniae* BC936 and *E. coli* U3790 isolates [107]. Cunha et al. reported that

UA isolated from *Miconia ligustroides* was active against *Bacillus cereus* with a MIC value of 20 μg/mL. The ester methylation and acetylation of UA improved the inhibitory activity against *Streptococcus pneumonia* [108]. Furthermore, UA derivatives demonstrated broad-spectrum antibacterial activities against both Gram-negative and Gram-positive bacteria. Do Nascimento and colleagues [109] synthesized two semi-synthetic compounds by modifying the UA structure at C-3. They investigated how UA and its derivatives affected the susceptibility of certain bacterial pathogens to aminoglycoside antibiotics, including neomycin, amikacin, kanamycin, and gentamicin. The most notable synergistic effect was observed with derivative 3β-formyloxy-urs-12-en-28-oic acid (**43**) (Figure 23) at a concentration of 32 μg/mL against *Shigella flexneri* and *E. coli*, a multidrug-resistant clinical isolate from sputum.

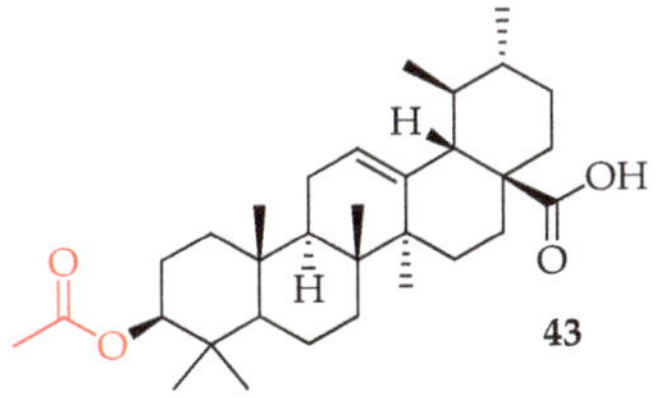

43

Compounds	MIC (μg/mL)		
	K. pneumoniae (ATCC 10031)	*S. flexneri* (ATCC 12022)	*E coli (ATCC 25922)*
UA	64	64	64
43	64	32	32

Figure 23. UA derivative **43** and its antibacterial outcomes compared to UA.

Zhao et al. extracted UA from the *Ilex hainanensis* Merr. leaves and synthesized seven UA-based derivatives. They assessed their antibacterial efficacy by measuring their MIC against both Gram-positive (*Streptococcus mutans* ATCC 25175) and Gram-negative (*Fusobacterium nucleatum* ATCC 10953) bacterial strains. Among the synthesized derivatives, compound **44** (Figure 24) demonstrated a notable effect against *S. mutans*, with a MIC of 9.7 μg/mL, but showed minimal antibacterial activity against *F. nucleatum* [110]. Oloyede et al. investigated the antibacterial properties of UA by examining how reactive oxygen species and oxidative stress contribute to its effectiveness against *Pseudomonas aeruginosa*, *S. aureus*, and *E. coli*. They found that the viability of bacteria treated with UA decreased over time with MIC of 256 mg/mL for *E. coli and P. aeruginosa*, and 64 mg/mL for *S. aureus*. Interestingly, when bacteria were treated with UA in the presence of 2,20-bipyrydyl, cell viability increased. The study also observed a significant ($p < 0.05$) increase in superoxide anion production in bacteria treated with UA. Furthermore, the ratio of NAD+/NADH significantly increased ($p < 0.05$) in these bacteria. Moreover, UA treatment led to a significant decrease in reduced glutathione levels and an increase in glutathione disulphide, malondialdehyde, and fragmented DNA in *E. coli*, *P. aeruginosa*, and *S. aureus*. These findings strongly indicate that UA shows promise as an effective antibacterial agent [27].

Previous studies indicate that several triterpenoids demonstrate synergistic effects with various classes of antibiotics, highlighting the potential of plant-derived compounds to enhance antibiotic efficacy against multidrug-resistant pathogens. To elucidate the mechanism by which triterpenoids combat these resistant bacteria. Wang and colleagues analyzed the SAR of UA against *S. aureus*. They investigated how UA could affect both bacterial and mammalian membranes. They employed 2D proteomic analysis to study how methicillin-resistant *S. aureus* responds at the proteomic level to treatment with UA [111]. Another study by Pandey et al. explored the antibacterial effect of UA derived from *Ocimum sanctum* against *E. coli*. They observed dose-dependent enhancement in its activity at concentrations of 15, 20, and 25 mg/mL. At these concentrations, the effectiveness of

UA showed comparable efficacy to the standard drug albendazole. The study utilized both disk diffusion and well diffusion methods to screen UA's antibacterial efficacy. In vitro antimicrobial tests indicated that UA exhibited promising antibacterial properties [112]. Furthermore, Park et al. [113] explored the antibacterial potential of three distinct saponin triterpenoids, including UA, employing diverse methodologies. They employed quantitative real-time PCR (qPCR) and microarray analysis to investigate the expression of genes linked to key metabolic pathways in *S. mutans* UA159 after incubation with UA. An oligonucleotide array containing 5363 probes was designed to examine 1928 of the 1963 genes in the *S. mutans* UA159 genome. Genes exhibiting a 2-fold change in expression due to the treatment were identified, and qPCR was used to analyze a selection of target genes involved in central metabolism. The gene expression patterns of UA-treated cells, as revealed by microarray analysis, indicated alterations in the antimicrobial mechanism. This finding suggests that UA-treated cells exhibit a promising antimicrobial mechanism worthy of further investigation.

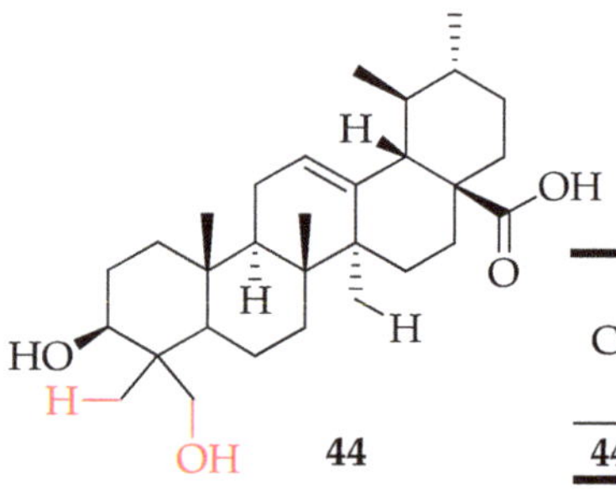

44

Compounds	MIC (μg/mL)	
	S. mutans (ATCC 25175)	*F. nucleatum* (ATCC 10953)
44	9.7	9.7

Figure 24. UA derivative **44** and its antibacterial outcomes compared to UA.

Qian et al. [114] evaluated the antimicrobial mechanism of UA against carbapenem-resistant *Klebsiella pneumoniae* (CRKP). Their findings indicate that UA is effective against CRKP at a minimum inhibitory concentration (MIC) of 0.8 mg/mL. UA was found to compromise the integrity of CRKP cell membranes, inhibit biofilm formation and the expression of biofilm-related genes, and inactivate CRKP cells within biofilms. This study investigated the antibacterial properties and mechanisms of UA against CRKP, using the agar dilution method to determine UA's MIC. To assess UA's impact on the cell membrane, researchers monitored changes in intracellular pH, ATP content, and cell membrane potential. The results suggest that UA could be a promising treatment for multidrug-resistant *K. pneumoniae* infections when used alongside other antibiotics.

To find treatments that inhibit the development of biofilms, numerous researchers have reported intriguing results. Nine derivatives of UA were evaluated for their in vitro antibacterial efficacy against both planktonic and biofilm cells of gram-positive pathogens like *Enterococcus faecalis*, *S. epidermidis*, and *S. aureus*. The researchers assessed the antibiofilm properties of these analogues, including UA, using the crystal violet method, and measured their antibacterial effectiveness through absorbance (OD600) at different concentrations (5, 25, and 100 μM). Additionally, they evaluated the in vitro cytotoxicity of similar molecules on African green monkey (VERO) cells using the MTT assay at the same concentrations. They observed that a C-3 substitution in the UA chemical structure enhanced antibiofilm activity. Notably, among all the promising UA analogues, compound **45** (Figure 25) emerged as the most active molecule with minimal or no toxic effects against mammalian cells [115].

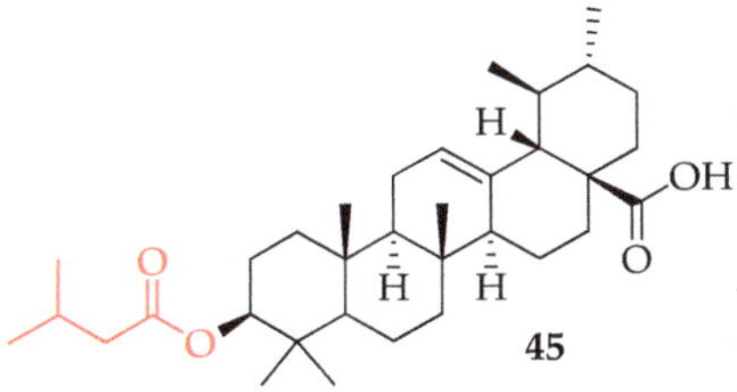

45

Compounds	VERO Cells Viability (%) of Compounds		
	100 μM	25 μM	5 μM
UA	13 ± 12	32 ± 7	37 ± 4
45	72 ± 26	105 ± 10	113 ± 32

Figure 25. UA derivative **45** and its antibacterial outcomes compared to UA.

The few UA derivatives exhibit significant antibacterial activity against a wide range of pathogenic bacteria, including both Gram-positive and Gram-negative strains. Studies have shown that these compounds can effectively inhibit the growth of antibiotic-resistant strains, making them promising candidates for addressing the growing issue of antibiotic resistance. Additionally, UA derivatives may enhance the efficacy of conventional antibiotics when used in combination, potentially leading to synergistic effects. Overall, the diverse antibacterial properties of UA derivatives underscore their potential as effective natural agents for treating bacterial infections. The summary of the antibacterial activity of UA derivatives is shown in Table 3 below, including the method of modification, the tested bacterial strains, and the observed effects.

Table 3. The summary of the antibacterial activity of compounds (**43**–**45**), including the method of modification, the tested bacterial strains, and the observed effects.

Compounds	Modification Method	Bacterial Strain	Effects	Ref.
43	UA was reacted with acetic anhydride (Ac_2O) in pyridine at room temperature for 24 h to yield compound **54**	*K. pneumoniae* (ATCC 10031) *Shigella flexneri* (ATCC 12022) *E. coli* (ATCC 25922)	Enhanced antibacterial activity against *Shigella flexneri* and *E. coli*, a multidrug-resistant clinical isolate from sputum	[109]
44	Hybridization of UA with hydrazide and 1,3,4-oxadiazole groups	*S. mutans* ATCC 25175, *Fusobacterium nucleatum* ATCC 10953	Showed significant antibacterial activity against *S. mutans*	[116]
45	The commercial anhydride was added to UA in pyridine (CH_2Cl_2, 2 mL) to form an ester derivative	*E. faecalis*, *S. epidermidis* and *S. aureus*	An antibiofilm activity against *S. aureus* without any effect on mammalian cells.	[115]

4.3.2. Antiviral Activity

UA and its derivatives have shown promising antiviral activities against a variety of viruses such as HIV, influenza, etc. UA can inhibit Hepatitis B Virus (HBV) replication and suppress HBx-mediated pathways, which are crucial for the virus's lifecycle. This includes the suppression of RhoA activation, beclin-1 promoter activation, and autophagy induction, as well as reversing HBx-induced drug resistance [117].

Human Immunodeficiency Virus (HIV)

It is estimated that approximately 36.7 million people worldwide were living with AIDS at the end of 2017. Year after year, morbidity and mortality rates have risen dramatically. More than thirty drugs targeting various stages of the HIV viral life cycle have been approved so far for the management of HIV/AIDS. However, serious issues such as the emergence of extensively drug-resistant bacteria and negative side effects remain [118]. Hence, there is a necessity to develop anti-HIV/AIDS drugs that exhibit potent therapeutic effects and favorable pharmacokinetic profiles, with minimal or no adverse effects. Several pentacyclic triterpenoids and their saponin derivatives have shown anti-HIV activity [119].

UA and its hydrogen malonate derivative **46** (Figure 26), extracted from the stems of *Cynomorium songaricum*, exhibit HIV-1 protease inhibition with EC_{50} values in the micromolar range. Additionally, the glutaryl hemiester compound **47** (Figure 26) of UA has demonstrated anti-HIV-1 protease activity at a concentration of 4 Mm [120].

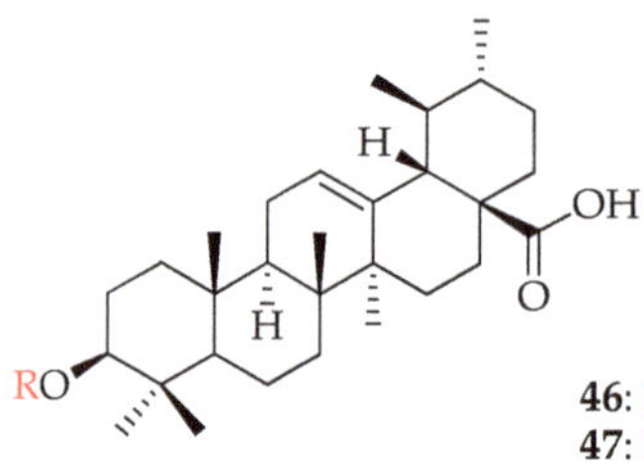

46: R = $COCH_2COOH$
47: R = $CO(CH_2)_3COOH$

Figure 26. UA derivatives (**46**, **47**) extracted from stems of *Cynomorium songaricum*.

Zhu et al. [118], developed a series of derivatives of UA, utilizing them as P2 ligands, along with phenyl sulfonamide as P2′ ligands, to investigate their SAR as inhibitors of HIV-1 protease. The results indicated that these derivatives exhibited micromolar inhibitory activity. Specifically, compound **48** (Figure 27) demonstrated potent inhibition of HIV-1 protease with IC_{50} = 0.12 μM), which was reported to be 67 times more effective than the parent compound UA (IC_{50} = 8.0 μM). These findings suggest that P2 ligands may not effectively complement the residues of the protease S2 subsite. Further research is recommended to explore pentacyclic terpenoid fragments, like those in UA, as potentially superior inhibitors of HIV targets beyond HIV-1.

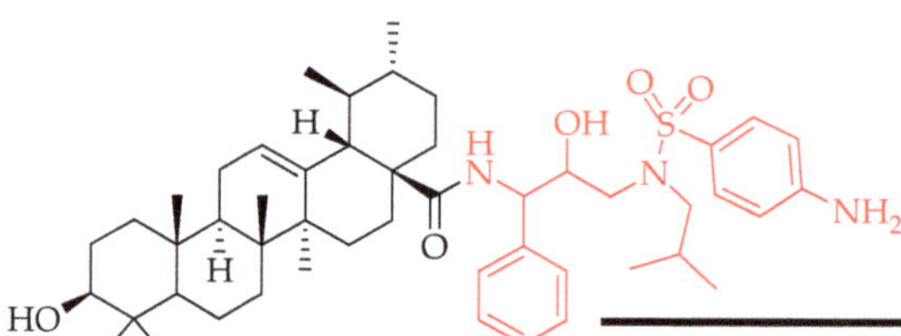

48

Compound	IC_{50}(μM)	CC_{50}(μM)	SI
48	0.12 ± 0.04	> 100	> 833
DRV	0.57 ± 0.17 nM	> 100	>175,000

Figure 27. UA derivative **48** and its antiviral outcomes compared to model drug.

Influenza Virus

Several viral changes have led to the formation of consistent strains of influenza A viruses (IAVs) within vulnerable human populations: (H1N1, H1N2, H2N2, and H3N2) [121]. Because of genetic changes caused by antigenic shifts and occasional antigenic drifts, IAVs exhibit high pathogenicity and are responsible for annual epidemics and occasional global pandemics of respiratory diseases. The highly pathogenic avian influenza (HPAI) H5N1 virus, specifically, has posed significant health and economic risks worldwide. Interestingly, certain protease inhibitors, such as pentacyclic triterpenoids, have demonstrated effective inhibition of IAVs through straightforward modifications of established natural pentacyclic triterpenoids or through innovative discovery methods [122]. Li et al. [122] synthesized derivatives of UA (**49** and **50**) (Figure 28) in their search for an effective inhibitor against IAVs. Compounds **49** and **50** were evaluated for their ability to inhibit the H5N1 virus and two other strains using a cytopathic effect reduction assay in A549 cells. Additionally, compounds **49** and **50** were subjected to an MTT assay on A549 cells to determine their cytotoxic effects relative to their antiviral activity. The results indicated that these derivatives demonstrated effective inhibition against the H5N1 virus at micromolar concentrations, although their antiviral potency was comparable to or slightly less than that of the standard drug (oseltamivir). Compound **50** was found to interfere with viral hemagglutinin, thereby preventing infection by H1, H3, and H5 types of influenza A viruses. Furthermore, the antiviral efficacy observed in experimental assays correlated well with docking studies, suggesting that compound **50** merits further optimization and development as a promising new lead compound.

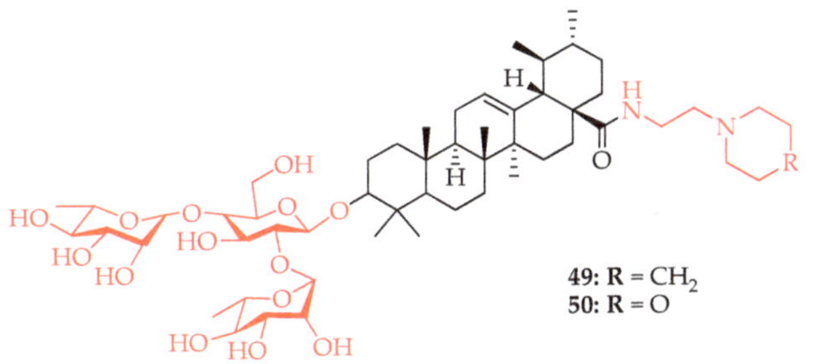

49: **R** = CH_2
50: **R** = O

Compound	CC_{50}(μM)	IC_{50}(μM)		
	H5N1c	PR/8 (H1N1)	JX/312 (H3N2)	
49	> 200	6.62 ± 0.73	21.33 ± 1.05	25.59 ± 1.22
50	> 200	4.13 ± 0.51	18.18 ± 0.83	20.12 ± 0.78
Oseltamivir	> 200	4 .18 ± 0.46	4.61 ± 0.84	4.25 ± 0.36

Figure 28. UA derivatives and their antiviral outcomes compared to reference drug.

Liao et al. [123] prepared a range of pentacyclic triterpene saponins modified at C-28 through conjugation with diverse amide derivatives. They assessed the antiviral properties of these compounds against the influenza A/Duck/Guangdong/99 virus (H5N1) using MDCK cells. Among these derivatives, compound **51** (Figure 29) significantly inhibited influenza A virus replication in a dose-dependent manner, aligning well with cytopathic effect reduction results. The SAR analysis indicated that introducing specific amide structures at the COOH position of UA could notably enhance both antiviral activity and selective index. The study highlighted that attaching a methoxy group or a Cl atom to the phenyl ring at the ortho- or para-position was essential for improving inhibitory activity. Mechanism studies showed that these triterpenoids could bind tightly to the viral envelope hemagglutinin, blocking the virus's attachment to host cells, consistent with docking studies.

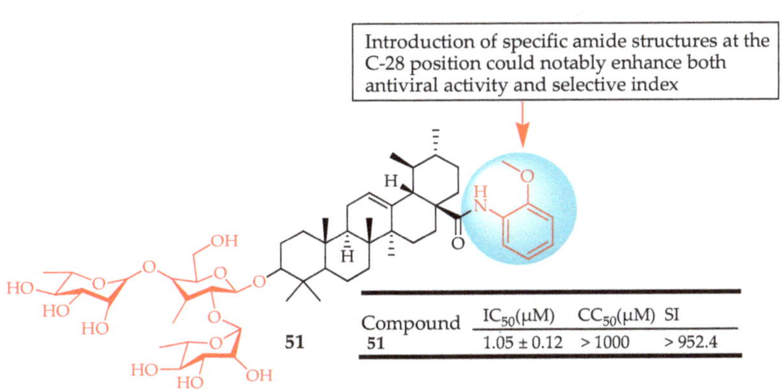

Compound	IC_{50}(μM)	CC_{50}(μM)	SI
51	1.05 ± 0.12	> 1000	> 952.4

Figure 29. UA derivative **51** and its antiviral outcomes.

A new codrug, referred to as compound **52** in Figure 30, which combines lamivudine and UA through an ester bond, had the dual action of anti-hepatitis B virus activity and hepatoprotective effects against acute liver injury [124]. The antiviral screening of the cyanoethyloximino derivative (**53**) of UA against human papillomavirus type 11 showed a selectivity index of 30, with no observed cellular cytotoxicity [14].

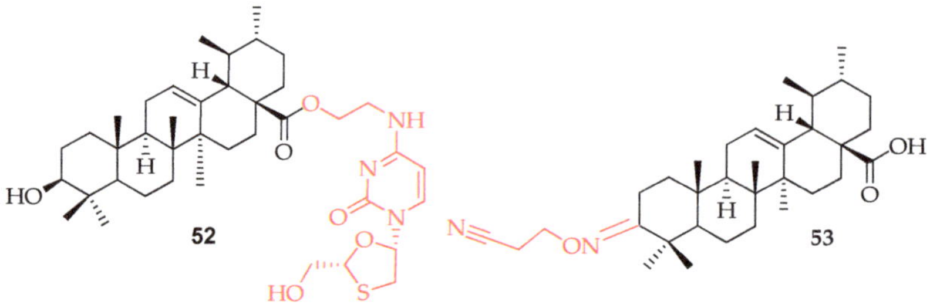

Figure 30. UA derivatives **52**, **53** linked with lamivudine at C-28 and cyanoethyloximino at C-3.

It has been observed that UA derivatives exhibit significant antiviral activity against a range of viral pathogens, demonstrating their potential application as therapeutic agents for treating viral infections. These compounds exert their antiviral effects through various mechanisms, including the inhibition of viral entry into host cells, disruption of viral replication, and modulation of the host immune response. Studies have shown that UA derivatives can interfere with viral enzymes, such as proteases. Overall, the diverse antiviral mechanisms of UA derivatives highlight their potential use for the development of effective therapeutics against various viral diseases. Table 4 below summarizes the antiviral activity of various UA derivatives, including the method of modification, the tested viruses, and the observed effects.

Table 4. The antiviral activity of various UA derivatives, including the method of modification, the tested viruses, and the observed effects.

Compounds	Modification Method	Target Virus	Notes	Ref.
48	Modified UA as P2 ligands and phenylsulfonamide as P2′ ligands	HIV-1	Demonstrated HIV-1 protease inhibition, exhibiting 67 times greater inhibitory activity compared to its precursor, UA	[118]
49, 50	Attached the privileged fragment 2-(piperidin-1-yl)ethan-1-amine or its bioisosteric surrogate 2-(1,3- oxazinan-3-yl)ethan-1-amine into UA by a crucial amide linker	H5N1, PR/8 (H1N1), JX/312 (H3N2)	50 Inhibited infection of H1-, H3-, and H5-typed influenza A viruses by interfering with the viral hemagglutinin	[122]
51	Modified the C-28 position of UA saponins via conjugation with a series of amide derivatives	H5N1	Inhibited influenza A virus replication	[123]
52	Coupled lamivudine and UA with ethyl chloroacetate through an amide and ester linkage		Had the dual action of anti-hepatitis B virus activity and hepatoprotective effects against acute liver injury	[124]
53	UA was oxidized using Jones' reagent. The resulting compound was then reacted with hydroxylamine hydrochloride ($NH_2OH{\cdot}HCl$). The intermediate was further reacted with acrylonitrile (CH_2CHCN).	Human papillomavirus type 11	Inhibited human papillomavirus type 11	[14]

4.3.3. Antioxidant Properties

UA acts as a potent antioxidant by scavenging reactive oxygen species (ROS) and upregulating endogenous antioxidant enzymes [111]. This helps protect cells from oxidative stress-induced damage, which is implicated in various chronic diseases, including neurodegenerative disorders. It can act effectively as a radical scavenger, a chain-breaking antioxidant, or a chelator of metals that generate radicals. It is widely recognized that many commonly used drugs, such as anticancer agents, non-steroidal anti-inflammatory drugs, antiretroviral agents, antipsychotics, and analgesics, can induce harmful free-radical toxicity. The metabolism of these drugs can produce reactive intermediates that directly reduce molecular oxygen, leading to the formation of reactive oxygen species [125].

In a study by Do Nascimento et al. [109] compound **54** (Figure 31) demonstrated antioxidant properties by inhibiting DPPH. They effectively scavenged the DPPH radical, with IC_{50} values of $5.97 \times 10^{-2} \pm 1 \times 10^{-3}$ mg/mL and $0.73 \pm 9.3 \times 10^{-2}$ mg/mL, respectively. In comparison, Trolox and Vitamin C, used as positive controls in this study, had IC_{50} values of $2.6 \times 10^{-3} \pm 2.3 \times 10^{-4}$ mg/mL and $4.3 \times 10^{-2} \pm 1.9 \times 10^{-2}$ mg/mL. Popov et al. [116] developed new hybrid derivatives of UA (**55** and **56**) (Figure 31), incorporating hydrazide and 1,3,4-oxadiazole groups, which demonstrated significant antioxidant activity.

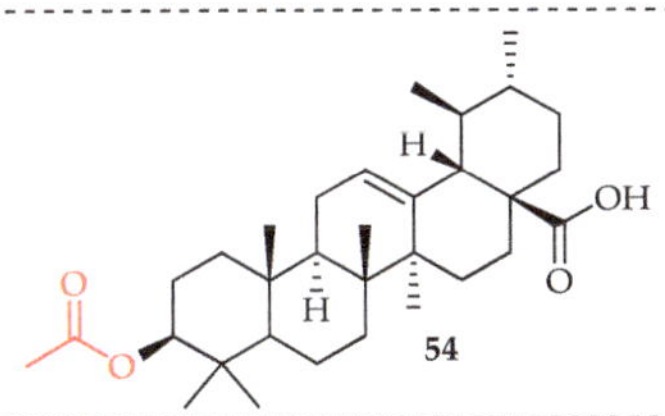

Samples	IC_{50} (mg/mL)
UA	$5.97 \times 10^{-2} \pm 1 \times 10^{-32}$
54	$0.73 \pm 9.3 \times 10^{-2}$
Trolox	$2.6 \times 10^{-3} \pm 2.3 \times 10^{-4}$
Vitamin C	$4.3 \times 10^{-2} \pm 1.9 \times 10^{-2}$

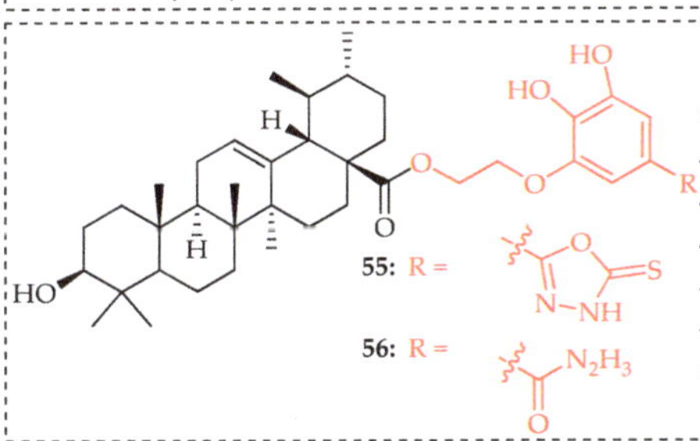

Compound	IC_{50}(μM) DPPH	ABTS
Ascorbic acid	23.8 ± 1.30	39.38 ± 2.14
UA	Inactive	Not studied
55	18.6 ± 0.57	10.19 ± 0.45
56	13.8 ± 0.49	5.21 ± 0.26

Figure 31. UA derivatives (**54–56**) and their antioxidant outcomes compared to UA/reference drugs.

The reported UA derivatives possess potent antioxidant properties, which are attributed to their ability to scavenge free radicals and reduce oxidative stress in biological systems. Table 5 summarizes the antioxidant activity of UA derivatives, including the method of modification, the antioxidant assays, and the observed effects.

Table 5. The antioxidant activity of UA derivatives (**54–56**), including the method of modification, the tested models or assays, and the observed effects.

Compounds	Modification Method	Antioxidant Assay	Notes	Ref.
54	UA was reacted with acetic anhydride (Ac_2O) in pyridine at room temperature for 24 h to yield compound **54**	DPPH Radical Scavenging Assay	Strong antioxidant activity	[109]
55, 56	Hybridization of UA with hydrazide and 1,3,4-oxadiazole groups	DPPH Radical and ABTS Radical Scavenging Assay	High antioxidant activity compared to ascorbic acid	[116]

4.3.4. Antidiabetic Activity

UA and its derivatives hold significant promise as antidiabetic agents due to their multifaceted mechanisms of action, including improving insulin sensitivity, reducing gluconeogenesis, anti-inflammatory and antioxidant effects, and activating AMPK [126]. In recent years, researchers have investigated structural modifications of UA to develop new derivatives with improved antidiabetic properties.

In a research conducted by Wu et al. [28] various derivatives of UA displayed notable inhibitory effects, particularly compounds **57–60** (Figure 32), with IC_{50} values of 2.66 ± 0.84, 1.01 ± 0.44, 3.26 ± 0.22, and 3.24 ± 0.21 μM, respectively. These compounds exhibited greater potency against α-glucosidase compared to acarbose, the positive control. To understand their inhibitory mechanisms, kinetic studies were conducted. Compound **57** was identified as a non-competitive inhibitor with an inhibition constant (Ki) of 2.67 ± 0.19 μM. On the other hand, compounds **58–60** were found to be mixed-type inhibitors through kinetic inhibition studies. Furthermore, the practical pharmacological effects of synthesized compounds **57** and **58** were demonstrated by their ability to lower postprandial blood glucose levels in normal Kunming mice.

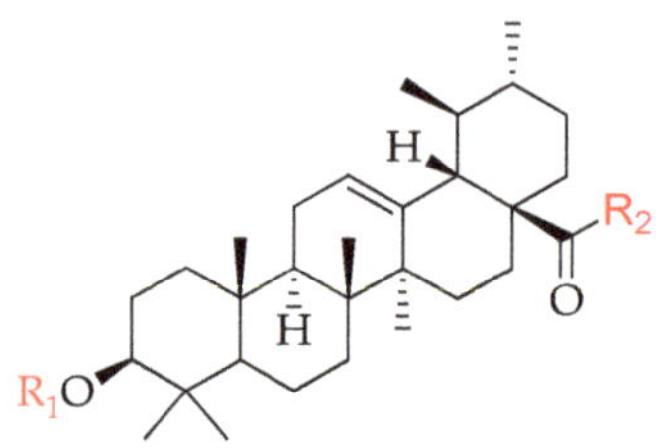

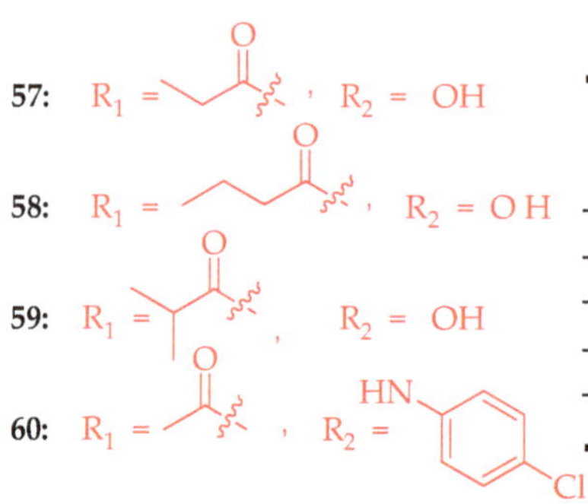

Compounds	α-Glucosidase inhibitory activity	
	%inhibition	IC_{50}(μM)
57	68.89 ± 3.58	2.66 ± 0.40
58	99.84 ± 5.09	1.01 ± 0.14
59	69.31 ± 3.91	3.26 ± 0.52
60	64.52 ± 2.38	3.24 ± 0.21
UA	48.65 ± 6.85	5.04 ± 0.80

Figure 32. UA derivatives (**57–60**) and their antidiabetic outcomes compared to UA.

Guzman Avila et al. [29] synthesized seven derivatives of UA. Among them, compounds **61**, **62**, and **63** (Figure 33) showed substantial inhibitory effects on the PTP-1B enzyme in a reversible manner. Compound **63** exhibited the highest activity, demonstrating significant effects both in vitro and in vivo. Furthermore, acetyl and crotonyl esters were identified as the most potent derivatives in experimental setups. Molecular docking analysis indicated that acetyl and crotonyl derivatives exhibited better binding scores compared to the parent compound, UA.

The findings from Wu et al.'s study indicated significant inhibitory activity among most analogues of UA, particularly analogues **64** and **65** (Figure 34), which displayed IC_{50} values of 1.27 ± 0.27 μM and 1.28 ± 0.27 μM, respectively. These values were lower compared to other synthesized analogues and the control. Among these, analogues with electronegative (-F, -Cl, -Br) substitutions at the para position were more active than those with substitutions at the ortho position, particularly analogues **64** and **65**. 2D-QSAR and molecular docking analysis were conducted to demonstrate that the C-3 position could interact with the hydrophobic region of the active pocket, forming hydrogen bonds to enhance the binding affinity of the ligand to the homology-modelling protein. Consequently, these findings offer insights into the correlation between binding mechanisms and bioactivity, aiding in the design of improved inhibitors derived from UA analogues [127].

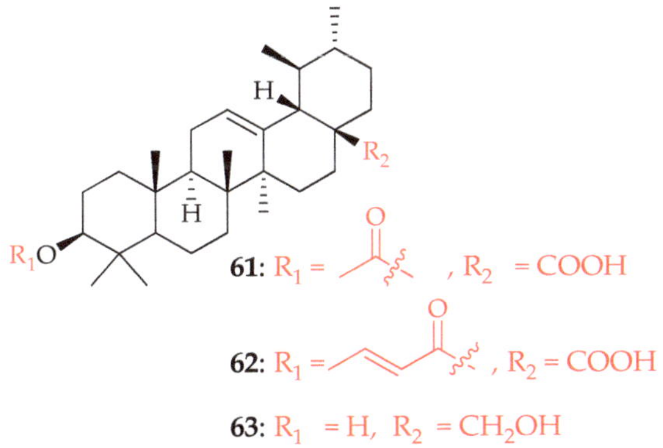

Compounds	α-Glucosidase inhibitory activity	
	%Reversibility	IC_{50}(μM)
61	94.3 ± 5.0	5.6 ± 0.2
62	99.3 ± 1.0	4.7 ± 0.2
63	88.3 ± 1.1	4.6 ± 0.2

Figure 33. UA derivatives (**61–63**) and their antidiabetic outcomes.

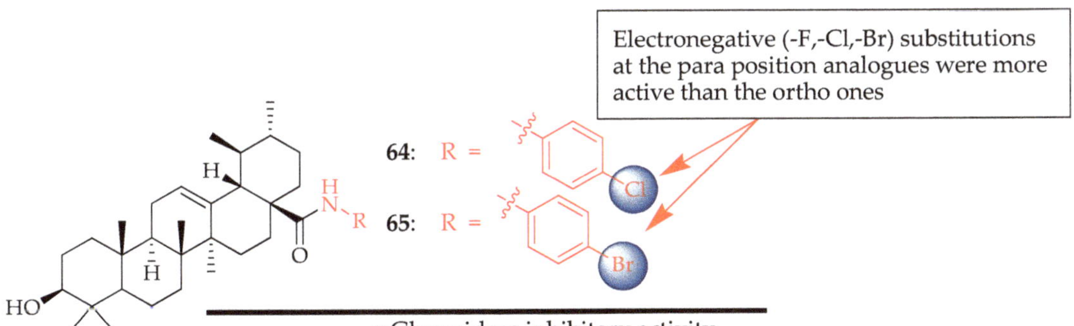

Compounds	α-Glucosidase inhibitory activity
	IC_{50}(μM)
64	1.27 ± 0.27
65	1.28 ± 0.27

Figure 34. UA derivatives (**64, 65**) and their antidiabetic outcomes.

In another study conducted by the same researchers [128], compounds **66** and **67** (Figure 35) exhibited significant inhibition of 2-NBDG uptake under both sodium-dependent and sodium-independent conditions. This inhibition was achieved by reducing the expression of SGLT-1 and GLUT-2 in the Caco-2 cell model. Subsequent in vivo studies demonstrated that compound **66** notably alleviated hyperglycemia by enhancing serum insulin levels, total protein, and albumin. Moreover, it effectively normalized fasting blood glucose levels, body weight, and food intake, bringing them closer to those of healthy rats. Compounds **66** and **67** also demonstrated hypolipidemic effects by reducing total cholesterol and triglyceride levels. Additionally, compound **66** exhibited antioxidant properties, as evidenced by increased levels of glutathione and superoxide dismutase, along with decreased levels of malondialdehyde in the liver and kidneys of diabetic rats.

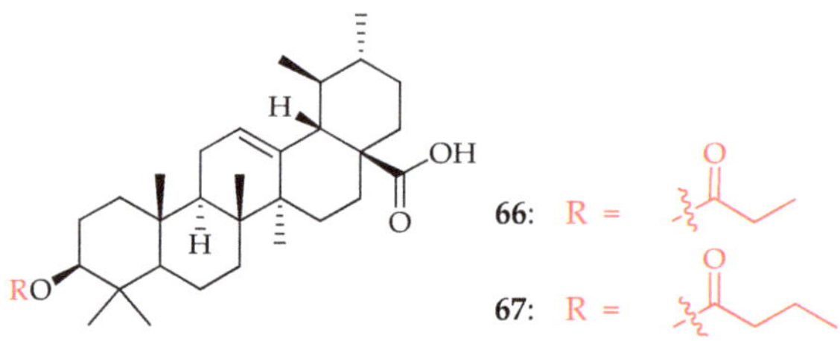

Compounds	Cell toxicity on Caco-2 Cells Inhibition Rate %
66	7.84 ± 4.15
67	2.29 ± 6.08
UA	9.86 ± 2.68

Figure 35. UA derivative (**66**, **67**) and their antidiabetic outcomes compared to UA.

Huang et al. [129] developed and synthesized a novel series of UA derivatives aimed at potentially serving as anti-diabetic agents through the inhibition of α-glucosidase. Their findings from half-maximal inhibitory concentration assays indicated that all tested compounds exhibited greater potency against α-glucosidase compared to acarbose. Notably, compounds **68–71** (Figure 36), which featured specific long hydrophilic groups at the C-3 or C-8 positions, demonstrated inhibitory activity ranging from twelve to thirty-seven times higher than the parent compound UA. However, compounds bearing free carboxyl groups at both the C-3 and C-28 positions showed reduced enzyme inhibition activity. Additionally, UA derivatives conjugated with hydrophobic groups displayed diminished inhibitory effects against Baker's yeast α-glucosidase. Mechanistically, compounds **68** and **69** were found to inhibit α-glucosidase through a mixed-type inhibition, while compounds **70** and **71** exhibited a non-competitive inhibition mechanism. Moreover, the correlation between IC_{50} values and binding free energies indicated that docking simulations provided valuable predictive insights. These results suggest that UA derivatives modified with polar and hydrophilic moieties could represent a promising new class of compounds worthy of further investigation in animal studies or clinical trials as potential anti-diabetic agents.

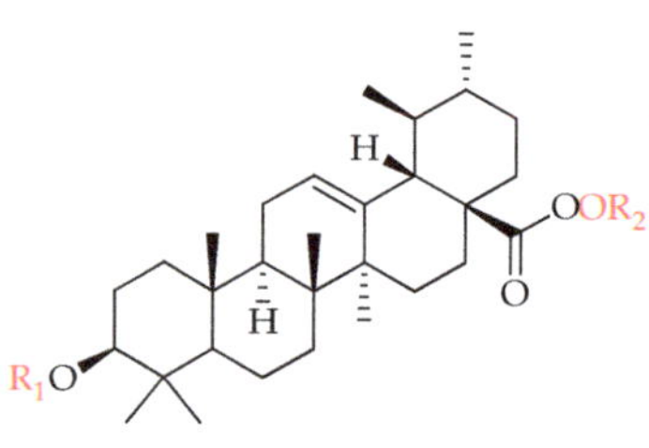

68: $R_1 = CO(CH_2)_2COOH$
$R_2 = Bn$
69: $R_1 = CO(CHC_2)_3COOH$
$R_2 = Bn$
70: $R_1 = OCCH_2CH_3$
$R_2 = CH_2COOH$
71: $R_1 = OC(CH_2)_2CH_3$
$R_2 = CH_2COOH$

a-Glucosidase inhibitory activity	
Compounds	IC_{50}
68	0.149 ± 0.00729
69	0.223 ± 0.023
70	0.466 ± 0.016
71	0.298 ± 0.021
UA	5.52 ± 0.054

Figure 36. UA derivatives (**68–71**) and their antidiabetic outcomes compared to UA.

UA derivatives demonstrate promising antidiabetic activity through several mechanisms that enhance glucose metabolism and improve insulin sensitivity. These compounds have been shown to increase glucose uptake in muscle and adipose tissues by upregulating glucose transporter proteins, such as SGLT-1 and GLUT-2. Additionally, UA derivatives can inhibit α-glucosidase activity, and the PTP-1B enzymes in a reversible manner. Overall, the multifaceted actions of UA derivatives position them as valuable candidates for the development of novel therapeutic agents in diabetes management. Table 6 below summarizes the antidiabetic activity of various UA derivatives, including the method of modification, the tested models or assays, and the observed effects.

Table 6. The antidiabetic activity of various UA derivatives, including the method of modification, the tested models or assays, and the observed effects.

Compounds	Modification Method	Assay/Model Used	Notes	Ref.
57–60	UA was esterified in anhydrous pyridine with different anhydrides	α-Glucosidase Inhibition Assay	Strong inhibition of α-glucosidase compared to acarbose, the positive control	[28]
61–63	For compounds **61** and **62** the reaction was initiated by adding a base to the UA at 0 °C in (CH_2Cl_2) or (THF). Then, an acyl or alkyl halide was added at C-3, and the mixture was subjected to microwave irradiation and refluxed.For compound **63**, UA was reacted with ($LiAlH_4$) in tetrahydrofuran (THF) for 8 h	PTP-1B inhibition assay	Significant inhibitory activity on PTP-1B enzyme in a reversible manner	[29]
66, 67	UA was esterified in anhydrous pyridine with different anhydrides	Glucose Uptake in L6 Myotubes	Displays an inhibitory effect on 2-NBDG uptake through inhibiting SGLT-1 and GLUT-2 transporter protein expression in Caco-2 cells	[128]
68–71	Conjugation of hydrophilic and polar groups at C-3 and/or C-28 position	α-Glucosidase Inhibition Assay	Inhibited α-glucosidase through a mixed-type inhibition, while compounds **70** and **71** exhibited a non-competitive inhibition mechanism	[129]

4.3.5. Conclusions

The synthesis of UA derivatives is currently of great interest to medicinal and organic chemists because of its strong pharmacological effects. The structural modification of UA significantly enhances its biological activities. Ongoing research in this field continues to uncover new derivatives with promising pharmacological properties aiding in the design of more effective therapeutic agents. Most identified derivatives of UA have shown greater potency than both standard drugs and the original compound, UA.

After reviewing the wide range of pharmacological activities of UA derivatives, it was noted that the anticancer properties of UA derivatives have garnered significant attention over the past decade, as most of the derivatives discussed in this study originate from the development of anticancer drugs. UA has been observed to impact numerous targets throughout different stages of cancer progression, including apoptosis, proliferation, angiogenesis, and metastasis. Compounds **8–42** (Figures 8–22) are representative UA-based compounds that demonstrate enhanced anticancer effects in comparison to either UA itself or the model drug.

In anti-inflammatory terms, UA derivatives suppress the activation of NF-κB, a transcription factor that plays a crucial role in regulating the expression of various pro-inflammatory cytokines and enzymes. They can downregulate cyclooxygenase-2 (COX-2) and inducible nitric oxide synthase (iNOS), enzymes involved in the production of inflammatory mediators. Compounds **2–7** (Figures 2–7) exemplify UA derivatives that exhibit superior anti-inflammatory effects compared to UA and the standard drugs used as controls.

The antidiabetic activities of the UA derivatives include the inhibition of α-glucosidase, an enzyme involved in carbohydrate digestion, thereby reducing postprandial blood glucose spikes. They enhance insulin-signaling pathways, improving glucose uptake in peripheral tissues. Compounds **57–71** (Figures 32–36) are representative UA-based compounds with enhanced antidiabetic activity.

UA exhibits significant antibacterial activity against Gram-negative and Gram-positive bacteria such as S. aureus, including methicillin-resistant *S. aureus* (MRSA). It disrupts bacterial cell walls and inhibits bacterial enzymes essential for survival and replication. Compounds **43–45** (Figures 23–25) are representative UA-based compounds with enhanced antibacterial activity.

In the field of antivirals, the derivatives of UA showed strong antiviral activity, mainly against HIV, influenza, and herpes. UA derivatives have demonstrated activity against HIV by inhibiting key enzymes such as reverse transcriptase and protease, essential for viral replication. UA has been shown to inhibit the replication of influenza viruses. It interferes with the viral entry into host cells and the replication of viral RNA. Studies have demonstrated that UA can reduce the production of pro-inflammatory cytokines, which are typically elevated during influenza infection. Compounds **46–53** (Figures 26–30) are representative UA-based compounds with antiviral activity. However, UA derivatives against other viral pathogens such as HSV and HCV have not been reported. Experiments show that the introduction of ester at the C3 or C28 position of UA can enhance the pharmacological activity, and further modification of the position of C3 may be an effective strategy to obtain compounds with stronger activity.

In summary, the structural properties of derivatives of UA modifications at the C3 position or within the ring A and C-28 positions of the UA skeleton have been widely reported. Additionally, to discover the potential of UA derivatives, further development and more evaluation of UA derivatives for other pharmacological activities are necessary, similar to the efforts focused on anticancer UA derivatives. This review can be useful to researchers working in the field of medicinal chemistry, as it will aid in the design and development of novel UA-based compounds with potent therapeutic activities.

Author Contributions: Conceptualization, V.K. and B.A.A.; Methodology, V.K. and B.A.A.; Software, V.K. and B.A.A.; Validation, V.K. and B.A.A.; Investigation, V.K. and B.A.A.; Resources, V.K. and B.A.A.; Writing—original draft preparation, V.K.; Writing—review and editing, V.K. and B.A.A.; Supervision, B.A.A.; Funding acquisition, B.A.A. All authors have read and agreed to the published version of the manuscript.

Funding: This research was funded by the Govan Mbeki Research and Development Council (GMRDC), University of Fort Hare; South Africa Medical Research Council (SAMRC).

Institutional Review Board Statement: Not applicable.

Informed Consent Statement: Not applicable.

Data Availability Statement: Not applicable.

Conflicts of Interest: The authors declare no conflicts of interest. The funders had no role in the design of the study; in the collection, analyses, or interpretation of data; in the writing of the manuscript; or in the decision to publish the results.

References

1. Huang, X.; Shen, Q.K.; Guo, H.Y.; Quan, Z.S.; Li, X. Research, Development and Pharmacological Activity of Fusidic Acid and Its Derivatives. *J. Mol. Struct.* **2023**, *1291*, 135942. [CrossRef]
2. Rodrigues, T.; Reker, D.; Schneider, P.; Schneider, G. Counting on Natural Products for Drug Design. *Nat. Chem.* **2016**, *8*, 531–541. [CrossRef]
3. Newman, D.J.; Cragg, G.M. Natural Products as Sources of New Drugs over the Nearly Four Decades from 01/1981 to 09/2019. *J. Nat. Prod.* **2020**, *83*, 770–803. [CrossRef] [PubMed]
4. Eder, J.; Sedrani, R.; Wiesmann, C. The Discovery of First-in-Class Drugs: Origins and Evolution. *Nat. Rev. Drug Discov.* **2014**, *13*, 577–587. [CrossRef] [PubMed]
5. Di Fabio, G.; Romanucci, V.; De Marco, A.; Zarrelli, A. Triterpenoids from *Gymnema sylvestre* and Their Pharmacological Activities. *Molecules* **2014**, *19*, 10956–10981. [CrossRef]
6. Sharma, H.; Kumar, P.; Deshmukh, R.R.; Bishayee, A.; Kumar, S. Pentacyclic Triterpenes: New Tools to Fight Metabolic Syndrome. *Phytomedicine* **2018**, *50*, 166–177. [CrossRef] [PubMed]

7. Amiri, S.; Dastghaib, S.; Ahmadi, M.; Mehrbod, P.; Khadem, F.; Behrouj, H.; Aghanoori, M.R.; Machaj, F.; Ghamsari, M.; Rosik, J.; et al. Betulin and Its Derivatives as Novel Compounds with Different Pharmacological Effects. *Biotechnol. Adv.* **2020**, *38*, 107409. [CrossRef]
8. Luo, J.; Hu, Y.L.; Wang, H. Ursolic Acid Inhibits Breast Cancer Growth by Inhibiting Proliferation, Inducing Autophagy and Apoptosis, and Suppressing Inflammatory Responses via the PI3K/AKT and NF-κB Signaling Pathways In Vitro. *Exp. Ther. Med.* **2017**, *14*, 3623–3631. [CrossRef]
9. Woźniak, Ł.; Skąpska, S.; Marszałek, K. Ursolic Acid—A Pentacyclic Triterpenoid with a Wide Spectrum of Pharmacological Activities. *Molecules* **2015**, *20*, 20614–20641. [CrossRef]
10. Alam, P.; Al-Yousef, H.M.; Siddiqui, N.A.; Alhowiriny, T.A.; Alqasoumi, S.I.; Amina, M.; Hassan, W.H.B.; Abdelaziz, S.; Abdalla, R.H. Anticancer Activity and Concurrent Analysis of Ursolic Acid, β-Sitosterol, and Lupeol in Three Different *Hibiscus* Species (Aerial Parts) by Validated HPTLC Method. *Saudi Pharm. J.* **2018**, *26*, 1060–1067. [CrossRef]
11. Chan, W.E.C.; Soon, Y.C.; Tan, J.B.L.; Yong, S.K.; Hui, Y.W. Ursolic Acid: An Overview on Its Cytotoxic Activities against Breast and Colorectal Cancer Cells. *J. Integr. Med.* **2019**, *17*, 155–160. [CrossRef] [PubMed]
12. Tohmé, M.J.; Giménez, M.C.; Peralta, A.; Colombo, M.I.; Delgui, L.R. Ursolic Acid: A Novel Antiviral Compound Inhibiting Rotavirus Infection In Vitro. *Int. J. Antimicrob. Agents* **2019**, *54*, 601–609. [CrossRef] [PubMed]
13. Kong, L.; Li, S.; Liao, Q.; Zhang, Y.; Sun, R.; Zhu, X.; Zhang, Q.; Wang, J.; Wu, X.; Fang, X.; et al. Oleanolic Acid and Ursolic Acid: Novel Hepatitis C Virus Antivirals that Inhibit NS5B Activity. *Antiviral Res.* **2013**, *98*, 44–53. [CrossRef] [PubMed]
14. Kazakova, O.B.; Giniyatullina, G.V.; Yamansarov, E.Y.; Tolstikov, G.A. Betulin and Ursolic Acid Synthetic Derivatives as Inhibitors of Papilloma Virus. *Bioorg. Med. Chem. Lett.* **2010**, *20*, 4088–4090. [CrossRef]
15. Zhao, J.; Zheng, H.; Sui, Z.; Jing, F.; Quan, X.; Zhao, W.; Liu, G. Ursolic Acid Exhibits Anti-Inflammatory Effects through Blocking TLR4-MyD88 Pathway Mediated by Autophagy. *Cytokine* **2019**, *123*, 154726. [CrossRef]
16. Lee, J.Y.; Choi, J.K.; Jeong, N.H.; Yoo, J.; Ha, Y.S.; Lee, B.; Choi, H.; Park, P.H.; Shin, T.Y.; Kwon, T.K.; et al. Anti-Inflammatory Effects of Ursolic Acid-3-Acetate on Human Synovial Fibroblasts and a Murine Model of Rheumatoid Arthritis. *Int. Immunopharmacol.* **2017**, *49*, 118–125. [CrossRef] [PubMed]
17. Rai, S.N.; Zahra, W.; Singh, S.S.; Birla, H.; Keswani, C.; Dilnashin, H.; Rathore, A.S.; Singh, R.; Singh, R.K.; Singh, S.P. Anti-Inflammatory Activity of Ursolic Acid in MPTP-Induced Parkinsonian Mouse Model. *Neurotox. Res.* **2019**, *36*, 452–462. [CrossRef]
18. Habtemariam, S. Antioxidant and Anti-Inflammatory Mechanisms of Neuroprotection by Ursolic Acid: Addressing Brain Injury, Cerebral Ischemia, Cognition Deficit, Anxiety, and Depression. *Oxid. Med. Cell. Longev.* **2019**, *2019*, 8512048. [CrossRef]
19. Yenigün, S.; Başar, Y.; İpek, Y.; Behçet, L.; Özen, T.; Demirtaş, İ. Determination of Antioxidant, DNA Protection, Enzyme Inhibition Potential and Molecular Docking Studies of a Biomarker Ursolic Acid in Nepeta Species. *J. Biomol. Struct. Dyn.* **2024**, *42*, 5799–5816. [CrossRef]
20. Zhao, L.; Duan, X.; Cao, W.; Ren, X.; Ren, G.; Liu, P.; Chen, J. Effects of Different Drying Methods on the Characterization, Dissolution Rate and Antioxidant Activity of Ursolic Acid-Loaded Chitosan Nanoparticles. *Foods* **2021**, *10*, 2470. [CrossRef]
21. Mahlo, S.M.; McGaw, L.J.; Eloff, J.N. Antifungal Activity and Cytotoxicity of Isolated Compounds from Leaves of *Breonadia salicina*. *J. Ethnopharmacol.* **2013**, *148*, 909–913. [CrossRef] [PubMed]
22. Shu, C.; Zhao, H.; Jiao, W.; Liu, B.; Cao, J.; Jiang, W. Antifungal Efficacy of Ursolic Acid in Control of *Alternaria alternata* Causing Black Spot Rot on Apple Fruit and Possible Mechanisms Involved. *Sci. Hortic.* **2019**, *256*, 108636. [CrossRef]
23. Zahari, R.; Halimoon, N.; Ahmad, M.F.; Ling, S.K. Antifungal Compound Isolated from *Catharanthus roseus* L. (Pink) for Biological Control of Root Rot Rubber Diseases. *Int. J. Anal. Chem.* **2018**, *2018*, 8150610. [CrossRef]
24. Shaik, A.B.; Ahil, S.B.; Govardhanam, R.; Senthi, M.; Khan, R.; Sojitra, R.; Kumar, S.; Srinivas, A. Antifungal Effect and Protective Role of Ursolic Acid and Three Phenolic Derivatives in the Management of Sorghum Grain Mold Under Field Conditions. *Chem. Biodivers.* **2016**, *13*, 1158–1164. [CrossRef] [PubMed]
25. Innocente, A.; Casanova, B.B.; Klein, F.; Lana, A.D.; Pereira, D.; Muniz, M.N.; Sonnet, P.; Gosmann, G.; Fuentefria, A.M.; Gnoatto, S.C. Synthesis of Isosteric Triterpenoid Derivatives and Antifungal Activity. *Chem. Biol. Drug Des.* **2014**, *83*, 344–349. [CrossRef] [PubMed]
26. Spivak, A.Y.; Khalitova, R.R.; Nedopekina, D.A.; Gubaidullin, R.R. Antimicrobial Properties of Amine- and Guanidine-Functionalized Derivatives of Betulinic, Ursolic and Oleanolic Acids: Synthesis and Structure/Activity Evaluation. *Steroids* **2020**, *154*, 108530. [CrossRef] [PubMed]
27. Oloyede, H.O.B.; Ajiboye, H.O.; Salawu, M.O.; Ajiboye, T.O. Influence of Oxidative Stress on the Antibacterial Activity of Betulin, Betulinic Acid and Ursolic Acid. *Microb. Pathog.* **2017**, *111*, 338–344. [CrossRef] [PubMed]
28. Wu, P.P.; Zhang, K.; Lu, Y.J.; He, P.; Zhao, S.Q. In Vitro and In Vivo Evaluation of the Antidiabetic Activity of Ursolic Acid Derivatives. *Eur. J. Med. Chem.* **2014**, *80*, 502–508. [CrossRef]
29. Guzmán-Ávila, R.; Flores-Morales, V.; Paoli, P.; Camici, G.; Ramírez-Espinosa, J.J.; Cerón-Romero, L.; Navarrete-Vázquez, G.; Hidalgo-Figueroa, S.; Yolanda Rios, M.; Villalobos-Molina, R.; et al. Ursolic Acid Derivatives as Potential Antidiabetic Agents: In Vitro, In Vivo, and In Silico Studies. *Drug Dev. Res.* **2018**, *79*, 70–80. [CrossRef]
30. Alkreathy, H.M.; Ahmad, A. *Catharanthus roseus* Combined with Ursolic Acid Attenuates Streptozotocin-Induced Diabetes through Insulin Secretion and Glycogen Storage. *Oxid. Med. Cell. Longev.* **2020**, *2020*, 8565760. [CrossRef]
31. Wang, J.; Zhao, J.; Yan, Y.; Liu, D.; Wang, C.; Wang, H. Inhibition of Glycosidase by Ursolic Acid: In Vitro, In Vivo and In Silico Study. *J. Sci. Food Agric.* **2020**, *100*, 986–994. [CrossRef] [PubMed]

32. Kalaycıoğlu, Z.; Uzaşçı, S.; Dirmenci, T.; Erim, F.B. α-Glucosidase Enzyme Inhibitory Effects and Ursolic and Oleanolic Acid Contents of Fourteen Anatolian *Salvia* Species. *J. Pharm. Biomed. Anal.* **2018**, *155*, 284–287. [CrossRef] [PubMed]
33. Fontana, G.; Bruno, M.; Notarbartolo, M.; Labbozzetta, M.; Poma, P.; Spinella, A.; Rosselli, S. Cytotoxicity of Oleanolic and Ursolic Acid Derivatives Toward Hepatocellular Carcinoma and Evaluation of NF-κB Involvement. *Bioorg. Chem.* **2019**, *90*, 103054. [CrossRef] [PubMed]
34. Zhang, L.H.; Jin, L.L.; Liu, F.; Jin, C.; Jin, C.M.; Wei, Z.Y. Evaluation of Ursolic Acid Derivatives with Potential Anti-*Toxoplasma gondii* Activity. *Exp. Parasitol.* **2020**, *216*, 107935. [CrossRef] [PubMed]
35. Frolova, T.S.; Lipeeva, A.V.; Baev, D.S.; Baiborodin, S.I.; Orishchenko, K.E.; Kochetov, A.V.; Sinitsyna, O.I. Fluorescent Labeling of Ursolic Acid with FITC for Investigation of Its Cytotoxic Activity Using Confocal Microscopy. *Bioorg. Chem.* **2019**, *87*, 876–887. [CrossRef]
36. Jiang, W.; Huang, R.Z.; Zhang, J.; Guo, T.; Zhang, M.T.; Huang, X.C.; Zhang, B.; Liao, Z.X.; Sun, J.; Wang, H.S. Discovery of Antitumor Ursolic Acid Long-Chain Diamine Derivatives as Potent Inhibitors of NF-κB. *Bioorg. Chem.* **2018**, *79*, 265–276. [CrossRef] [PubMed]
37. Chen, H.; Gao, Y.; Wang, A.; Zhou, X.; Zheng, Y.; Zhou, J. Evolution in Medicinal Chemistry of Ursolic Acid Derivatives as Anticancer Agents. *Eur. J. Med. Chem.* **2015**, *92*, 648–655. [CrossRef] [PubMed]
38. Wu, J.; Zhang, Z.H.; Zhang, L.H.; Jin, X.J.; Ma, J.; Piao, H.R. Design, Synthesis, and Screening of Novel Ursolic Acid Derivatives as Potential Anti-Cancer Agents That Target the HIF-1α Pathway. *Bioorg. Med. Chem. Lett.* **2019**, *29*, 853–858. [CrossRef] [PubMed]
39. Zhang, L.H.; Zhang, Z.H.; Li, M.Y.; Wei, Z.Y.; Jin, X.J.; Piao, H.R. Synthesis and Evaluation of the HIF-1α Inhibitory Activities of Novel Ursolic Acid Tetrazole Derivatives. *Bioorg. Med. Chem. Lett.* **2019**, *29*, 1440–1445. [CrossRef]
40. Wang, W.Y.; Wu, W.Y.; Li, A.L.; Liu, Q.S.; Sun, Y.; Gu, W. Synthesis, Anticancer Evaluation and Mechanism Studies of Novel Indolequinone Derivatives of Ursolic Acid. *Bioorg. Chem.* **2021**, *109*, 104705. [CrossRef]
41. Bai, K.K.; Yu, Z.; Chen, F.L.; Li, F.; Li, W.Y.; Guo, Y.H. Synthesis and Evaluation of Ursolic Acid Derivatives as Potent Cytotoxic Agents. *Bioorg. Med. Chem. Lett.* **2012**, *22*, 2488–2493. [CrossRef] [PubMed]
42. Dwivedi, G.R.; Maurya, A. Drug Resistance Reversal Potential of Ursolic Acid Derivatives against Nalidixic Acid- and Multidrug-Resistant *Escherichia coli*. *Chem. Biol. Drug Des.* **2014**, *83*, 601–612. [CrossRef] [PubMed]
43. Wei, Z.Y.; Chi, K.Q.; Wang, K.S.; Wu, J.; Liu, L.P.; Piao, H.R. Design, Synthesis, Evaluation, and Molecular Docking of Ursolic Acid Derivatives Containing a Nitrogen Heterocycle as Anti-Inflammatory Agents. *Bioorg. Med. Chem. Lett.* **2018**, *28*, 1797–1803. [CrossRef]
44. Huang, Q.; Chen, H.; Ren, Y.; Wang, Z.; Zeng, P.; Li, X.; Wang, J.; Zheng, X. Anti-Hepatocellular Carcinoma Activity and Mechanism of Chemopreventive Compounds: Ursolic Acid Derivatives. *Pharm. Biol.* **2016**, *54*, 3189–3196. [CrossRef] [PubMed]
45. Khusnutdinova, E.; Petrova, A.; Zileeva, Z.; Kuzmina, U.; Zainullina, L.; Vakhitova, Y.; Babkov, D.; Kazakova, O. Novel A-Ring Chalcone Derivatives of Oleanolic and Ursolic Amides with Anti-Proliferative Effect Mediated Through ROS-Triggered Apoptosis. *Int. J. Mol. Sci.* **2021**, *22*, 9796. [CrossRef] [PubMed]
46. Sylla, B.; Lavoie, S.; Legault, J.; Gauthier, C.; Pichette, A. Synthesis, Cytotoxicity and Anti-Inflammatory Activity of Rhamnose-Containing Ursolic and Betulinic Acid Saponins. *RSC Adv.* **2019**, *9*, 39743–39757. [CrossRef] [PubMed]
47. Chu, C.; Song, K.; Zhang, Y.; Yang, M.; Fan, B.; Huang, H.; Chen, G. Biotransformation of Ursolic Acid by *Circinella muscae* and Their Anti-Neuroinflammatory Activities of Metabolites. *Nat. Prod. Res.* **2022**, *36*, 2777–2782. [CrossRef] [PubMed]
48. Antonio, E.; Junior, O.D.R.A.; Marcano, R.G.D.J.V.; Diedrich, C.; da Silva Santos, J.; Machado, C.S.; Khalil, N.M.; Mainardes, R.M. Chitosan Modified Poly (Lactic Acid) Nanoparticles Increased the Ursolic Acid Oral Bioavailability. *Int. J. Biol. Macromol.* **2021**, *172*, 133–142. [CrossRef]
49. Shao, J.; Fang, Y.; Zhao, R.; Chen, F.; Yang, M.; Jiang, J.; Chen, Z.; Yuan, X.; Jia, L. Evolution from Small Molecule to Nano-Drug Delivery Systems: An Emerging Approach for Cancer Therapy of Ursolic Acid. *Asian J. Pharm. Sci.* **2020**, *15*, 685–700. [CrossRef]
50. Khan, K.; Aqil, M.; Imam, S.S.; Ahad, A.; Moolakkadath, T.; Sultana, Y.; Mujeeb, M. Ursolic Acid Loaded Intra Nasal Nano Lipid Vesicles for Brain Tumour: Formulation, Optimization, In-Vivo Brain/Plasma Distribution Study and Histopathological Assessment. *Biomed. Pharmacother.* **2018**, *106*, 1578–1585. [CrossRef]
51. Cargnin, S.T.; Gnoatto, S.B. Ursolic Acid from Apple Pomace and Traditional Plants: A Valuable Triterpenoid with Functional Properties. *Food Chem.* **2017**, *220*, 477–489. [CrossRef]
52. Kashyap, D.; Singh, H.; Sharma, A.K. Ursolic Acid (UA): A Metabolite with Promising Therapeutic Potential. *Life Sci.* **2016**, *146*, 201–213. [CrossRef] [PubMed]
53. Yu, M.; Li, R.; Zhang, J. Repositioning of Antibiotic Levofloxacin as a Mitochondrial Biogenesis Inhibitor to Target Breast Cancer. *Biochem. Biophys. Res. Commun.* **2016**, *471*, 639–645. [CrossRef]
54. Farwick, M.; Köhler, T.; Schild, J.; Mentel, M.; Maczkiewitz, U.; Pagani, V.; Bonfigli, A.; Rigano, L.; Bureik, D.; Gauglitz, G.G. Pentacyclic Triterpenes from *Terminalia arjuna* Show Multiple Benefits on Aged and Dry Skin. *Skin Pharmacol. Physiol.* **2014**, *27*, 71–81. [CrossRef] [PubMed]
55. López-Hortas, L.; Pérez-Larrán, P.; González-Muñoz, M.J.; Falqué, E.; Domínguez, H. Recent Developments on the Extraction and Application of Ursolic Acid: A Review. *Food Res. Int.* **2018**, *103*, 130–149. [CrossRef]
56. Ramos, A.A.; Pereira-Wilson, C.; Collins, A.R. Protective Effects of Ursolic Acid and Luteolin against Oxidative DNA Damage Include Enhancement of DNA Repair in Caco-2 Cells. *Mutat. Res./Fundam. Mol. Mech. Mutagen.* **2010**, *692*, 6–11. [CrossRef] [PubMed]

57. Checker, R.; Sandur, S.K.; Sharma, D.; Patwardhan, R.S.; Jayakumar, S.; Kohli, V.; Sethi, G.; Aggarwal, B.B.; Sainis, K.B. Potent Anti-Inflammatory Activity of Ursolic Acid, a Triterpenoid Antioxidant, Is Mediated Through Suppression of NF-κB, AP-1 and NF-AT. *PLoS ONE* **2012**, *7*, e31318. [CrossRef]
58. Takada, K.; Nakane, T.; Masuda, K.; Ishii, H. Ursolic Acid and Oleanolic Acid, Members of Pentacyclic Triterpenoid Acids, Suppress TNF-α-Induced E-Selectin Expression by Cultured Umbilical Vein Endothelial Cells. *Phytomedicine* **2010**, *17*, 1114–1119. [CrossRef]
59. Khwaza, V.; Oyedeji, O.O.; Aderibigbe, B.A. Ursolic Acid-Based Derivatives as Potential Anti-Cancer Agents: An Update. *Int. J. Mol. Sci.* **2020**, *21*, 5920. [CrossRef]
60. Zhang, T.Y.; Li, C.S.; Cao, L.T.; Bai, X.Q.; Zhao, D.H.; Sun, S.M. New Ursolic Acid Derivatives Bearing 1,2,3-Triazole Moieties: Design, Synthesis and Anti-Inflammatory Activity In Vitro and In Vivo. *Mol. Divers.* **2022**, *26*, 1129–1139. [CrossRef]
61. Zhang, T.Y.; Li, C.S.; Li, P.; Bai, X.Q.; Guo, S.Y.; Jin, Y.; Piao, S.J. Synthesis and Evaluation of Ursolic Acid-Based 1,2,4-Triazolo[1,5-a]Pyrimidines Derivatives as Anti-Inflammatory Agents. *Mol. Divers.* **2022**, *26*, 27–38. [CrossRef]
62. Wu, J.; Ma, S.; Wei, T.Z.Z.; Guo, H.W.F.; Piao, C.Z.H. Synthesis and Biological Evaluation of Ursolic Acid Derivatives Containing an Aminoguanidine Moiety. *Med. Chem. Res.* **2019**, *28*, 959–973. [CrossRef]
63. Qi, Z.; Xie, P.; Wang, Z.; Zhou, H.; Tao, R.; Popov, S.A.; Yang, G.; Shults, E.E.; Wang, C. Synthesis of Novel Ursolic Acid-Gallate Hybrids via 1,2,3-Triazole Linkage and Its Anti-Oxidant and Anti-Inflammatory Activity Study. *Arab. J. Chem.* **2024**, *17*, 105762. [CrossRef]
64. Hawash, M.; Jaradat, N.; Hameedi, S.; Mousa, A. Design, Synthesis and Biological Evaluation of Novel Benzodioxole Derivatives as COX Inhibitors and Cytotoxic Agents. *BMC Chem.* **2020**, *14*, 54. [CrossRef]
65. Xie, Y.D.; Xu, Y.H.; Liu, J.P.; Wang, B.; Shi, Y.H.; Wang, W.; Wang, X.P.; Sun, M.; Xu, X.Y.; Bian, X.L. 1,3-Benzodioxole-Based Fibrate Derivatives as Potential Hypolipidemic and Hepatoprotective Agents. *Bioorg. Med. Chem. Lett.* **2021**, *43*, 127898. [CrossRef]
66. Li, C.; Zhang, T.; Zhang, Q.; Liu, X.; Zou, J.; Bai, X. Screening of Ursolic Acid Analogs with HIF-1α and COX-2-Inhibiting Effects. *Chem. Nat. Compd.* **2022**, *58*, 882–887. [CrossRef]
67. Zhang, R.X.; Li, Y.; Tian, D.D.; Liu, Y.; Nian, W.; Zou, X.; Chen, Q.Z.; Zhou, L.Y.; Deng, Z.L.; He, B.C. Ursolic Acid Inhibits Proliferation and Induces Apoptosis by Inactivating Wnt/β-Catenin Signaling in Human Osteosarcoma Cells. *Int. J. Oncol.* **2016**, *49*, 1973–1982. [CrossRef] [PubMed]
68. Cheng, W.; Dahmani, F.Z.; Zhang, J.; Xiong, H.; Wu, Y.; Yin, L.; Zhou, J.; Yao, J. 2 Anti-angiogenic activity and antitumor efficacy of amphiphilic twin drug from ursolic acid and low molecular weight heparin. *Nanotechnology* **2017**, *28*, 075102. [CrossRef]
69. Jiang, K.; Chi, T.; Li, T.; Zheng, G.; Fan, L.; Liu, Y.; Chen, X.; Chen, S.; Jia, L.; Shao, J. Smart pH-Responsive Nano-Carrier as a Drug Delivery System for the Targeted Delivery of Ursolic Acid: Suppresses Cancer Growth and Metastasis by Modulating P53/MMP-9/PTEN/CD44 Mediated Multiple Signaling Pathways. *Nanoscale* **2017**, *9*, 9428–9439. [CrossRef]
70. Gupta, A.P. *Anticancer Curcumin: Natural Analogues and Structure-Activity Relationship*, 1st ed.; Elsevier: Amsterdam, The Netherlands, 2017; Volume 54.
71. Prasad, S.; Yadav, V.R.; Sung, B.; Reuter, S.; Kannappan, R.; Deorukhkar, A.; Diagaradjane, P.; Wei, C.; Baladandayuthapani, V.; Krishnan, S.; et al. Ursolic Acid Inhibits Growth and Metastasis of Human Colorectal Cancer in an Orthotopic Nude Mouse Model by Targeting Multiple Cell Signaling Pathways: Chemosensitization with Capecitabine. *Clin. Cancer Res.* **2012**, *18*, 4942–4953. [CrossRef] [PubMed]
72. Li, W.; Zhang, H.; Nie, M.; Tian, Y.; Chen, X.; Chen, C.; Chen, H.; Liu, R. Ursolic Acid Derivative FZU-03,010 Inhibits STAT3 and Induces Cell Cycle Arrest and Apoptosis in Renal and Breast Cancer Cells. *Acta Biochim. Biophys. Sin.* **2017**, *49*, 367–373. [CrossRef]
73. Wang, W.J.; Sui, H.; Qi, C.; Li, Q.; Zhang, J.; Wu, S.F.; Mei, M.Z.; Lu, Y.Y.; Wan, Y.T.; Chang, H.; et al. Ursolic Acid Inhibits Proliferation and Reverses Drug Resistance of Ovarian Cancer Stem Cells by Downregulating ABCG2 through Suppressing the Expression of Hypoxia-Inducible Factor-1α In Vitro. *Oncol. Rep.* **2016**, *36*, 428–440. [CrossRef]
74. Zong, L.; Cheng, G.; Liu, S.; Pi, Z.; Liu, Z.; Song, F. Reversal of Multidrug Resistance in Breast Cancer Cells by a Combination of Ursolic Acid with Doxorubicin. *J. Pharm. Biomed. Anal.* **2019**, *165*, 268–275. [CrossRef] [PubMed]
75. Obeagu, E.I.; Ubosi, N.I.; Obeagu, G.U.; Egba, S.I.; Bluth, M.H. Understanding Apoptosis in Sickle Cell Anemia Patients: Mechanisms and Implications. *Medicine* **2024**, *103*, E36898. [CrossRef]
76. Moghadam, A.R.; da Silva Rosa, S.C.; Samiei, E.; Alizadeh, J.; Field, J.; Kawalec, P.; Thliveris, J.; Akbari, M.; Ghavami, S.; Gordon, J.W. Autophagy Modulates Temozolomide-Induced Cell Death in Alveolar Rhabdomyosarcoma Cells. *Cell Death Discov.* **2018**, *4*, 52. [CrossRef] [PubMed]
77. Alizadeh, J.; Zeki, A.A.; Mirzaei, N.; Tewary, S.; Rezaei Moghadam, A.; Glogowska, A.; Nagakannan, P.; Eftekharpour, E.; Wiechec, E.; Gordon, J.W.; et al. Mevalonate Cascade Inhibition by Simvastatin Induces the Intrinsic Apoptosis Pathway via Depletion of Isoprenoids in Tumor Cells. *Nat. Publ. Gr.* **2017**, *7*, 1–14. [CrossRef]
78. Chuang, W.; Lin, P.; Lin, H.; Chen, Y. The Apoptotic Effect of Ursolic Acid on SK-Hep-1 Cells is Regulated by the PI3K/Akt, p38, and JNK MAPK Signaling Pathways. *Molecules* **2016**, *21*, 460. [CrossRef]
79. Sun, Q.; He, M.; Zhang, M.; Zeng, S.; Chen, L.; Zhou, L.; Xu, H. Ursolic Acid: A Systematic Review of its Pharmacology, Toxicity and Rethink on its Pharmacokinetics Based on PK-PD Model. *Fitoterapia* **2020**, *147*, 104735. [CrossRef] [PubMed]
80. Weng, H.; Tan, Z.J.; Hu, Y.P.; Shu, Y.J.; Bao, R.F.; Jiang, L.; Wu, X.S.; Li, M.L.; Ding, Q.; Wang, X.A.; et al. Ursolic Acid Induces Cell Cycle Arrest and Apoptosis of Gallbladder Carcinoma Cells. *Cancer Cell Int.* **2014**, *14*, 96. [CrossRef] [PubMed]

81. Fan, H.; Geng, L.; Yang, F.; Dong, X.; He, D.; Zhang, Y. Ursolic Acid Derivative Induces Apoptosis in Glioma Cells through Down-Regulation of cAMP. *Eur. J. Med. Chem.* **2019**, *176*, 61–67. [CrossRef]
82. Mendes, V.I.S.; Bartholomeusz, G.A.; Ayres, M.; Gandhi, V.; Salvador, J.A.R. Synthesis and Cytotoxic Activity of Novel A-Ring Cleaved Ursolic Acid Derivatives in Human Non-Small Cell Lung Cancer Cells. *Eur. J. Med. Chem.* **2016**, *123*, 317–331. [CrossRef]
83. Nedopekina, D.A. Mitochondria-Targeted Betulinic and Ursolic Acid Derivatives: Synthesis and Anticancer Activity. *MedChemComm* **2017**, *8*, 1934–1945. [CrossRef]
84. Liu, M.; Yang, S.; Hu, L.J.D.; Xue, W.; Eb, A.O. Synthesis and Evaluation as Potential Antitumor Agents of Novel Ursolic Acid Derivatives. *Med. Chem. Res.* **2016**, *25*, 2267–2279. [CrossRef]
85. Gou, W.; Luo, N.; Wei, H.; Wu, H.; Yu, X.; Duan, Y.; Bi, C.; Ning, H.; Hou, W.; Li, Y. Ursolic Acid Derivative UA232 Evokes Apoptosis of Lung Cancer Cells Induced by Endoplasmic Reticulum Stress. *Pharm. Biol.* **2020**, *58*, 707–715. [CrossRef]
86. Meng, Y.; Xu, C.; Yu, T.; Li, W.; Li, Q. Synthesis and Antitumor Activity Evaluation of Ursolic Acid Derivatives. *J. Asian Nat. Prod. Res.* **2020**, *22*, 359–369. [CrossRef] [PubMed]
87. Jin, X.Y.; Chen, H.; Li, D.D.; Li, A.L.; Wang, W.Y.; Gu, W. Design, Synthesis, and Anticancer Evaluation of Novel Quinoline Derivatives of Ursolic Acid with Hydrazide, Oxadiazole, and Thiadiazole Moieties as Potent MEK Inhibitors. *J. Enzyme Inhib. Med. Chem.* **2019**, *34*, 955–972. [CrossRef]
88. Gu, W.; Jin, X.Y.; Li, D.D.; Wang, S.F.; Tao, X.B.; Chen, H. Design, Synthesis and In Vitro Anticancer Activity of Novel Quinoline and Oxadiazole Derivatives of Ursolic Acid. *Bioorg. Med. Chem. Lett.* **2017**, *27*, 4128–4132. [CrossRef]
89. Meng, Y.Q.; Zhang, L.F.; Liu, D.Y.; Liu, L.W.; Zhang, Y.; Zhao, M.J. Synthesis and Antitumor Activity Evaluation of Novel Ursolic Acid Derivatives. *J. Asian Nat. Prod. Res.* **2016**, *18*, 280–288. [CrossRef]
90. Csuk, R.; Deigner, H.P. The Potential of Click Reactions for the Synthesis of Bioactive Triterpenes. *Bioorg. Med. Chem. Lett.* **2019**, *29*, 949–958. [CrossRef] [PubMed]
91. Popov, S.A.; Semenova, M.D.; Baev, D.S.; Frolova, T.S.; Shestopalov, M.A.; Wang, C.; Qi, Z.; Shults, E.E.; Turks, M. Synthesis and Cytotoxicity of Hybrids of 1,3,4- or 1,2,5-Oxadiazoles Tethered from Ursane and Lupane Core with 1,2,3-Triazole. *Steroids* **2020**, *162*, 108698. [CrossRef]
92. Zhang, T.; He, B.; Yuan, H.; Feng, G.; Chen, F.; Wu, A.; Zhang, L.; Lin, H.; Zhuo, Z.; Wang, T. Synthesis and Antitumor Evaluation in Vitro of NO-Donating Ursolic Acid-Benzylidene Derivatives. *Chem. Biodivers.* **2019**, *16*, e1900111. [CrossRef]
93. Wang, W.; Lei, L.; Liu, Z.; Wang, H.; Meng, Q. Design, Synthesis, and Biological Evaluation of Novel Nitrogen Heterocycle-Containing Ursolic Acid Analogs as Antitumor Agents. *Molecules* **2019**, *24*, 877. [CrossRef] [PubMed]
94. Spivak, A.; Khalitova, R.; Nedopekina, D.; Dzhemileva, L.; Yunusbaeva, M.; Odinokov, V.; D'yakonov, V.; Dzhemilev, U. Synthesis and Evaluation of Anticancer Activities of Novel C-28 Guanidine-Functionalized Triterpene Acid Derivatives. *Molecules* **2018**, *23*, 3000. [CrossRef] [PubMed]
95. Li, W.; Zhang, H.; Nie, M.; Wang, W.; Liu, Z.; Chen, C.; Chen, H.; Liu, R.; Baloch, Z.; Ma, K. A novel synthetic ursolic acid derivative inhibits growth and induces apoptosis in breast cancer cell lines. *Oncol. Lett.* **2018**, *15*, 2323–2329. [CrossRef] [PubMed]
96. Butler, M.S.; Gigante, V.; Sati, H.; Paulin, S.; Al-Sulaiman, L.; Rex, J.H.; Fernandes, P.; Arias, C.A.; Paul, M.; Thwaites, G.E.; et al. Analysis of the clinical pipeline of treatments for drug-resistant bacterial infections: Despite progress, more action is needed. *Antimicrob. Agents Chemother.* **2022**, *66*, e01991-21. [CrossRef]
97. Vardakas, K.Z.; Rafailidis, P.I.; Konstantelias, A.A.; Falagas, M.E. Predictors of mortality in patients with infections due to multi-drug resistant Gram-negative bacteria: The study, the patient, the bug or the drug? *J. Infect.* **2013**, *66*, 401–414. [CrossRef]
98. Chung, P.Y.; Navaratnam, P.; Chung, L.Y. Synergistic antimicrobial activity between pentacyclic triterpenoids and antibiotics against *Staphylococcus aureus* strains. *Ann. Clin. Microbiol. Antimicrob.* **2011**, *10*, 25. [CrossRef] [PubMed]
99. Ríos, J.L.; Máñez, S. New pharmacological opportunities for betulinic acid. *Planta Med.* **2018**, *84*, 8–19. [CrossRef]
100. Chung, P.Y.; Chung, L.Y.; Navaratnam, P. Potential targets by pentacyclic triterpenoids from *Callicarpa farinosa* against methicillin-resistant and sensitive *Staphylococcus aureus*. *Fitoterapia* **2014**, *94*, 48–54. [CrossRef]
101. e Silva, M.D.L.; David, J.P.; Silva, L.C.; Santos, R.A.; David, J.M.; Lima, L.S.; Reis, P.S.; Fontana, R. Bioactive oleanane, lupane and ursane triterpene acid derivatives. *Molecules* **2012**, *17*, 12197–12205. [CrossRef]
102. Siewert, B.; Pianowski, E.; Csuk, R. Esters and amides of maslinic acid trigger apoptosis in human tumor cells and alter their mode of action with respect to the substitution pattern at C-28. *Eur. J. Med. Chem.* **2013**, *70*, 259–272. [CrossRef] [PubMed]
103. Chouaïb, K.; Hichri, F.; Nguir, A.; Daami-Remadi, M.; Elie, N.; Touboul, D.; Jannet, H.B. Semi-synthesis of new antimicrobial esters from the natural oleanolic and maslinic acids. *Food Chem.* **2015**, *183*, 8–17. [CrossRef]
104. Swidorski, J.J.; Liu, Z.; Sit, S.Y.; Chen, J.; Chen, Y.; Sin, N.; Venables, B.L.; Parker, D.D.; Nowicka-Sans, B.; Terry, B.J.; et al. Inhibitors of HIV-1 maturation: Development of structure-activity relationship for C-28 amides based on C-3 benzoic acid-modified triterpenoids. *Bioorg. Med. Chem. Lett.* **2016**, *26*, 1925–1930. [CrossRef] [PubMed]
105. Zhou, M.; Zhang, R.-H.; Wang, M.; Xu, G.-B.; Liao, S.-G. Prodrugs of triterpenoids and their derivatives. *Eur. J. Med. Chem.* **2017**, *131*, 222–236. [CrossRef] [PubMed]
106. Wojnicz, D.; Tichaczek-Goska, D.; Kicia, M. Pentacyclic triterpenes combined with ciprofloxacin help to eradicate the biofilm formed in vitro by *Escherichia coli*. *Indian J. Med. Res. Suppl.* **2015**, *141*, 343–353. [CrossRef]
107. Liu, G.; Qin, P.; Cheng, X.; Wu, L.; Zhao, W.; Gao, W. Evaluation of the mechanistic basis for the antibacterial activity of ursolic acid against *Staphylococcus aureus*. *Front. Microbiol.* **2024**, *15*, 1389242. [CrossRef] [PubMed]

108. Cunha, W.R.; de Matos, G.X.; Souza, M.G.M.; Tozatti, M.G.; Andrade e Silva, M.L.; Martins, C.H.; Silva, R.D.; Da Silva Filho, A.A. Evaluation of the antibacterial activity of the methylene chloride extract of *Miconia ligustroides*, isolated triterpene acids, and ursolic acid derivatives. *Pharm. Biol.* **2010**, *48*, 166–169. [CrossRef] [PubMed]
109. Do Nascimento, P.G.; Lemos, T.L.; Bizerra, A.M.; Arriaga, Â.M.; Ferreira, D.A.; Santiago, G.M.; Braz-Filho, R.; Costa, J.G.M. Antibacterial and antioxidant activities of ursolic acid and derivatives. *Molecules* **2014**, *19*, 1317–1327. [CrossRef]
110. Zhao, W.W.; Zan, K.; Wu, J.Y.; Gao, W.; Yang, J.; Ba, Y.Y.; Wu, X.; Chen, X.Q. Antibacterial triterpenoids from the leaves of *Ilex hainanensis* Merr. *Nat. Prod. Res.* **2019**, *33*, 2435–2439. [CrossRef]
111. Wang, C.M.; Jhan, Y.L.; Tsai, S.J.; Chou, C.H. The pleiotropic antibacterial mechanisms of ursolic acid against methicillin-resistant *Staphylococcus aureus* (MRSA). *Molecules* **2016**, *21*, 884. [CrossRef]
112. Pandey, P.; Garg, A.; Singh, V.; Shukla, A. Evaluation of anthelmintic and antimicrobial activity of ursolic acid obtained from Tulsi (*Ocimum sanctum*). *Asian J. Pharm. Pharmacol.* **2016**, *2*, 67–71.
113. Park, S.N.; Lim, Y.K.; Choi, M.H.; Cho, E.; Bang, I.S.; Kim, J.M.; Ahn, S.J.; Kook, J.K. Antimicrobial mechanism of oleanolic and ursolic acids on *Streptococcus mutans* UA159. *Curr. Microbiol.* **2018**, *75*, 11–19. [CrossRef] [PubMed]
114. Qian, W.; Wang, W.; Zhang, J.; Wang, T.; Liu, M.; Yang, M.; Sun, Z.; Li, X.; Li, Y. Antimicrobial and antibiofilm activities of ursolic acid against carbapenem-resistant *Klebsiella pneumoniae*. *J. Antibiot.* **2020**, *73*, 382–391. [CrossRef] [PubMed]
115. da Silva, G.N.S.; Primon-Barros, M.; Macedo, A.J.; Gnoatto, S.C.B. Triterpene Derivatives as Relevant Scaffold for New Antibiofilm Drugs. *Biomolecules* **2019**, *9*, 58. [CrossRef] [PubMed]
116. Popov, S.A.; Wang, C.; Qi, Z.; Shul'ts, E.E.; Turks, M. Synthesis and Antioxidant Activity of New N-Containing Hybrid Derivatives of Gallic and Ursolic Acids. *Chem. Nat. Compd.* **2021**, *57*, 1042–1046. [CrossRef]
117. Chang, C.D.; Lin, P.Y.; Hsu, J.L.; Shih, W.L. Ursolic Acid Suppresses Hepatitis B Virus X Protein-Mediated Autophagy and Chemotherapeutic Drug Resistance. *Anticancer Res.* **2016**, *36*, 5097–5107. [CrossRef] [PubMed]
118. Zhu, M.; Du, X.N.; Li, Y.G.; Zhang, G.N.; Wang, J.X.; Wang, Y.C. Design, Synthesis and Biological Evaluation of Novel HIV-1 Protease Inhibitors with Pentacyclic Triterpenoids as P2-Ligands. *Bioorg. Med. Chem. Lett.* **2019**, *29*, 357–361. [CrossRef]
119. Xiao, S.; Tian, Z.; Wang, Y.; Si, L.; Zhang, L.; Zhou, D. Anti-HIV Activity Has Been Identified for a Variety of Pentacyclic Triterpenoids, as Well as Their Saponin or Modifying Agents. *Med. Res. Rev.* **2018**, *38*, 951–976. [CrossRef]
120. Xiao, S.; Tian, Z.; Wang, Y.; Si, L.; Zhang, L.; Zhou, D. Recent Progress in the Antiviral Activity and Mechanism Study of Pentacyclic Triterpenoids and Their Derivatives. *Med. Res. Rev.* **2018**, *38*, 951–976. [CrossRef]
121. Yoo, S.J.; Kwon, T.; Lyoo, Y.S. Challenges of Influenza A Viruses in Humans and Animals and Current Animal Vaccines as an Effective Control Measure. *Clin. Exp. Vaccine Res.* **2018**, *7*, 1–15. [CrossRef]
122. Li, H.; Li, Z.; Wang, H.; Luo, Z.; Zhang, L.; Zhou, D. Incorporation of Privileged Structures into 3-O-β-Chacotriosyl Ursolic Acid Can Enhance Inhibiting the Entry of the H5N1 Virus. *Bioorg. Med. Chem. Lett.* **2019**, *29*, 2675–2680. [CrossRef] [PubMed]
123. Liao, Y.; Dai, Z.; Xu, Y.; Teng, Y.; Wu, B. Structure-Aided Optimization of 3-O-β-Chacotriosyl Ursolic Acid as Novel H5N1 Entry Inhibitors with High Selective Index. *Bioorg. Med. Chem.* **2019**, *27*, 4048–4058. [CrossRef] [PubMed]
124. Zhong, Y.; Dai, Z.; Xu, Y.; Teng, Y.; Wu, B. Synthesis, Stability and Pharmacological Evaluation of a Novel Codrug Consisting of Lamivudine and Ursolic Acid. *Eur. J. Pharm. Sci.* **2012**, *45*, 110–115. [CrossRef] [PubMed]
125. Samsonowicz, M.; Kalinowska, M.; Gryko, K. Enhanced Antioxidant Activity of Ursolic Acid by Complexation with Copper (II): Experimental and Theoretical Study. *Materials* **2021**, *14*, 268. [CrossRef] [PubMed]
126. Busuioc, A.C.; Costea, G.V.; Botezatu, A.V.D.; Furdui, B.; Dinica, R.M. Cucumis metuliferus L. Fruits Extract with Antioxidant, Anti-Inflammatory, and Antidiabetic Properties as Source of Ursolic Acid. *Separations* **2023**, *10*, 274. [CrossRef]
127. Wu, P.; He, P.; Zhao, S.; Huang, T.; Lu, Y.; Zhang, K. Synthesis and Evaluation of Novel Triterpene Analogues of Ursolic Acid as Potential Antidiabetic Agent. *PLoS ONE* **2015**, *10*, e0138767. [CrossRef] [PubMed]
128. Wu, P.; He, P.; Zhao, S.; Huang, T.; Lu, Y.; Zhang, K. Effects of Ursolic Acid Derivatives on Caco-2 Cells and Their Alleviating Role in Streptozocin-Induced Type 2 Diabetic Rats. *Molecules* **2014**, *19*, 12559–12576. [CrossRef] [PubMed]
129. Huang, T.; Wu, P.; Cheng, A.; Qin, J.; Zhang, K.; Zhao, S. A Hydrophilic Conjugate Approach Toward the Design and Synthesis of Ursolic Acid Derivatives as Potential Antidiabetic Agent. *RSC Adv.* **2015**, *5*, 44234–44246. [CrossRef]

molecules

MDPI

Review

Turmeric Essential Oil Constituents as Potential Drug Candidates: A Comprehensive Overview of Their Individual Bioactivities

Adriana Monserrath Orellana-Paucar [1,2]

[1] Nutrition and Dietetics School, Faculty of Medical Sciences, University of Cuenca, Cuenca 010204, Ecuador; adriana.orellanap@ucuenca.edu.ec

[2] Pharmacology and Nutritional Sciences Interdisciplinary Research Group, Faculty of Medical Sciences, University of Cuenca, Cuenca 010204, Ecuador

Abstract: The therapeutic properties of turmeric essential oil have been extensively documented in both preclinical and clinical studies. Research indicates that its primary active compounds are promising candidates for addressing a wide range of pathologies, exhibiting anticancer, anti-inflammation, antioxidant, cardiovascular, hypoglycemic, dermatological, hepatoprotective, neurological, antiparasitic, antiviral, insecticidal, antifungal, and antivenom activities. While numerous compounds possess similar potential applications, the isolated active constituents of turmeric essential oil stand out due to their unique pharmacological profiles and absence of toxicity. This literature review meticulously compiles and analyzes the bioactivities of these constituents, emphasizing their molecular mechanisms of action, reported pharmacological effects, and potential therapeutic applications. The aim of this review is to provide a comprehensive synthesis of currently available clinical and preclinical findings related to individual turmeric essential oil compounds, while also identifying critical knowledge gaps. By summarizing these findings, this work encourages further research into the isolated compounds from turmeric oil as viable drug candidates, ultimately contributing to the development of innovative therapeutic strategies.

Keywords: turmeric; *Curcuma longa*; turmeric oil; curcuma oil; bioactivity; toxicity

1. Introduction

Curcuma longa L., commonly known as turmeric, belongs to the Zingiberaceae family and is a native Southeast Asian herb. Its dried rhizome powder has been used for centuries as food, spice, or medicine. Due to its significant biological activities, turmeric is considered an attractive source of drug candidates for preventing or treating various diseases. Most of these pharmacological properties are attributed to the extensively studied curcuminoids [1–4]. Turmeric rhizomes contain around 2–5% curcuminoids, including curcumin, demethoxycurcumin, and bisdemethoxycurcumin [5].

In addition to curcuminoids, turmeric exhibits a wide variety of chemical constituents with diverse pharmacological activities attributed to its active constituents, including antioxidant, anticancer, anti-inflammatory, cardiovascular, immunomodulatory, hepatoprotection, neuroprotective, antimicrobial, antivenom, and chemo-preventive action, among others [5,6].

Turmeric essential oil, responsible for the spice's aromatic taste and smell, is isolated from *Curcuma longa* rhizomes and does not contain curcuminoids. Dried turmeric rhizome typically includes 3–6% essential oil [7]. Turmeric rhizome essential oil (TEO) is traditionally obtained by hydro-distillation using the conventional Soxhlet technique.

The chemical composition of TEO exhibits a remarkable consistency on a global scale; however, the concentration of individual compounds varies significantly based on factors such as the geographical origin of the crops, the specific part of the plant utilized, and the methods employed during the drying process. Table 1 illustrates the variation in the content of the essential oil extracted from the rhizome, highlighting differences attributable to geographical location [8–11].

Table 1. Variations in major compound content of turmeric essential oil.

	India	Korea	Ecuador
ar-turmerone	16.7–25.7%	19.54–32.24%	1.08–45.5%
α-turmerone	30.1–32.0%	3.72–6.50%	13.4–19.8%
β-turmerone	14.7–18.4%	2.86–5.60%	7.35%
α-zingiberene	1.5–4.2%	-	5.3%

The primary constituents of TEO with documented pharmacological activities are terpenoids, specifically monoterpenes and sesquiterpenes (Figure 1). Sesquiterpenoids are synthesized by the assembly of three isoprenoid units. Many sesquiterpenoid carbon skeletons originate from the common precursor farnesyl pyrophosphate, undergoing various cyclization processes that are frequently followed by skeletal rearrangements. Consequently, the predominant categories of sesquiterpenes identified in TEO include bisabolane, elemane, germacrane, and guaiane types [12,13].

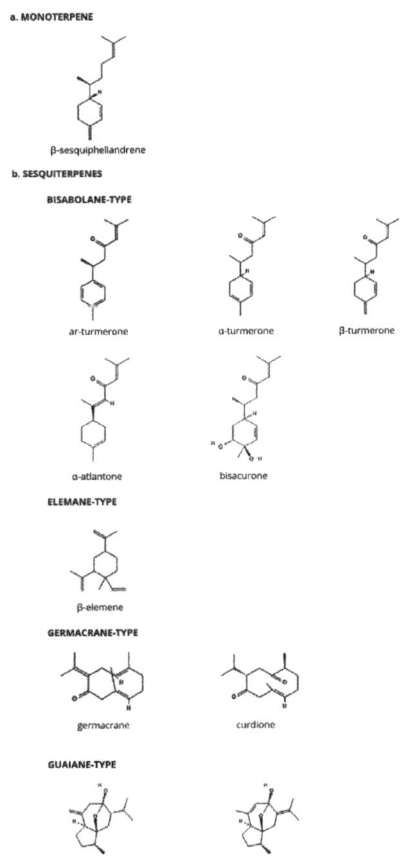

Figure 1. The main chemical constituents of turmeric essential oil with reported bioactive properties.

2. Bioactivities of Turmeric Essential Oil Constituents

2.1. Anticancer Activity

Cancer is a chronic and often fatal disease with a high global mortality rate and generally poor survival outcomes. Cancer-related deaths can result from the heterogeneous nature of cancerous cells or the failure of pharmacological treatments [14]. Interestingly, ar-turmerone, germacrone, and β-elemene have shown potential as anticancer agents.

Ar-turmerone has been shown to induce apoptosis in human lymphoma and lymphoblast cells through the activation of caspase-3 [15,16]. This bisabolane sesquiterpenoid also downregulates the secretion of growth factor and the phosphorylation of epidermal growth factor [17]. Additionally, ar-turmerone significantly inhibits the TPA-induced upregulation of MMP-9 and COX-2 expression in human breast cancer cells, effectively blocking critical signaling pathways such as NF-kB, PI3K/Akt, and ERK1/2. Importantly, ar-turmerone suppresses TPA-induced invasion, migration, and colony formation in these cells, underscoring its promising therapeutic potential [18]. Furthermore, ar-turmerone induces a highly selective apoptotic process in human leukemia Molt 4B and HL-60 cells [19]. Both α-turmerone and ar-turmerone also enhance the proliferation of peripheral blood mononuclear cells (PBMCs) and stimulate cytokine production. Notably, α-turmerone induces apoptosis in MDA-MB-231 cells and human leukemia cells, as evidenced by a significant reduction in the levels of procaspases-3, -8, and -9 [20].

Regarding benign prostatic hyperplasia, germacrone has been shown to inhibit androgens by selectively targeting the steroid 5-alpha reductase in vitro. This inhibitory effect is attributed to the structural similarity between the α,β-unsaturated carbonyl of germacrone and testosterone. Key factors contributing to its androgenic activity include the conformation of the cyclodecadiene ring and the presence of the α,β-unsaturated ketone/hydroxyl moiety in the germacrone molecule [21]. Additionally, germacrone induces apoptosis in a concentration-dependent manner, with treated cells exhibiting elevated levels of LC3B-II protein and distinctive punctate patterns, indicative of the initiation of protective autophagy. Moreover, germacrone suppresses the phosphorylation of Akt and mTOR in prostate cancer cells [22].

On the other hand, β-elemene has demonstrated efficacy in overcoming drug resistance in tumor cells. It inhibits the proliferation of A549/DDP cells in a manner that is dependent on both time and dosage. Furthermore, β-elemene enhances the sensitivity of these cells to cisplatin, effectively reversing drug resistance. Notably, β-elemene induces a reduction in mitochondrial membrane potential, an increase in intracellular reactive oxygen species (ROS) concentration, and a decrease in cytoplasmic glutathione levels. The combined treatment with β-elemene and cisplatin results in elevated protein expression of cytochrome c, caspase-3, and Bad, while concomitantly decreasing the protein levels of Bcl-2 and procaspase-3. This suggests the involvement of a procaspase-3-β-elemene pathway that impacts mitochondrial membrane potential, initiating apoptosis through the release of cytochrome c into the cytoplasm and modulating apoptosis-related genes [23].

Collectively, these findings suggest the potential efficacy of turmeric essential oil constituents against cancer cells. However, it is important to note that the primary limitations of these studies stem from their preclinical nature. Therefore, further clinical research is necessary to confirm the positive effects of these isolated compounds on human health.

2.2. Anti-Inflammatory Properties

Inflammation is a complex biological and pathological response that typically arises as a protective mechanism against harmful stimuli, such as infections and tissue injuries, with the aim of maintaining homeostasis within the body. Inflammation can be broadly classified into two categories: acute and chronic. Acute inflammation is a transient and generally beneficial response; however, when inflammation persists over an extended period, it can evolve into chronic inflammation, which is associated with various persistent health conditions, including obesity, diabetes, arthritis, pancreatitis, cardiovascular disorders, neurodegenerative diseases, metabolic disorders, and certain types of cancer [24].

While the anti-inflammatory properties of turmeric have traditionally been attributed to curcumin, bisabolene sesquiterpenes have emerged as a significant class of anti-inflammatory agents [25]. For instance, ar-turmerone has been shown to inhibit CD8+ T cells in the epidermis, leading to the reduced expression of NF-κB and COX-2, as well as the inhibition of p38 MAPK phosphorylation [26]. Additionally, ar-turmerone effectively inhibits critical inflammatory cytokines, including IFN-γ and IL-2, in CD4+ T cells without adversely affecting their proliferation rates upon stimulation [27].

Ar-turmerone also mitigates skin inflammation by lowering the levels of TNF-α and IL-6 while downregulating the mRNA synthesis of IL-17, IL-22, and IL-23. Furthermore, ar-turmerone decreases the production of TNF-α, IL-1β, IL-6, and MCP-1 in Aβ-stimulated microglial cells by inhibiting the NF-κB, JNK, and p38 MAPK signaling pathways [28–30].

In murine models, germacrone demonstrated anti-inflammatory effects by significantly reducing the expression of pro-inflammatory cytokines IL-6 and TNF-α while promoting the expression of anti-inflammatory mediators such as TGF-β1 and IL-10 [31]. It has been suggested that germacrone plays a crucial neuroprotective role by modulating autophagy through regulation of the PI3K III/Beclin-1/Bcl-2 and PI3K I/Akt/mTOR pathways [32].

Curcumol inhibits the LPS-induced nitric oxide (NO) production by suppressing the expression of iNOS mRNA and protein levels, although it does not affect iNOS activity. Furthermore, curcumol reduces the LPS-induced production of TNF-α, IL-1β, and IL-6 at both transcriptional and translational levels, accompanied by a decrease in JNK phosphorylation [33].

The anti-inflammatory potential of these turmeric essential oil constituents has been demonstrated both *in vitro* and in experimental animal models. While historical reports indicate the use of TEO to treat inflammatory diseases [34], further investigation through randomized and controlled clinical studies is warranted to elucidate the underlying mechanisms of action.

2.3. Antioxidant Action

Free radicals are generated through the accumulation of reactive oxygen species (ROS) resulting from exposure to oxidizing substances. Free radicals can contribute to the development of various chronic and degenerative diseases. However, the risk of such diseases can be mitigated by employing external antioxidants or enhancing the production of endogenous oxidants [35]. *In vitro* studies have demonstrated the potent antioxidant capacity of ar-turmerone in scavenging free radicals [36]. Additionally, turmerone Q has been shown to inhibit lipopolysaccharide-induced NO production [37].

A comparative analysis of the chemical composition and antioxidant activity of essential oils highlighted the significant impact of sample processing, storage, distribution, and preservation on the quality of antioxidant properties. This research compared the antioxidant capabilities of essential oils and crude extracts from the Zingiberaceae family, including turmeric, revealing notable variations in antioxidant activity based on the extraction method employed [38]. Furthermore, the study examined the chemical composition and antioxidant activity of both fresh and dried turmeric samples, finding that the essential oil from fresh turmeric exhibited superior antioxidant activity. Chemical analysis identified α-turmerone as the predominant constituent of this TEO [39].

Antioxidants play a vital role in human physiology and food preservation. Research on turmeric has demonstrated its effectiveness in controlling lipid peroxidation in hamburger and chicken meat during cooking processes [40,41]. Given the antioxidant activity of isolated turmeric compounds, such as ar-turmerone, turmerone Q, and α-turmerone, further characterization of these compounds is essential for potential pharmacological and nutraceutical applications.

2.4. Cardiovascular Activity

Endothelial dysfunction and vascular inflammation are key contributors to atherosclerosis, which is the leading cause of cardiovascular disease and a significant risk factor for mortality worldwide [42]. Curdione, a sesquiterpene derived from turmeric essential oil, has demonstrated protective effects against cardiovascular diseases. This compound exhibits potent anticoagulant and anti-thrombotic properties, effectively inhibiting platelet activation. Curdione modulates the expression of vinculin and Talin1 through its interaction with β1-tubulin, thereby influencing the integrin signaling pathway and subsequently restraining platelet activation. Notably, β-1 tubulin serves as a critical target for curdione, suppressing the thrombin-induced activation of human platelets [43]. Furthermore, curdione reduces P-selectin expression in platelet-activating factor (PAF) by elevating cyclic adenosine monophosphate (cAMP) levels and decreasing intracellular calcium mobilization [44].

Similarly, ar-turmerone has been shown to inhibit platelet aggregation triggered by collagen and arachidonic acid, although it does not significantly affect aggregation induced by PAF or thrombin [45]. Additionally, β-elemene has been found to attenuate atherosclerosis and enhance plaque stability through its antioxidative and anti-inflammatory features. In murine models, β-elemene protects against endothelial dysfunction by significantly improving plasma nitrite and nitrate levels, as well as promoting the phosphorylation of endothelial nitric oxide synthase (eNOS) [46]. Moreover, a derivative of β-elemene has demonstrated protective effects on endothelial cells from H_2O_2-induced injury by engaging antioxidant mechanisms and activating the PI3K/Akt/eNOS/NO signaling pathways [47].

2.5. Hypoglycemic Action

Type 2 diabetes mellitus is the most prevalent chronic metabolic disorder impacting global health. The primary therapeutic approach for managing this condition involves the use of antidiabetic medications aimed at controlling glucose levels. However, the chronic administration of these drugs can lead to clinically significant side effects and drug interactions. Consequently, there is a growing interest in alternative drug candidates with hypoglycemic properties [48].

Terpenes and terpenoids are recognized for their antidiabetic activities, which inhibit the action of enzymes responsible for insulin resistance, thereby restoring physiological plasma glucose and insulin levels [49]. The antidiabetic effects of curdione and germacrone have been demonstrated in glucose consumption assays using HepG2 Cells [50]. Additionally, studies in murine models revealed the hypoglycemic potential of ar-turmerone through the activation of peroxisome proliferator-activated receptor gamma (PPAR-g), suggesting a synergistic effect between curcuminoids and sesquiterpenoids such as ar-turmerone [51].

Collectively, these findings indicate that curdione, germacrone, and ar-turmerone offer protective effects against chronic conditions such as insulin resistance and diabetes. However, most research to date has been conducted using cell and animal models, necessitating further clinical trials to establish their therapeutic efficacy. Future studies should focus on prolonged intervention periods and specific endpoints for evaluating health outcomes to comprehensively assess the long-term safety and efficacy of these turmeric essential oil compounds.

2.6. Dermatological Application

Turmeric essential oil is widely utilized in cosmetic and pharmaceutical applications due to its antimicrobial, anti-inflammatory, antioxidant, and insect-repelling properties. The major TEO component, ar-turmerone, has alleviated skin inflammation in both *in vitro* and *in vivo* psoriasis models [26,52]. Given that psoriasis is an immune-mediated inflammatory skin disorder, ar-turmerone appears to exert its effects through a dose-dependent suppression of cell proliferation, promotion of apoptosis, and reduction in interleukin (IL)-1β, IL-6, and IL-8 induced by TNF-α in HaCaT cells, as evidenced by the decreased expression levels of Shh, Gli1, and SMO [52]. Additionally, ar-turmerone inhibits CD8+ T cell migration into the epidermis and lowers the expression of NF-κB and COX-2, along with the phosphorylation of p38 MAPK. In imiquimod-induced murine models, the topical application of ar-turmerone reduced the levels of TNF-α and IL-6 while downregulating the mRNA synthesis of IL-17, IL-22, and IL-23 [26].

Moreover, ar-turmerone has the potential to serve as a therapeutic agent for hyperpigmentation disorders by inhibiting the expression of tyrosinase and by inactivating α-MSH- and IBMX-induced melanin synthesis and tyrosinase activity [53].

Germacrone-type sesquiterpenes have been shown to regulate the UVB-induced mRNA upregulation and protein expression levels of MMP-1, MMP-2, and MMP-3 in human keratinocytes, indicating their potential as photoprotective and anti-aging agents [54]. Furthermore, germacrone may address skin conditions such as acne, hirsutism, and androgenic alopecia due to its inhibitory action on steroid 5-alpha reductase *in vitro* [21]. These findings underscore the promising dermatological applications of ar-turmerone and germacrone as natural bioactive compounds.

2.7. Hepatoprotection

Chronic liver diseases can lead to significant injuries, contributing to conditions such as cirrhosis and liver cancer. These chronic injuries stimulate the release of inflammatory cytokines and reactive oxygen species (ROS), while damaged hepatocytes secrete extracellular matrix protein, resulting in fibrosis. The hepatoprotective effect of TEO sesquiterpenes have been demonstrated in a murine model of D-galactosamine-induced liver injury where ar-, α-, and β-turmerone effectively suppressed the elevated levels of lactate dehydrogenase (LDH), alanine aminotransferase (ALT), and aspartate aminotransferase (AST) [55].

Ar-turmerone and bisacurone have also shown protective effects against ethanol-induced hepatocyte injury, a common cause of alcohol-related liver damage [56]. *In vitro* studies have indicated that turmeric essential oil sesquiterpenes, including ar-turmerone, β-sesquiphellandrene, and curcumenol, exhibited cytotoxic activity through the inhibition of cell growth and the induction of apoptosis in the HepG2 cell line [57].

Curcumol has been shown to effectively inhibit hepatic stellate cells (HSCs), reducing the secretion and expression of POSTN, and inhibiting the NF-kB signaling pathway along with the production of pro-inflammatory factors [58].

Collectively, ar-turmerone, α-turmerone, β-turmerone bisacurone, β-sesquiphellandrene, curcumenol, and curcumol appear to exert hepatoprotective effects by modulating various signaling pathways. Further investigations are warranted to elucidate the molecular mechanisms underlying their protective actions against hepatic pathologies.

2.8. Neurological Action

The neuroprotective properties of turmeric essential oil and its constituents are closely associated with their anti-inflammatory and antioxidant activities at the neuronal level [59]. β-elemene has been shown to reduce the expression of pro-inflammatory cytokines, such as tumor necrosis factor-a (TNF-α), interleukin-1β (IL-1β), and IL-6, while mitigating the translocation of nuclear factor-kB (NF-κB) p65 from the cytoplasm to the nucleus in BV-2 cells exposed to lipopolysaccharide. Additionally, β-elemene inhibits the activation of RAC1, mixed-lineage protein kinase 3 (MLK3), and p38 mitogen-activated protein kinase (MAPK), while increasing the phosphorylation of the RAC1 Ser71 site [60]. Germacrone has also improved motor dysfunction, spatial learning issues, and memory deficits induced by traumatic brain injury in murine models, with this mechanism of action involving Nrf2 upregulation and downregulation of the pro-inflammatory protein p-p65 [61].

Ar-turmerone and its analogs have demonstrated the ability to inhibit dopaminergic neurodegeneration by activating nuclear factor erythroid 2-related factor 2 (Nrf2) in dopaminergic neurons. Furthermore, ar-turmerone inhibits acetylcholinesterase activity and mitigates dopaminergic neurodegeneration through significant anti-inflammatory action in microglial BV2 cells [62,63]. Given that Parkinson's disease (PD) is characterized by the loss of dopaminergic neurons in the substantia nigra due to the inflammatory activation of microglia, ar-turmerone is a compelling candidate for the prevention and treatment of PD. Additionally, elevated levels of monoamine oxidase A (MAO-A) are linked to major depression [64], and ar-turmerone has been shown to exert antidepressant-like effects by reducing MAO-A levels and alleviating stress in a murine model [65].

The neuroprotective effects of ar-turmerone are further supported by its ability to enhance the survival of primary cerebellar granule neuronal cultures by restraining caspase-3 cleavage. Conversely, in cancer cell lines, ar-turmerone promotes apoptosis and inhibits cell proliferation, indicating a degree of target specificity that may correlate with a lower likelihood of adverse effects [66]. Therefore, further development of ar-turmerone as a potential therapeutic agent for neurological disorders is strongly warranted.

Moreover, the regenerative capacity of endogenous neural stem cells is crucial in the context of neurodegenerative diseases. Ar-turmerone has been shown to promote the dose-dependent differentiation and proliferation of neural stem cells *in vitro* and *in vivo* [67]. Similarly, β-elemene has been reported to stimulate neurite outgrowth and axonal regeneration in ventral spinal cord motoneuronal cells and primary cortical neurons by inhibiting the RhoA signaling pathway, effectively preventing the activation of RhoA kinase, and enhancing the expression of GAP43 [68]. Thus, both ar-turmerone and β-elemene exhibit the potential to regenerate neuronal tissue and demonstrate neuroprotective properties, positioning them as promising candidates for the prevention and treatment of neurodegenerative diseases.

Regarding anticonvulsant activity, bisabolene sesquiterpenoids, including ar-, α-, β-turmerone, and α-atlantone, have displayed anticonvulsant properties in zebrafish and murine models [69]. Further evaluation of ar-turmerone revealed its ability to control seizures in the intravenous pentylenetetrazole (PTZ) and 6-Hz murine models, as well as its ability to decrease the expression of c-fos and brain-derived neurotrophic factor (bdnf), two genes associated with seizure activity in zebrafish. Additionally, the neurological safety of ar-turmerone was assessed in mice using the beam walking test, revealing no adverse effects on balance or motor function. Notably, brain concentration analysis confirmed the ability of ar-turmerone to cross the blood–brain barrier and persist in brain tissue for up to 24 h following intraperitoneal administration [70].

Likewise, curcumol has been shown to enhance GABA-induced currents in cultured mouse hippocampal neurons and human embryonic kidney cells in a concentration-dependent manner. In murine models of seizures induced by PTZ and kainate, curcumol increased the latency period for both clonic and tonic seizures, reduced mortality rates, and decreased seizure susceptibility, indicating that curcumol exerts its anticonvulsant effects by enhancing GABAergic inhibition [71].

This comprehensive body of evidence underscores the potential of TEO constituents, particularly ar-turmerone, α-turmerone, β-turmerone, α-atlantone, β-elemene, and curcumol, as therapeutic agents for neurological disorders, warranting further investigation into their mechanisms of action and clinical applications.

2.9. Antiparasitic Properties

In vitro studies have demonstrated that ar-turmerone exhibits activity against *Plasmodium falciparum* 3D7 (chloroquine-sensitive), with its efficacy being contingent upon the specific stage of the parasite's life cycle. Notably, ar-turmerone has been shown to inhibit the transition from the ring stage to the trophozoite stage during the intraerythrocytic life cycle of the parasite's development. This compound displays high cytotoxic specificity, suggesting its potential as a promising non-toxic candidate for antimalarial drug development, warranting further research into the molecular mechanisms underlying its antiplasmodial action [72].

Additionally, turmerones have demonstrated a dose-dependent capacity to inhibit the growth of *Leishmania amazonensis* promastigotes [73]. However, comprehensive research is essential to elucidate the mechanisms that govern their antileishmanial effects.

2.10. Antiviral Activity

Influenza is a viral respiratory illness associated with seasonal outbreaks and sporadic pandemics, affecting approximately 10% of the global population annually and resulting in nearly half a million deaths [74]. While vaccine efficacy is generally high, it remains suboptimal in elderly populations [75]. Consequently, there is an urgent need for new influenza vaccines and antiviral therapies. The severity of influenza can be exacerbated by the disruption of cytokine regulation induced by the virus. Bisabolene sesquiterpenoids from turmeric oil have been proposed as potential modulators of this dysregulation, as they may inhibit the expression of virus-induced inflammatory cytokines by regulating the NF-κB/MAPK and RIG-1/STAT-1/2 signaling pathways in vitro [76].

Moreover, germacrone has been shown to inhibit the replication of H1N1 and H3N2 influenza A viruses, as well as influenza B virus, in a dose-dependent manner. *In vitro* studies indicate that germacrone reduces viral protein expression, RNA synthesis, and the production of infectious progeny virus. Additionally, this compound inhibits viral attachment during the early stages of the replication cycle. *In vivo*, germacrone has demonstrated protective effects against lethal infection in mice, significantly reducing viral titers in lung tissue. A synergistic effect was observed when germacrone was combined with oseltamivir in both *in vitro* and *in vivo* models [77].

Furthermore, germacrone exhibits antiviral activity against pseudorabies virus (PRV), a member of the Herpesviridae family responsible for various acute infections in animals, particularly pigs. Given the significant public health implications, there is an urgent need for innovative therapeutic options to effectively manage the transmission and severity of PRV infections, as current treatments have shown limited efficacy. In this context, germacrone emerges as a promising candidate, demonstrating the ability to inhibit PRV replication *in vitro* in a dose-dependent manner [78].

Consequently, both bisabolane sesquiterpenes and germacrone represent promising avenues for further development as therapeutic agents or adjuncts in the treatment of influenza and pseudorabies virus infections.

2.11. Insecticidal Action

Synthetic insecticides are the predominant method for vector control; however, their widespread use has led to the emergence of resistant strains and significant environmental contamination. Ar-turmerone has demonstrated larvicidal properties and the ability to deter biting by *Aedes aegypti* L. and *Anopheles quadrimaculatus* mosquitoes [79]. Additionally, ar-turmerone exhibits notable larvicidal activity against *Culex pipiens pallens*, inducing disruptions in the myofibrils of ventral muscle cells in larvae. This effect is mediated through an increase in detoxifying enzymes, including carboxylesterase (CarE), glutathione-S-transferase (GST), and cytochrome P450 monooxidases (P450) [80].

Given these findings, long-term studies are essential to elucidate the specificity of ar-turmerone's insecticidal action and to objectively assess its safety for both the environment and human health.

2.12. Antifungal Properties

Dermatophytosis, caused by pathogenic keratin-digesting fungi known as dermatophytes, affects both humans and animals [81]. Timely and effective treatment is crucial to prevent substantial cosmetic and health issues. However, the presence of adverse effects and the emergence of drug-resistant strains underscore the necessity for novel therapeutic agents. In this context, ar-turmerone has demonstrated *in vitro* antidermatophytic activity against the genera *Trichophyton*, *Microsporum*, and *Epidermophyton* [82]. Further clinical assessment of the antifungal properties of ar-turmerone will provide valuable insights into its molecular mechanisms of action, safety profile, and overall efficacy.

2.13. Antivenom Activity

The antivenom activity of turmeric essential oil appears to be closely linked to the anti-inflammatory properties of ar-turmerone. This compound has been shown to inhibit lymphocyte proliferation and their natural killer activity. In murine models, ar-turmerone neutralized the hemorrhagic effects induced by *Bothrops jararaca* venom and the lethal impact of *Crotalus durissus terrificus* venom. Moreover, numerous immunological studies have demonstrated that ar-turmerone can inhibit lymphocyte proliferation and the natural killer activity of human lymphocytes [83].

Further investigation into ar-turmerone and its pharmacological targets is essential to fully comprehend its potential for antivenom applications. Additionally, the mechanisms by which this compound operates and its safety in humans require additional exploration.

Table 2 summarizes published research studies concerning the anticancer, anti-inflammatory, antioxidant, cardiovascular, hypoglycemic, dermatological, hepatoprotective, neurological, antiparasitic, antiviral, insecticidal, antifungal, and antivenom properties of the constituents derived from turmeric essential oil.

Table 2. Summary of research on the bioactive properties of turmeric essential oil constituents.

Bioactivity	Compound	Study Design	Sample/Subject	Dose	Route	Effect	Reference
Anticancer	Ar-turmerone	*In vitro*	U937 cells	61–84%	NA	Apoptosis induction through caspase-3 activation involving Bax and p53 proteins, not Bcl-2 and p21	[15]
						Cell death mediated through activation of mitochondrial cytochrome c and caspase-3	
		In vivo	P388D1 lymphoblast cell implanted tumors in mouse model	200–300 mg/kg	i.p.	Immune activity enhancement and inhibition of P388D1 lymphocytic leukemia	[16]
						Increase in T-lymphocyte and B-lymphocyte proliferation activities	
						IL-2 production activity increase	
		In vitro	Human breast MDA-MB-231 cells	10–30 mM	NA	Inhibition of MMP-9 and COX-2 via NF-kB	[18]
						Suppression of TPA-induced invasion and migration	
		In vitro	Human leukemia Molt 4B and H60 cells	30 μg/mL	NA	Selective apoptosis in human leukemia cells	[19]
	Ar-turmerone and α-turmerone	*In vitro*	Human cancer cell lines: HepG2, MCF-7, MDA-MB-231; human skin fibroblast cell line: Hs-68	11.0–41.8 μg/mL	NA	Inhibition of cancer cell proliferation and apoptosis induction	[20]
						Stimulation of immune cell proliferation and cytokine production	
	Germacrone	*In vitro*	Prostate cancer cell lines: PC-3 and 22RV1	30 to 480 mM	NA	Apoptosis and autophagy induction in prostate cancer cells	[22]
						Inhibition of Akt/mTOR signaling pathway, leading to cell death	
	β-elemene	*In vitro*	A549/DDP lung cancer cells	20 μg/mL	NA	Reversal of lung cancer pharmacoresistance via mitochondrial apoptosis pathway	[23]
						Enhancement of cisplatin sensitivity and apoptosis induction in A549/DDP cells	

Table 2. *Cont.*

Bioactivity	Compound	Study Design	Sample/Subject	Dose	Route	Effect	Reference
Anti-inflammation	Ar-turmerone	*In vitro*	CD4+ T cells	10 mM	NA	Suppression of IFN-g and IL-2 production in T cells.	[27]
						Anti-inflammatory effects without affecting IL-4, IL-5, or T-cell expansion	
		In vitro	BV-2 microglial cells	5 μM	NA	Suppression of LPS-induced neuroinflammatory molecules in microglia	[28]
		In vitro	BV2 microglial and HT-22 hippocampal cells	5–20 μM	NA	Inhibition of neuroinflammatory molecules and ROS production in microglial cells	[30]
						Protection of hippocampal cells from neuronal toxicity	
						Suppression of NF-κB, JNK, and p38 MAPK signaling pathways	
	Turmerones (including ar-turmerone)	*In vitro/In vivo*	QR-32 cells/mouse	0.2–100 nM/500 ppp	NA/p.o.	Significant tumor growth reduction in mice	[29]
						Inhibition of inflammation-related carcinogenesis in mouse model	
						Maintenance of a reducing environment at inflammatory lesions	
						Suppression of iNOS and 8-OHdG expression	
	Germacrone	*In vivo*	Human type II-like alveolar epithelial cells A549/rats	50–150 μM/10 mg/kg	NA/i.p.	Cell apoptosis reduction and promotion of cell viability	[31]
						Attenuation of LPS-induced pathological changes and pulmonary edema in rats	
						Decrease in IL-6 and TNF-α and increase in TGF-β1 and IL-10	
		In vitro	PC12 cells	20–80 μM	NA	Inhibition of autophagy in PC12 cells, improving cell viability	[32]
						Control of PC12 cell injury caused by OGDR	

Table 2. *Cont.*

Bioactivity	Compound	Study Design	Sample/Subject	Dose	Route	Effect	Reference
	Curcumol	*In vitro*	Murine macrophage RAW264.7 cell line	12.5–200 μM	NA	Inhibition of NO production, TNF-α, IL-1β, and IL-6	[33]
						Suppression of JNK-mediated AP-1 pathway, targeting inflammation mediators	
Antioxidant	Turmerone Q	*In vitro*	RAW264.7 cell line	Not provided	NA	Inhibition of NO production in macrophages	[37]
Cardiovascular	Curdione	*In vitro/In vivo*	Human platelets	100 μM	NA	Inhibition of platelet activation by targeting b1-tubulin and vinculin	[43]
						Downregulation of Talin1 and b1-tubulin proteins	
		In vitro/In vivo	Human platelets/mouse	20–1000 μM/50–200 mg/kg	NA/p.o.	Inhibition of PAF and thrombin-induced platelet aggregation	[44]
						Increase in cAMP levels and suppression of intracellular Ca^{2+} mobilization in platelets	
	Ar-turmerone	*In vitro*	Rabbit platelets	100 μg/mL	NA	Inhibition of platelet aggregation induced by collagen and arachidonic acid	[45]
						More potent activity than aspirin against collagen-induced platelet aggregation	
	β-elemene	*In vivo*	C57BL/6 mice	Not provided	intragastrical	Enhancement of antioxidative defense and reduced lipid peroxidation in atherosclerosis	[46]
						Increase in plasma nitrite and nitrate levels and eNOS phosphorylation in $ApoE^{-/-}$ mice	
		In vitro	Human umbilical vein endothelial cells	0.1, 1, and 10 μmol/L	NA	Antioxidant activity superior to vitamin E	[47]
						Protection against oxidative stress by inhibiting ROS production and signaling pathways	

Table 2. *Cont.*

Bioactivity	Compound	Study Design	Sample/Subject	Dose	Route	Effect	Reference
Hypoglycemic	Ar-turmerone	*In vivo*	Type-2 diabetic KK-Ay mice	0.1–0.5 g/100 g of diet	p.o.	Control of blood glucose increase	[49]
						Stimulation of human adipocyte differentiation and PPAR-γ ligand-binding activity	
Dermatological	Ar-turmerone	*In vivo*	IMQ-induced psoriasis-like BALBc mice	0.4–40 mg/kg/day	topical	Inhibition of CD8 T cells, NF-kB, and proinflammatory cytokines	[26]
						Reduction in TNF-a, IL-6, IL-17, IL-22, and IL-23 levels	
		In vitro	HaCaT cells	5–30 µM	NA	Reduction in cell proliferation and inflammatory cytokine expression	[52]
		In vitro	B16F10 murine melanoma cells	5–40 µM	NA	Inhibition of a-MSH and IBMX-induced melanogenesis by suppressing CREB	[53]
						Expression reduction in tyrosinase, TRP-1, and TRP-2 in cells	
	Germacrone	*In vitro*	HaCaT cells	5–10 µM	NA	Inhibition of UVB-induced MMP upregulation in keratinocytes	[54]
Hepatoprotection	Ar-, α-, and β-turmerone	*In vivo*	Wistar rats	0.5%	p.o.	Reduced liver injury markers in rats	[55]
						Downregulation of LDH, ALT, and AST increased levels triggered by D-GalN treatment	
	Ar-turmerone and bisacurone	*In vitro*	Hepatocytes isolated from Sprague–Dawley rats	1–6 µM	NA	Preventive effects against ethanol-induced injury in primary cells	[56]
	Ar-turmerone, β-sesquiphellandrene and curcumenol	*In vitro*	Hepatoma cell line (HepG2)	15–2000 µg/mL	NA	Inhibition of hepatoma cell growth	[57]
	Curcumol	*In vitro*	Human hepatic stellate cells (HSCs)	20–45 µM	NA	Inhibition of HSC migration and adhesion by regulating NF-kB	[58]
		In vivo	ICR mice	30 mg/kg	p.o.	Reduction in periostin (POSTN) secretion and expression in HSCs	

Table 2. *Cont.*

Bioactivity	Compound	Study Design	Sample/Subject	Dose	Route	Effect	Reference
Neurological	β-elemene	*In vitro*	Microglial cell line BV-2	1–25 μM	NA	Alleviated sepsis-associated encephalopathy by inhibiting RAC1/MLK3/p38 pathway	[60]
		In vivo	C57BL6 mice	10–40 mg/kg	i.p.	Reduced p38 MAPK phosphorylation and pro-inflammatory cytokines in hippocampus	
						Improved learning and memory in septic mice	
		In vivo	Sprague–Dawley rats	80–320 μg/kg	Not specified	Enhancement of neurite outgrowth and GAP-43 expression	[68]
						Inhibition of RhoA kinase activation, promoting locomotor recovery	
						Lesion cavity area reduction and sparing of white matter	
						Significant upregulation of GAP-43 expression	
	Germacrone	*In vivo*	C57BL6 mice	5–20 mg/kg	i.p.	Enhanced motor function and memory, reduced neuroinflammation and oxidative stress	[61]
						Reduced neuronal apoptosis and microglial activation in a dose-dependent manner	
						Increased Nrf2 expression and inhibition of p-p65 expression	

Table 2. *Cont.*

Bioactivity	Compound	Study Design	Sample/Subject	Dose	Route	Effect	Reference
	Ar-turmerone	*In vitro*	Murine microglial BV2 cells	20 µM	NA	Protection of dopaminergic neurons through Nrf2 activation	[62]
						Inhibition of microglial activation and neurodegeneration prevention	
		In vitro	Human breast MDA-MB-231 cells	50–250 µM	NA	Acetylcholinesterase inhibition	[63]
		In vivo	ICR mice	1.25–5.0 mg/kg	p.o.	Reduced immobility time in mouse forced swimming test and tail suspension test	[65]
						Increased levels of monoamines in various brain regions	
						Decreased MAO-A activity in the frontal cortex and hippocampus	
		In vitro	Neural stem cells	1.56–25 µg/mL	NA	Induction of neural stem cell proliferation	[67]
		In vivo	Wistar rats	3 mg	intracerebroventricular	Enhanced neuronal differentiation of neural stem cells	
						Mobilization of proliferating neural stem cells from SVZ and hippocampus	
						Promotion of endogenous neural stem cell mobilization in the rat brain	
		In vitro	Zebrafish	46 µM	p.o.	Anticonvulsant properties in acute seizure models in mice	[69]
		In vivo	C57Bl6 and NMRI mice	0.01–50 mg/kg	i.p.	No motor function or balance effects observed in mice post-treatment	
						Rapid absorption and long permanence of ar-turmerone in mouse brains after administration	
	Ar-, α-, β-turmerone, and α-atlantone	*In vivo*	Zebrafish	11–46 µM	p.o.	Electrographic evaluation demonstrated anticonvulsant effects in zebrafish	[70]
			C57Bl6 mice	50 mg/kg	i.p.	Anticonvulsant activity in zebrafish and mouse models	

Table 2. *Cont.*

Bioactivity	Compound	Study Design	Sample/Subject	Dose	Route	Effect	Reference
	Curcumol	*In vitro*	Human embryonic kidney cells and primary cultures of mouse hippocampal neurons	10–300 μM	NA	Enhancement of GABAergic inhibition in hippocampus, suppressing neuronal excitability	[71]
		In vivo	C57BL6J mice	100 mg/kg	i.p.	Stimulation of GABA A receptors, reducing chemically induced seizure activity in mice	
						Increased GABAergic miniature inhibitory postsynaptic currents in hippocampal slices, affecting amplitude and frequency.	
Antiparasitic	Ar-turmerone	*In vitro*	*Plasmodium falciparum* 3D7	46.8–820.4 μM	NA	Parasite development delayed due to antiplasmodial effect and cytotoxic activity	[72]
	Turmerones	*In vitro*	*Leishmania amazonensis*'s promastigotes	2.75 μg/mL	p.o.	Significant cellular alterations in *L. amazonensis* promastigotes	[73]
Antiviral	Bisabolane-type sesquiterpenoids	*In vitro*	A549 and MDCK cells	25–100 μg/mL	NA	Inhibition of H1N1 replication in A549 and MDCK cells	[76]
						Regulation of NF-κB/MAPK and RIG-1/STAT-1/2 signaling pathways	
						Reduction in pro-inflammatory cytokine production	
	Germacrone	*In vitro/In vivo*	Madin–Darby canine kidney cells (MDCKs)/BALBc mice	1.6–25 μM/ 50–100 mg/kg	NA/i.v.	Inhibition of H1N1, H3N2, and influenza B viruses	[77]
		In vitro	Vero and PK-1 cells	10–250 μM	NA	Inhibition of PRV replication in a dose-dependent manner	[78]
						Reduction in virus titer and PRV-gB protein level	
Insecticidal	Ar-turmerone	*In vivo*	*Aedes aegypti* mosquitoes	5–25 nmol/cm^2	p.o.	High biting deterrent activity against mosquitoes	[79]
		In vivo	*C. pipiens pallens* larvae	100 p.p.m.	p.o.	Induction of muscle and digestive tissue changes in larvae	[80]
						Larvicidal mechanism involving stomach poison action, unrelated to AChE	

Table 2. *Cont.*

Bioactivity	Compound	Study Design	Sample/Subject	Dose	Route	Effect	Reference
Antifungal	Ar-turmerone	*In vitro*	Dermatophytes	3.90–7.81 μg/mL	NA	Effective antidermatophytic activity	[82]
						Lower MIC values than standard ketoconazole	
Antivenom	Ar-turmerone	*In vivo*	Swiss albino mice	30–70 μg	i.p.	Neutralization of snake venom effects in mice and lymphocytes	[83]
						Inhibition of hemorrhagic activity and lethal effects of snake venoms	
						Blockage of human lymphocyte proliferation and cytotoxicity	

NA (not applicable.); i.p. (intraperitoneal); p.o. (oral); i.v. (intravenous).

3. Safety of the Bioactive Constituents of Turmeric Essential Oil

TEO exhibits a favorable safety profile when consumed in dietary contexts [7], with no documented cases of toxicity associated with its oral intake. The cytotoxic effects observed in laboratory settings are context-specific and dose-dependent, primarily occurring under conditions such as simulated oncological changes. Importantly, these effects do not translate to adverse outcomes in typical dietary consumption. While the potential cytotoxicity of turmeric essential oil components warrants further research, it is essential to recognize that such effects do not reflect the overall safety of the oil as a food additive or dietary supplement.

Currently, there is a notable lack of clinical studies assessing the individual toxicity of the various constituents of TEO. Notably, only one clinical report has documented a single case of a cutaneous allergic reaction potentially linked to the oral consumption of turmeric essential oil, although the specific association was not specifically analyzed [84]. Given that Ayurvedic medicine traditionally endorses the use of turmeric for treating allergies [85], there is an urgent need for clinical studies to establish the therapeutic range of turmeric essential oil and its active constituents for specific routes of administration. Defining these parameters will enhance our understanding of their safety and pharmacokinetics, thereby facilitating their integration into contemporary therapeutic practices.

4. Conclusions

This review provides a comprehensive overview of the intricate pharmacological characteristics of the components found in TEO and their potential applications for preventive and therapeutic purposes. Among its chemical constituents, sesquiterpenes represent the predominant group in turmeric essential oil, demonstrating a diverse array of noteworthy bioactivities, including anticancer, anti-inflammatory, antioxidant, cardiovascular, hypoglycemic, dermatological, hepatoprotection, immunological, antiparasitic, antiviral, insecticidal, antifungal, and antivenom properties.

The primary focus of this work was to elucidate the mechanisms that potentially underlie the attributes of monoterpenes, bisabolanes, germacranes, elemanes, and guaianes found in TEO. It is noteworthy that some of these isolated constituents exhibit similar effects or activity pathways, suggesting possible synergistic interactions when co administered. Furthermore, studies have reported additive effects when isolated compounds are utilized alongside commercially available pharmaceuticals, presenting an intriguing avenue for investigation. Such studies may offer the potential to reduce medication dosages, particularly in the context of chronic conditions, thereby minimizing adverse effects, enhancing therapeutic outcomes, and improving medication adherence.

Most of the studies discussed in this review are preclinical in nature. Therefore, further clinical investigations are imperative to achieve a more comprehensive understanding of the pharmacokinetic profile, therapeutic index, efficacy, and safety of the compounds isolated from turmeric essential oil.

Funding: This research was funded by the Research Vice-Chancellorship of the University of Cuenca, Ecuador.

Institutional Review Board Statement: Not applicable.

Informed Consent Statement: Not applicable.

Data Availability Statement: Not applicable.

Conflicts of Interest: A.M.O.-P. holds patents on turmeric oil's application for treating neurodegenerative disorders. The author declares no conflict of interest.

References

1. Tsuda, T. Curcumin as a Functional Food-Derived Factor: Degradation Products, Metabolites, Bioactivity, and Future Perspectives. *Food Funct.* **2018**, *9*, 705–714. [CrossRef]
2. Abd El-Hack, M.E.; El-Saadony, M.T.; Swelum, A.A.; Arif, M.; Abo Ghanima, M.M.; Shukry, M.; Noreldin, A.; Taha, A.E.; El-Tarabily, K.A. Curcumin, the Active Substance of Turmeric: Its Effects on Health and Ways to Improve Its Bioavailability. *J. Sci. Food Agric.* **2021**, *101*, 5747–5762. [CrossRef] [PubMed]
3. Kotha, R.R.; Luthria, D.L. Curcumin: Biological, Pharmaceutical, Nutraceutical, and Analytical Aspects. *Molecules* **2019**, *24*, 2930. [CrossRef] [PubMed]
4. Sharifi-Rad, J.; El Rayess, Y.; Rizk, A.A.; Sadaka, C.; Zgheib, R.; Zam, W.; Sestito, S.; Rapposelli, S.; Neffe-Skocińska, K.; Zielińska, D.; et al. Turmeric and Its Major Compound Curcumin on Health: Bioactive Effects and Safety Profiles for Food, Pharmaceutical, Biotechnological and Medicinal Applications. *Front. Pharmacol.* **2020**, *11*, 1021. [CrossRef] [PubMed]
5. Nair, A.; Amalraj, A.; Jacob, J.; Kunnumakkara, A.B.; Gopi, S. Non-Curcuminoids from Turmeric and Their Potential in Cancer Therapy and Anticancer Drug Delivery Formulations. *Biomolecules* **2019**, *9*, 13. [CrossRef]
6. Orellana-Paucar, A.M.; Machado-Orellana, M.G. Pharmacological Profile, Bioactivities, and Safety of Turmeric Oil. *Molecules* **2022**, *27*, 5055. [CrossRef]
7. EFSA Panel on Additives and Products or Substances used in Animal Feed (FEEDAP); Bampidis, V.; Azimonti, G.; Bastos, M.L.; Christensen, H.; Durjava, K.; Kouba, M.; López-Alonso, M.; López Puente, S.; Marcon, F.; et al. Safety and Efficacy of Turmeric Extract, Turmeric Oil, Turmeric Oleoresin and Turmeric Tincture from Curcuma Longa L. Rhizome When Used as Sensory Additives in Feed for All Animal Species. *EFSA J.* **2020**, *18*, e06146. [CrossRef]
8. Hwang, K.W.; Son, D.; Jo, H.W.; Kim, C.H.; Seong, K.C.; Moon, J.K. Levels of Curcuminoid and Essential Oil Compositions in Turmerics (*Curcuma Longa* L.) Grown in Korea. *Appl. Biol. Chem.* **2016**, *59*, 209–215. [CrossRef]
9. Sharma, R.K.; Misra, B.P.; Sarma, T.C.; Bordoloi, A.K.; Pathak, M.G.; Leclercq, P.A. Essential Oils of *Curcuma Longa* L. from Bhutan. *J. Essent. Oil Res.* **1997**, *9*, 589–592. [CrossRef]
10. Sacchetti, G.; Maietti, S.; Muzzoli, M.; Scaglianti, M.; Manfredini, S.; Radice, M.; Bruni, R. Comparative Evaluation of 11 Essential Oils of Different Origin as Functional Antioxidants, Antiradicals and Antimicrobials in Foods. *Food Chem.* **2005**, *91*, 621–632. [CrossRef]
11. Pino, J.A.; Fon-Fay, F.M.; Pérez, J.C.; Falco, A.S.; Hernández, I.; Rodeiro, I.; Fernández, M.D. Chemical Composition and Biological Activities of Essential Oil from Turmeric (*Curcuma Longa* L.) Rhizomes Grown in Amazonian Ecuador. *Cienc. Químicas* **2018**, *49*, 1–8.
12. Aggarwal, B.B.; Yuan, W.; Li, S.; Gupta, S.C. Curcumin-Free Turmeric Exhibits Anti-Inflammatory and Anticancer Activities: Identification of Novel Components of Turmeric. *Mol. Nutr. Food Res.* **2013**, *57*, 1529–1542. [CrossRef] [PubMed]
13. Zhang, H.A.; Kitts, D.D. Turmeric and Its Bioactive Constituents Trigger Cell Signaling Mechanisms That Protect against Diabetes and Cardiovascular Diseases. *Mol. Cell. Biochem.* **2021**, *476*, 3785–3814. [CrossRef] [PubMed]
14. Hausman, D.M. What Is Cancer? *Perspect. Biol. Med.* **2019**, *62*, 778–784. [CrossRef]
15. Lee, Y. Activation of Apoptotic Protein in U937 Cells by a Component of Turmeric Oil. *BMB Rep.* **2009**, *42*, 96–100. [CrossRef]
16. Kim, D.; Suh, Y.; Lee, H.; Lee, Y. Immune Activation and Antitumor Response of Ar-Turmerone on P388D1 Lymphoblast Cell Implanted Tumors. *Int. J. Mol. Med.* **2013**, *31*, 386–392. [CrossRef]
17. Sun, M.; Ma, W.N.; Guo, Y.; Hu, Z.G.; He, L.C. Simultaneous Screening of Four Epidermal Growth Factor Receptor Antagonists from Curcuma Longa via Cell Membrane Chromatography Online Coupled with HPLC-MS. *J. Sep. Sci.* **2013**, *36*, 2096–2103. [CrossRef]
18. Park, S.Y.; Kim, Y.H.; Kim, Y.; Lee, S.J. Aromatic-Turmerone Attenuates Invasion and Expression of MMP-9 and COX-2 through Inhibition of NF-KB Activation in TPA-Induced Breast Cancer Cells. *J. Cell Biochem.* **2012**, *113*, 3653–3662. [CrossRef] [PubMed]
19. Aratanechemuge, Y.; Komiya, T.; Moteki, H.; Katsuzaki, H.; Imai, K.; Hibasami, H. Selective Induction of Apoptosis by Ar-Turmerone Isolated from Turmeric (*Curcuma Longa* L) in Two Human Leukemia Cell Lines, but Not in Human Stomach Cancer Cell Line. *Int. J. Mol. Med.* **2002**, *9*, 481–484. [CrossRef]
20. Yue, G.G.L.; Chan, B.C.L.; Hon, P.M.; Lee, M.Y.H.; Fung, K.P.; Leung, P.C.; Lau, C.B.S. Evaluation of in Vitro Anti-Proliferative and Immunomodulatory Activities of Compounds Isolated from Curcuma Longa. *Food Chem. Toxicol.* **2010**, *48*, 2011–2020. [CrossRef]
21. Srivilai, J.; Khorana, N.; Waranuch, N.; Wisuitiprot, W.; Suphrom, N.; Suksamrarn, A.; Ingkaninan, K. Germacrene Analogs Are Anti-Androgenic on Androgen-Dependent Cells. *NPC Nat. Prod. Commun.* **2016**, *11*, 1225–1228. [CrossRef]
22. Yu, Z.; Xu, J.; Shao, M.; Zou, J. Germacrone Induces Apoptosis as Well as Protective Autophagy in Human Prostate Cancer Cells. *Cancer Manag. Res.* **2020**, *12*, 4009–4016. [CrossRef] [PubMed]
23. Yao, C.C.; Tu, Y.R.; Jiang, J.; Ye, S.F.; Du, H.X.; Zhang, Y. β-Elemene Reverses the Drug Resistance of Lung Cancer A549/DDP Cells via the Mitochondrial Apoptosis Pathway. *Oncol. Rep.* **2014**, *31*, 2131–2138. [CrossRef] [PubMed]
24. Medzhitov, R. Inflammation 2010: New Adventures of an Old Flame. *Cell* **2010**, *140*, 771–776. [CrossRef]
25. Del Prete, D.; Millán, E.; Pollastro, F.; Chianese, G.; Luciano, P.; Collado, J.A.; Munoz, E.; Appendino, G.; Taglialatela-Scafati, O. Turmeric Sesquiterpenoids: Expeditious Resolution, Comparative Bioactivity, and a New Bicyclic Turmeronoid. *J. Nat. Prod.* **2016**, *79*, 267–273. [CrossRef] [PubMed]

26. Li, Y.L.; Du, Z.Y.; Li, P.H.; Yan, L.; Zhou, W.; Tang, Y.D.; Liu, G.R.; Fang, Y.X.; Zhang, K.; Dong, C.Z.; et al. Aromatic-Turmerone Ameliorates Imiquimod-Induced Psoriasis-like Inflammation of BALB/c Mice. *Int. Immunopharmacol.* **2018**, *64*, 319–325. [CrossRef]
27. Oh, S.; Han, A.R.; Park, H.R.; Jang, E.J.; Kim, H.K.; Jeong, M.G.; Song, H.; Park, G.H.; Seo, E.K.; Hwang, E.S. Suppression of Inflammatory Cytokine Production by Ar-Turmerone Isolated from Curcuma Phaeocaulis. *Chem. Biodivers.* **2014**, *11*, 1034–1041. [CrossRef]
28. Park, S.Y.; Kim, Y.H.; Kim, Y.; Lee, S.J. Aromatic-Turmerone's Anti-Inflammatory Effects in Microglial Cells Are Mediated by Protein Kinase A and Heme Oxygenase-1 Signaling. *Neurochem. Int.* **2012**, *61*, 767–777. [CrossRef]
29. Onuma, K.; Suenaga, Y.; Sakaki, R.; Yoshitome, S.; Sato, Y.; Ogawara, S.; Suzuki, S.; Kuramitsu, Y.; Yokoyama, H.; Murakami, A.; et al. Development of a Quantitative Bioassay to Assess Preventive Compounds against Inflammation-Based Carcinogenesis. *Nitric. Oxide* **2011**, *25*, 183–194. [CrossRef]
30. Park, S.Y.; Jin, M.L.; Kim, Y.H.; Kim, Y.; Lee, S.J. Anti-Inflammatory Effects of Aromatic-Turmerone through Blocking of NF-KB, JNK, and P38 MAPK Signaling Pathways in Amyloid β-Stimulated Microglia. *Int. Immunopharmacol.* **2012**, *14*, 13–20. [CrossRef]
31. An, J.; Sun, Y.; Zhang, Q.; Zhang, F.; Zhang, J.; Zhang, J. The Effects of Germacrone on Lipopolysaccharide-Induced Acute Lung Injury in Neonatal Rats. *Cell Mol. Biol.* **2014**, *60*, 8–12. [CrossRef]
32. Zhang, J.; Yuan, L.; Wang, S.; Liu, J.; Bi, H.; Chen, G.; Li, J.; Chen, L. Germacrone Protects against Oxygen-Glucose Deprivation/Reperfusion Injury by Inhibiting Autophagy Processes in PC12 Cells. *BMC Complement Med. Ther.* **2020**, *20*, 77. [CrossRef]
33. Chen, X.; Zong, C.; Gao, Y.; Cai, R.; Fang, L.; Lu, J.; Liu, F.; Qi, Y. Curcumol Exhibits Anti-Inflammatory Properties by Interfering with the JNK-Mediated AP-1 Pathway in Lipopolysaccharide-Activated RAW264.7 Cells. *Eur. J. Pharmacol.* **2014**, *723*, 339–345. [CrossRef]
34. Hewlings, S.J.; Kalman, D.S. Curcumin: A Review of Its' Effects on Human Health. *Foods* **2017**, *6*, 92. [CrossRef]
35. Alkadi, H. A Review on Free Radicals and Antioxidants. *Infect. Disord. Drug Targets* **2020**, *20*, 16–26. [CrossRef]
36. Zhao, J.; Zhang, J.S.; Yang, B.; Lv, G.P.; Li, S.P. Free Radical Scavenging Activity and Characterization of Sesquiterpenoids in Four Species of Curcuma Using a TLC Bioautography Assay and GC-MS Analysis. *Molecules* **2010**, *15*, 7547–7557. [CrossRef]
37. Yuan, T.; Zhang, C.; Qiu, C.; Xia, G.; Wang, F.; Lin, B.; Li, H.; Chen, L. Chemical Constituents from Curcuma Longa L. and Their Inhibitory Effects of Nitric Oxide Production. *Nat. Prod. Res.* **2017**, *32*, 1887–1892. [CrossRef]
38. Ivanović, M.; Makoter, K.; Razboršek, M.I. Comparative Study of Chemical Composition and Antioxidant Activity of Essential Oils and Crude Extracts of Four Characteristic Zingiberaceae Herbs. *Plants* **2021**, *10*, 501. [CrossRef]
39. Singh, G.; Kapoor, I.P.S.; Singh, P.; de Heluani, C.S.; de Lampasona, M.P.; Catalan, C.A.N. Comparative Study of Chemical Composition and Antioxidant Activity of Fresh and Dry Rhizomes of Turmeric (*Curcuma Longa* Linn.). *Food Chem. Toxicol.* **2010**, *48*, 1026–1031. [CrossRef]
40. Zhang, Y.; Henning, S.M.; Lee, R.P.; Huang, J.; Zerlin, A.; Li, Z.; Heber, D. Turmeric and Black Pepper Spices Decrease Lipid Peroxidation in Meat Patties during Cooking. *Int. J. Food Sci. Nutr.* **2015**, *66*, 260–265. [CrossRef]
41. Kanani, P.B.; Daneshyar, M.; Aliakbarlu, J.; Hamian, F. Effect of Dietary Turmeric and Cinnamon Powders on Meat Quality and Lipid Peroxidation of Broiler Chicken under Heat Stress Condition. *Vet. Res. Forum* **2017**, *8*, 163.
42. Fan, J.; Watanabe, T. Atherosclerosis: Known and Unknown. *Pathol. Int.* **2022**, *72*, 151–160. [CrossRef]
43. Zhang, D.; Qiao, W.; Zhao, Y.; Fang, H.; Xu, D.; Xia, Q. Curdione Attenuates Thrombin-Induced Human Platelet Activation: B1-Tubulin as a Potential Therapeutic Target. *Fitoterapia* **2017**, *116*, 106–115. [CrossRef]
44. Xia, Q.; Wang, X.; Xu, D.J.; Chen, X.H.; Chen, F.H. Inhibition of Platelet Aggregation by Curdione from Curcuma Wenyujin Essential Oil. *Thromb. Res.* **2012**, *130*, 409–414. [CrossRef]
45. Lee, H.S. Antiplatelet Property of Curcuma Longa L. Rhizome-Derived Ar-Turmerone. *Bioresour. Technol.* **2006**, *97*, 1372–1376. [CrossRef]
46. Liu, M.; Chen, X.; Ma, J.; Hassan, W.; Wu, H.; Ling, J.; Shang, J. β-Elemene Attenuates Atherosclerosis in Apolipoprotein E-Deficient Mice via Restoring NO Levels and Alleviating Oxidative Stress. *Biomed. Pharmacother.* **2017**, *95*, 1789–1798. [CrossRef]
47. Ahmad, K.A.; Ze, H.; Chen, J.; Khan, F.U.; Xuezhuo, C.; Xu, J.; Qilong, D. The Protective Effects of a Novel Synthetic β-Elemene Derivative on Human Umbilical Vein Endothelial Cells against Oxidative Stress-Induced Injury: Involvement of Antioxidation and PI3k/Akt/ENOS/NO Signaling Pathways. *Biomed. Pharmacother.* **2018**, *106*, 1734–1741. [CrossRef]
48. Padhi, S.; Nayak, A.K.; Behera, A. Type II Diabetes Mellitus: A Review on Recent Drug Based Therapeutics. *Biomed. Pharmacother.* **2020**, *131*, 110708. [CrossRef]
49. Panigrahy, S.K.; Bhatt, R.; Kumar, A. Targeting Type II Diabetes with Plant Terpenes: The New and Promising Antidiabetic Therapeutics. *Biologia* **2020**, *76*, 241–254. [CrossRef]
50. Zhou, C.X.; Zhang, L.S.; Chen, F.F.; Wu, H.S.; Mo, J.X.; Gan, L.S. Terpenoids from Curcuma Wenyujin Increased Glucose Consumption on HepG2 Cells. *Fitoterapia* **2017**, *121*, 141–145. [CrossRef]
51. Nishiyama, T.; Mae, T.; Kishida, H.; Tsukagawa, M.; Mimaki, Y.; Kuroda, M.; Sashida, Y.; Takahashi, K.; Kawada, T.; Nakagawa, K.; et al. Curcuminoids and Sesquiterpenoids in Turmeric (*Curcuma Longa* L.) Suppress an Increase in Blood Glucose Level in Type 2 Diabetic KK-Ay Mice. *J. Agric. Food Chem.* **2005**, *53*, 959–963. [CrossRef]
52. Yang, S.; Liu, J.; Jiao, J.; Jiao, L. Ar-Turmerone Exerts Anti-Proliferative and Anti-Inflammatory Activities in HaCaT Keratinocytes by Inactivating Hedgehog Pathway. *Inflammation* **2020**, *43*, 478–486. [CrossRef]

53. Park, S.Y.; Jin, M.L.; Kim, Y.H.; Kim, Y.; Lee, S.J. Aromatic-Turmerone Inhibits α-MSH and IBMX-Induced Melanogenesis by Inactivating CREB and MITF Signaling Pathways. *Arch. Dermatol. Res.* **2011**, *303*, 737–744. [CrossRef]
54. Park, J.-H.; Mohamed, M.; Shrestha, S. Germacrane Sesquiterpenes Isolated from the Rhizome of Curcuma Xanthorrhiza Roxb. Inhibit UVB-Induced Upregulation of MMP-1,-2, and-3 Expression in Human Keratinocytes Antioxidant Properties of Honey from Different Altitudes of Nepal Himalayas View Project Dissect IFT View Project. *Artic. Arch. Pharmacal Res.* 2014. [CrossRef]
55. Miyakoshi, M.; Yamaguchi, Y.; Takagaki, R.; Mizutani, K.; Kambara, T.; Ikeda, T.; Zaman, M.S.; Kakihara, H.; Takenaka, A.; Igarashi, K. Hepatoprotective Effect of Sesquiterpenes in Turmeric. *BioFactors* **2004**, *21*, 167–170. [CrossRef]
56. Megumi, C.; Muroyama, K.; Sasako, H.; Tsuge, N. Preventive Activity of Ar-Turmerone and Bisacurone Isolated from Turmeric Extract Against Ethanol-Induced Hepatocyte Injury. *Food Sci. Technol. Res.* **2017**, *23*, 275–281. [CrossRef]
57. Abdel-Lateef, E.; Mahmoud, F.; Hammam, O.; El-Ahwany, E.; El-Wakil, E.; Kandil, S.; Abu Taleb, H.; El-Sayed, M.; Hassenein, H. Bioactive Chemical Constituents of Curcuma Longa L. Rhizomes Extract Inhibit the Growth of Human Hepatoma Cell Line (HepG2). *Acta Pharmaceutica* **2016**, *66*, 387–398. [CrossRef]
58. Jia, Y.; Gao, L.; Yang, X.; Zhang, F.; Chen, A.; Wang, S.; Shao, J.; Tan, S.; Zheng, S. Blockade of Periostin-Dependent Migration and Adhesion by Curcumol via Inhibition of Nuclear Factor Kappa B Signaling in Hepatic Stellate Cells. *Toxicology* **2020**, *440*, 152475. [CrossRef]
59. Liju, V.B.; Jeena, K.; Kuttan, R. An Evaluation of Antioxidant, Anti-Inflammatory, and Antinociceptive Activities of Essential Oil from Curcuma Longa. L. *Indian J. Pharmacol.* **2011**, *43*, 526. [CrossRef]
60. Pan, C.; Si, Y.; Meng, Q.; Jing, L.; Chen, L.; Zhang, Y.; Bao, H. Suppression of the Rac1/MlK3/P38 Signaling Pathway by β-Elemene Alleviates Sepsis-Associated Encephalopathy in Mice. *Front. Neurosci.* **2019**, *13*, 443499. [CrossRef]
61. Zhuang, S.; Liu, B.; Guo, S.; Xue, Y.; Wu, L.; Liu, S.; Zhang, C.; Ni, X. Germacrone Alleviates Neurological Deficits Following Traumatic Brain Injury by Modulating Neuroinflammation and Oxidative Stress. *BMC Complement. Med. Ther.* **2021**, *21*, 6. [CrossRef]
62. Hori, Y.; Tsutsumi, R.; Nasu, K.; Boateng, A.; Ashikari, Y.; Sugiura, M.; Nakajima, M.; Kurauchi, Y.; Hisatsune, A.; Katsuki, H.; et al. Aromatic-Turmerone Analogs Protect Dopaminergic Neurons in Midbrain Slice Cultures through Their Neuroprotective Activities. *Cells* **2021**, *10*, 1090. [CrossRef]
63. Fujiwaraj, M.; Yagi, N.; Miyazawa, M. Acetylcholinesterase Inhibitory Activity of Volatile Oil from Peltophorum Dasyrachis Kurz Ex Bakar (Yellow Batai) and Bisabolane-Type Sesquiterpenoids. *J. Agric. Food Chem.* **2010**, *58*, 2824–2829. [CrossRef]
64. Meyer, J.H.; Ginovart, N.; Boovariwala, A.; Sagrati, S.; Hussey, D.; Garcia, A.; Young, T.; Praschak-Rieder, N.; Wilson, A.A.; Houle, S. Elevated Monoamine Oxidase A Levels in the Brain: An Explanation for the Monoamine Imbalance of Major Depression. *Arch. Gen. Psychiatry* **2006**, *63*, 1209–1216. [CrossRef] [PubMed]
65. Liao, J.C.; Tsai, J.C.; Liu, C.Y.; Huang, H.C.; Wu, L.Y.; Peng, W.H. Antidepressant-like Activity of Turmerone in Behavioral Despair Tests in Mice. *BMC Complement. Altern. Med.* **2013**, *13*, 299. [CrossRef]
66. Saga, Y.; Hatakenaka, Y.; Matsumoto, M.; Yoshioka, Y.; Matsumura, S.; Zaima, N.; Konishi, Y. Neuroprotective Effects of Aromatic Turmerone on Activity Deprivation-Induced Apoptosis in Cerebellar Granule Neurons. *Neuroreport* **2020**, *31*, 1302–1307. [CrossRef]
67. Hucklenbroich, J.; Klein, R.; Neumaier, B.; Graf, R.; Fink, G.R.; Schroeter, M.; Rueger, M.A. Aromatic-Turmerone Induces Neural Stem Cell Proliferation In Vitro and In Vivo. *Stem. Cell Res. Ther.* **2014**, *5*, 100. [CrossRef]
68. Wang, J.; Li, H.; Yao, Y.; Ren, Y.; Lin, J.; Hu, J.; Zheng, M.; Song, X.; Zhao, T.; Chen, Y.Y.; et al. β-Elemene Enhances GAP-43 Expression and Neurite Outgrowth by Inhibiting RhoA Kinase Activation in Rats with Spinal Cord Injury. *Neuroscience* **2018**, *383*, 12–21. [CrossRef] [PubMed]
69. Orellana-Paucar, A.M.; Serruys, A.S.K.; Afrikanova, T.; Maes, J.; De Borggraeve, W.; Alen, J.; León-Tamariz, F.; Wilches-Arizábala, I.M.; Crawford, A.D.; de Witte, P.A.M.; et al. Anticonvulsant Activity of Bisabolene Sesquiterpenoids of Curcuma Longa in Zebrafish and Mouse Seizure Models. *Epilepsy Behav.* **2012**, *24*, 14–22. [CrossRef] [PubMed]
70. Orellana-Paucar, A.M.; Afrikanova, T.; Thomas, J.; Aibuldinov, Y.K.; Dehaen, W.; De Witte, P.A.M.; Esguerra, C.V. Insights from Zebrafish and Mouse Models on the Activity and Safety of Ar-Turmerone as a Potential Drug Candidate for the Treatment of Epilepsy. *PLoS ONE* **2013**, *8*, e81634. [CrossRef]
71. Ding, J.; Wang, J.J.; Huang, C.; Wang, L.; Deng, S.; Xu, T.-L.; Ge, W.H.; Li, W.G.; Li, F. Curcumol from Rhizoma Curcumae Suppresses Epileptic Seizure by Facilitation of GABA(A) Receptors. *Neuropharmacology* **2014**, *81*, 244–255. [CrossRef]
72. Ali, A.H.; Agustar, H.K.; Hassan, N.I.; Latip, J.; Embi, N.; Sidek, H.M. Data on Antiplasmodial and Stage-Specific Inhibitory Effects of Aromatic (Ar)-Turmerone against Plasmodium Falciparum 3D7. *Data Brief* **2020**, *33*, 106592. [CrossRef]
73. Amaral, A.C.F.; Gomes, L.A.; Silva, J.R.D.A.; Ferreira, J.L.P.; Ramos, A.D.S.; Rosa, M.D.S.S.; Vermelho, A.B.; Rodrigues, I.A. Liposomal Formulation of Turmerone-Rich Hexane Fractions from Curcuma Longa Enhances Their Antileishmanial Activity. *Biomed. Res. Int.* **2014**, *2014*, 694934. [CrossRef] [PubMed]
74. Javanian, M.; Barary, M.; Ghebrehewet, S.; Koppolu, V.; Vasigala, V.K.R.; Ebrahimpour, S. A Brief Review of Influenza Virus Infection. *J. Med. Virol.* **2021**, *93*, 4638–4646. [CrossRef] [PubMed]
75. Schaffner, W.; Chen, W.H.; Hopkins, R.H.; Neuzil, K. Effective Immunization of Older Adults Against Seasonal Influenza. *Am. J. Med.* **2018**, *131*, 865–873. [CrossRef]

76. Ti, H.; Mai, Z.; Wang, Z.; Zhang, W.; Xiao, M.; Yang, Z.; Shaw, P. Bisabolane-Type Sesquiterpenoids from *Curcuma Longa* L. Exert Anti-Influenza and Anti-Inflammatory Activities through NF-KB/MAPK and RIG-1/STAT1/2 Signaling Pathways. *Food Funct.* **2021**, *12*, 6697–6711. [CrossRef]
77. Liao, Q.; Qian, Z.; Liu, R.; An, L.; Chen, X. Germacrone Inhibits Early Stages of Influenza Virus Infection. *Antiviral. Res.* **2013**, *100*, 578–588. [CrossRef]
78. He, W.; Zhai, X.; Su, J.; Ye, R.; Zheng, Y.; Su, S. Antiviral Activity of Germacrone against Pseudorabies Virus in Vitro. *Pathogens* **2019**, *8*, 258. [CrossRef] [PubMed]
79. Ali, A.; Wang, Y.H.; Khan, I.A. Larvicidal and Biting Deterrent Activity of Essential Oils of Curcuma Longa, Ar-Turmerone, and Curcuminoids Against Aedes Aegypti and Anopheles Quadrimaculatus (Culicidae: Diptera). *J. Med. Entomol.* **2015**, *52*, 979–986. [CrossRef]
80. Liu, J.; Fernandez, D.; Gao, Y.; Pierre, S.; Gao, Y.; Dai, G. Enzymology, Histological and Ultrastructural Effects of Ar-Turmerone on Culex Pipiens Pallens Larvae. *Insects* **2020**, *11*, 336. [CrossRef]
81. Gnat, S.; Nowakiewicz, A.; Łagowski, D.; Zięba, P. Host- and Pathogen-Dependent Susceptibility and Predisposition to Dermatophytosis. *J. Med. Microbiol.* **2019**, *68*, 823–836. [CrossRef]
82. Jankasem, M.; Wuthi-udomlert, M.; Gritsanapan, W. Antidermatophytic Properties of Ar -Turmerone, Turmeric Oil, and Curcuma Longa Preparations. *ISRN Dermatol.* **2013**, *2013*, 250597. [CrossRef] [PubMed]
83. Ferreira, L.A.F.; Henriques, O.B.; Andreoni, A.A.S.; Vital, G.R.F.; Campos, M.M.C.; Habermehl, G.G.; de Moraes, V.L.G. Antivenom and Biological Effects of Ar-Turmerone Isolated from Curcuma Longa (Zingiberaceae). *Toxicon* **1992**, *30*, 1211–1218. [CrossRef] [PubMed]
84. Joshi, J.P.; Ghaisas, S.; Vaidya, A.; Vaidya, R.; Kamat, D.V.; Bhagwat, A.; Bhide, S. Early Human Safety Study of Turmeric Oil (*Curcuma Longa* Oil) Administered Orally in Healthy Volunteers. *J. Assoc. Physicians India* **2003**, *51*, 1055–1060. [PubMed]
85. Prasad, S.; Aggarwal, B.B. Turmeric, the Golden Spice. In *Herbal Medicine: Biomolecular and Clinical Aspects*, 2nd ed.; CRC Press/Taylor & Francis: Boca Raton, FL, USA, 2011; pp. 263–288.

molecules

MDPI

Review

Defense Molecules of the Invasive Plant Species *Ageratum conyzoides*

Hisashi Kato-Noguchi * and Midori Kato

Department of Applied Biological Science, Faculty of Agriculture, Kagawa University, Miki 761-0795, Kagawa, Japan
* Correspondence: kato.hisashi@kagawa-u.ac.jp

Abstract: *Ageratum conyzoides* L. is native to Tropical America, and it has naturalized in many other tropical, subtropical, and temperate countries in South America, Central and Southern Africa, South and East Asia, Eastern Austria, and Europe. The population of the species has increased dramatically as an invasive alien species, and it causes significant problems in agriculture and natural ecosystems. The life history traits of *Ageratum conyzoides*, such as its short life cycle, early reproductive maturity, prolific seed production, and high adaptive ability to various environmental conditions, may contribute to its naturalization and increasing population. Possible evidence of the molecules involved in the defense of *Ageratum conyzoides* against its natural enemies, such as herbivore insects and fungal pathogens, and the allelochemicals involved in its competitive ability against neighboring plant species has been accumulated in the literature. The volatiles, essential oils, extracts, residues, and/or rhizosphere soil of *Ageratum conyzoides* show insecticidal, fungicidal, nematocidal, and allelopathic activity. The pyrrolizidine alkaloids lycopsamine and echinatine, found in the species, are highly toxic and show insecticidal activity. Benzopyran derivatives precocenes I and II show inhibitory activity against insect juvenile hormone biosynthesis and trichothecene mycotoxin biosynthesis. A mixture of volatiles emitted from *Ageratum conyzoides*, such as β-caryophyllene, β-bisabolene, and β-farnesene, may work as herbivore-induced plant volatiles, which are involved in the indirect defense function against herbivore insects. Flavonoids, such as nobiletin, eupalestin, 5′-methoxynobiletin, 5,6,7,3′,4′,5′-hexamethoxyflavone, and 5,6,8,3,4′,5′-hexamethoxyflavone, show inhibitory activity against the spore germination of pathogenic fungi. The benzoic acid and cinnamic acid derivatives found in the species, such as protocatechuic acid, gallic acid, *p*-coumaric acid, *p*-hydroxybenzoic acid, and ferulic acid, may act as allelopathic agents, causing the germination and growth inhibition of competitive plant species. These molecules produced by *Ageratum conyzoides* may act as defense molecules against its natural enemies and as allelochemicals against neighboring plant species, and they may contribute to the naturalization of the increasing population of *Ageratum conyzoides* in new habitats as an invasive plant species. This article presents the first review focusing on the defense function and allelopathy of *Ageratum conyzoides*.

Keywords: allelochemical; herbivore; invasive species; natural enemy; nematode; pathogen; precocene; pyrrolizidine alkaloid

1. Introduction

Ageratum conyzoides L., belonging to the family Asteraceae, is an annual or subshrub and grows to 20–150 cm in height. The stems are erect and round, covered with villi, and they branch well. The opposite leaves are simple, ovate, serrate, pubescent, 2–8 cm long, and 1–5 cm wide, with long petioles. It has a fibrous root system. The capitula are 4–6 cm in diameter, generated in panicles at the ends of the twigs, and a single capitulum contains 30–50 tubular florets. The corollas of the florets are white to mauve. The fruits are black and liner achenes, having aristate pappi [1–4] (Figure 1).

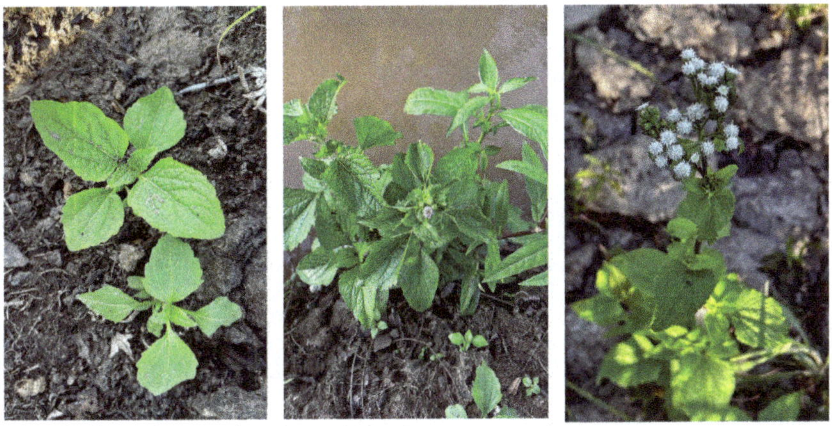

Figure 1. *Ageratum conyzoides*. Photos were kindly provided by Dr. Poonpaiboonpipat, T.

The native range of *Ageratum conyzoides* consists of Tropical America. The species is thought to have been introduced into different countries as an ornamental plant, but it has naturalized and spread in many tropical, subtropical, and temperate countries in South America, Central and Southern Africa, South and East Asia, Eastern Austria, and Europe [1–5]. Primary infestation may occur along road margins because the density of the species population is correlated with the distance from roads [2]. It was estimated that 40% of the geographical areas in the Eastern Ghats of India would be covered by *Ageratum conyzoides* by the end of 2100 [6].

The population of *Ageratum conyzoides* has been reported to have increased dramatically and it causes significant problems in agriculture in the introduced ranges. The infestation of *Ageratum conyzoides* has suppressed the production of more than 30 crops over 40 countries [6–9]. For example, the species reduced the production of direct-seed rice by 15–65%, soybean by 50–75%, maize by 15–65%, and groundnut by 45–70% [10]. *Ageratum conyzoides* also acts as a host for many crop diseases, such as okra enation leaf curl virus, capsicum chlorosis virus, cotton leaf curl virus, and tomato yellow leaf curl virus [11–13], and as a host of aphids that carry papaya ringspot virus [14]. The infestation of *Ageratum conyzoides* in grasslands reduced the production of grass fodder, causing a shortage in the fodder supply for livestock [15]. The infestation of *Ageratum conyzoides* has also been reported to significantly affect natural ecosystems. The species formed dense monocultural stands on forest floors and grasslands, reducing the species diversity by 32%, fresh biomass by 40%, and dry biomass by 49% in the introduced ranges [16]. Its infestation has been reported to threaten the survival of protective indigenous plant species on the Hawaiian islands, including *Isodendrion longifolium* and *Brighamia insignis* [4,17].

Its life history traits, such as its high growth rate, high reproduction rate, and high adaptivity, including phenotypic plasticity, contribute to the naturalization of this invasive plant species and to increasing its population in the introduced ranges [18–22]. *Ageratum conyzoides* has a short life cycle and early reproductive maturity. The species can complete its life cycle in less than 2 months, and it bears flowers when two leaves expand [23,24]. *Ageratum conyzoides* produces two generations a year under favorable growth conditions [24]. The species produces 40,000–95,000 seeds per plant [4,15,24]. The seeds are small and lightweight, and dispersed through water and wind, the attachment of the aristate pappus to stick to animals and human clothes, and the contaminant in crops and soil [3–5]. The average dispersal distance was recorded to be 2.4 km per year [25]. The seeds did not show any marked dormancy, and half of the seeds germinated [15,23,24,26–29].

Ageratum conyzoides thrives in open areas with high humidity and high soil fertility and at temperatures ranging between 20 °C and 25 °C [4,5]. Its chromosome number was reported to be 2n = 20 or 40 [1,4,30]. The species has great morphological variety and is highly adaptive to different moisture and temperature conditions and shade conditions [31]. The species has survived at temperatures between 15 °C and 30 °C [5]. The species was found in mountain areas at up to 1800 m elevation [28,32]. *Ageratum conyzoides* also maintains its dense population under dry and shaded conditions [33–35]. The species has infested protective forests, in which the forest floor was relatively dark, and destroyed the community of the native undergrowth species [34,35]. These observations suggest that the life history traits of *Ageratum conyzoides*, such as its short life cycle and early reproductive maturity, prolific seed production, and high adaptivity to various environmental conditions, may contribute to the invasiveness of the species.

Many of the invasive plant species are also reported to possess defense molecules, which are involved in defense functions against natural enemies, such as herbivores and pathogens, as well as allelochemicals involved in allelopathy against competitive plant species [19,20,36–39]. These compounds may also contribute to the invasiveness of *Ageratum conyzoides*. However, there has been no review article focusing on the defense molecules, including allelochemicals, of *Ageratum conyzoides* involved in such functions. This work provides an overview of the defense responses and allelopathy of the species, and the compounds involved in its defense functions. The action mechanisms of the molecules involved in the defense functions are also discussed. The literature has been searched using a combination of the predominant online search engines, i.e., Scopus, ScienceDirect, and Google Scholar, and all possible combinations of *Ageratum conyzoides* with the following terms: botany, biology, habitat, reproduction, adaptively, plasticity, invasiveness, impact, natural enemy, insecticidal activity, fungicidal activity, nematode, symbiosis, rhizobium, allelopathy, allelochemical, pharmacology, and second metabolite.

2. Defense Molecules against Herbivore Insects

One of the essential factors for plant species to survive invasion is their defense ability against herbivore insects as natural enemies. Herbivore insects sometimes cause significant damage to plant growth, development, and regeneration [40–42]. Therefore, some plant species have developed a chemical defense strategy against their natural enemies [19,20,43,44].

Aqueous extracts of *Ageratum conyzoides* stems and leaves increased the mortality of an adult polyphagous grasshopper (*Zonocerus variegatus*) [45]. Hexane extracts of *Ageratum conyzoides* leaves also increased the mortality of the adult insects of *Diaphania hyalinata*, *Musca domestica*, *Periplaneta americana*, and *Rhyzopertha dominica* [46]. The whole plant extracts of *Ageratum conyzoides*, using aqueous solutions, methanol, and other organic solvents, showed insecticidal activity against several crop pest insects, such as a stalk borer (*Chilo partelus*) [47], a rice weevil (*Sitophilus oryza*), a rice bug (*Leptocorisa chinensis*) [48], and a mosquito (*Anopheles gambiae*), which is the most important vector of malaria [49]. The essential oil of *Ageratum conyzoides* also showed insecticidal activity against a crop grain insect (*Tribolium castaneum*) [50] and inhibitory activity regarding the metamorphosis of a cowpea weevil (*Callosobruche naculatus*) [51]. The essential oil showed ovicidal activity and reduced the fertility of a cotton strainer (*Dysdercus angulatus*) [48].

Two isomeric pyrrolizine alkaloids, lycopsamine and echinatine, were found in extracts of *Ageratum conyzoides* [52]. Pyrrolizidine alkaloids consist of a necine base and a double five-membered ring with a nitrogen atom in the middle, esterified with mono- or dicarboxylic acids, called a necic acid [53]. Pyrrolizidine alkaloids have been found in more than 300 different compounds in the plant families of Asteraceae, Boraginaceae, Fabaceae, and Orchidaceae [54]. These compounds are synthesized from L-arginine, and the specific intermediate is a homospermidine (polyamine). Pyrrolizidine alkaloid *N*-oxides are some of the primary products of pyrrolizidine alkaloid biosynthesis [55]. These plant species may produce these pyrrolizidine alkaloids as chemical defense agents against herbivores, such as insects and mammals [56–59]. The compounds are highly toxic, showing highly hepatotoxic, genotoxic, cytotoxic, tumorigenic, and neurotoxic activity. After absorption by insects and mammals, the first step in the activation of pyrrolizidine alkaloids is dehydrogenation catalyzed by cytochrome P450 monooxygenases [60,61], and the activated compounds interrupt several types of metabolism in the cell functions of these insects and mammals [62,63]. Therefore, the pyrrolizidine alkaloids in *Ageratum conyzoides* may be involved in the insecticidal activity caused by the extracts and essential oil of the species, as described above, and contribute to the protection of the species from herbivore attacks (Figure 2).

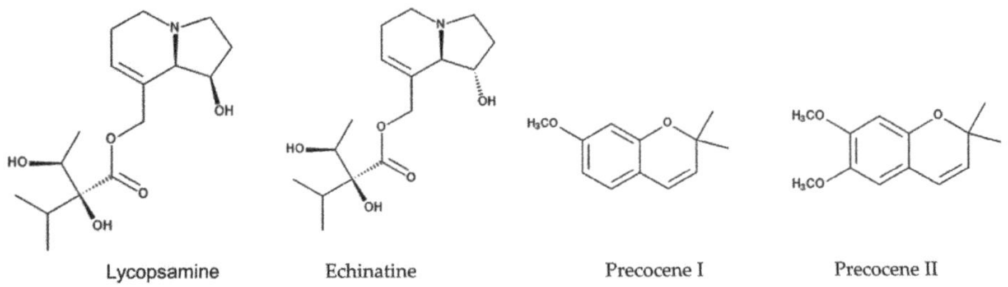

Figure 2. The compounds involved in the insecticidal activity of *Ageratum conyzoides*.

However, certain specialist herbivores have evolved tolerance to pyrrolizidine alkaloids. These specialists accumulate and store pyrrolizidine alkaloids in certain organs. The accumulated pyrrolizidine alkaloids are used for protection from their predators as poison and as precursors to synthesize mating pheromones. Some of these insects also transfer the pyrrolizidine alkaloids to their eggs for the protection of their offspring [53,64,65]. However, *Ageratum conyzoides* may seldom meet these specialist insects in its introduced ranges, because there may be no such coevolutionary history between these insects and *Ageratum conyzoides* in the introduced ranges.

The extracts and essential oil of *Ageratum conyzoides* were reported to contain two benzopyran derivatives, precocene I and precocene II (formerly named ageratochromene) [48,66,67]. These compounds are toxic and have shown anti-juvenile hormone activity, such as the inhibition of the reproduction of a bean beetle (*Epilachna varivestis*), the induction of diapause in a potato beetle (*Leptinotarsa decenlineata*) [66], and the inhibition of the metamorphosis of a moth (*Spodoptera manuritta*) [68]. The juvenile hormone is known to control several aspects of insect development, such as reproduction, diapause, and metamorphosis [69]. Precocene II was reported to inhibit the biosynthesis of the juvenile hormone [70]. In addition, precocene II was reported to cause morphological abnormalities in the pupae development of a crop pest beetle (*Epilachna vigintioctopunctata*) [71] and to interrupt mitochondrial function in rat cells [72]. These observations suggest that precocene I and precocene II may suppress insect growth and development due to the interruption of juvenile hormone biosynthesis and contribute to protection from herbivore insect attacks as defense molecules (Figure 2).

The intercropping of *Ageratum conyzoides* in citrus orchards increased the population of a predator mite, *Amblyseius newsami*, which hunts for a herbivore mite, *Panonychus citri*. *Panonychus citri* is the natural enemy of citrus and reduces citrus production significantly [68,73]. *Ageratum conyzoides* emits a mixture of volatiles, such as precocenes I and II, and three sesquiterpenes: β-caryophyllene, β-bisabolene, and β-farnesene (Figure 3). The concentrations of these volatiles in the air of *Ageratum conyzoides*-intercropping citrus orchards were greater than those in non-intercropping citrus orchards [67].

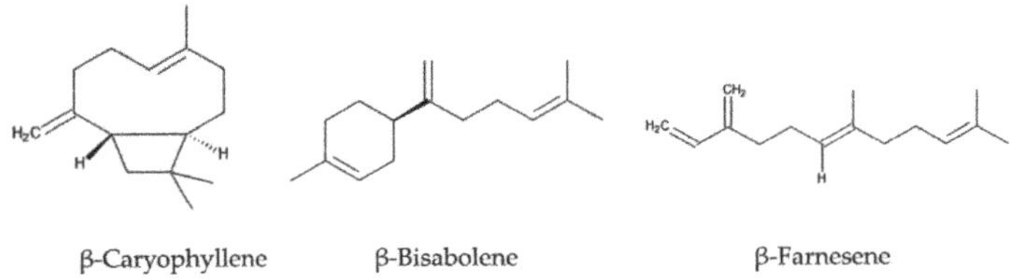

Figure 3. The compounds that act as HIPVs involved in indirect defense function.

When herbivore insects attack, certain plants emit a mixture of volatiles consisting of different chemical classes, called herbivore-induced plant volatiles (HIPVs) [70]. HIPVs stimulate predators to hunt herbivores as their prey. The predator insects sense HIPVs via the olfactory sensilla located on their antennae [74]. The responses of predator insects to HIPVs vary among predator species, and only a particular mixture of HIPVs (chemical competition and concentration) serve as signals for specific insects [75]. Then, the sensorial functions trigger the hunting behavior of these insects against the herbivores. HIPVs are considered to be involved in the indirect defense function of plants against herbivores [74,75]. The essential oil of *Ageratum conyzoides* and a volatile mixture of precocenes I and II, β-caryophyllene, β-bisabolene, and β-farnesene attracted *Amblyseius newsami* [67]. Therefore, the volatile mixture emitted from *Ageratum conyzoides* may serve as HIPVs involved in indirect defense function. β-Farnesene is known to act as a HIPV in several other plant species [75].

3. Defense Molecules against Nematodes

Plant-parasitic nematodes, such as root-knot nematodes *Meloidogyne* spp., are some of the major plant pathogens [76,77]. The host range of *Meloidogyne* spp. is wide, and their parasitism causes significant growth retardation in the host plant species. The nematodes creates galls in the plant roots and reduce the photosynthates and nutrients available to their host plants, leading to the loss of plant vigor and defense capabilities against other pathogen attacks [78–80]. Aqueous extracts of *Ageratum conyzoides* leaves increased the mortality of *Meloidogyne incognita* [81] and *Meloidogyne javanica* [82]. Its aqueous leaf extracts also suppressed the parasitic gall formation of *Meloidogyne incognita* [83]. Although the active compounds in the extracts have not yet been determined, these observations suggest that *Ageratum conyzoides* may possess certain compounds that have nematicidal activity. As described in Section 2, *Ageratum conyzoides* contains pyrrolizidine alkaloids, which are highly toxic to insects and mammals [60,61]. Therefore, these pyrrolizidine alkaloids may be involved in the nematicidal activity of the species.

4. Defense Molecules against Fungal Pathogens

The defense ability against fungal pathogens is one of the essential factors for plants to survive an invasion. Some *Fusarium* spp. are fungal plant pathogens, causing diseases such as rot, blights, cankers, and wilts in the host plant tissue [84–86]. *Fusarium* also produces a number of mycotoxins, such as trichothecenes and fumonisins [87,88]. Aqueous *n*-hexane and methanol extracts of whole plants of *Ageratum conyzoides* suppressed the growth of *Fusarium solani*, which causes rot and wilt diseases [89]. Methanol extracts of the aboveground parts of *Ageratum conyzoides* suppressed the growth of *Fusarium oxysporum*, which causes blight and wilt diseases [90]. In addition, extracts of the aerial parts of *Ageratum conyzoides* inhibited the growth of a rice blast fungus, *Pyricularia oryzae*, and a sugar beet root rot fungus, *Rhizoctonia solani*. Precocene II and four flavonoids, nobiletin, 5′-methoxynobiletin, eupalestin, and 5,6,7,3′,4′,5′-hexamethoxyflavone, were identified in the extracts as the active compounds, and the inhibitory activity of precocene II was the highest among them [91] (Figure 4).

The intercropping of *Ageratum conyzoides* in citrus orchards decreased the populations of the soil-pathogenic fungi *Phytophthora citrophthora*, *Pythium aphanidermatum*, and *Fusarium solani*. Precocenes I and II and three flavonoids, 5′-methoxynobiletin (5,6,7,8,3,4′,5′-heptamethoxyflavone), 5,6,7,3′,4′,5′-hexamethoxyflavone, and 5,6,8,3,4′,5′-hexamethoxyflavone, were found in the soil where *Ageratum conyzoides* was intercropped. These compounds inhibited the spore germination of these pathogenic fungi [92]. These observations suggest that *Ageratum conyzoides* possesses antifungal activity and precocenes I and II, as well as the mentioned flavonoids, may be involved in this activity.

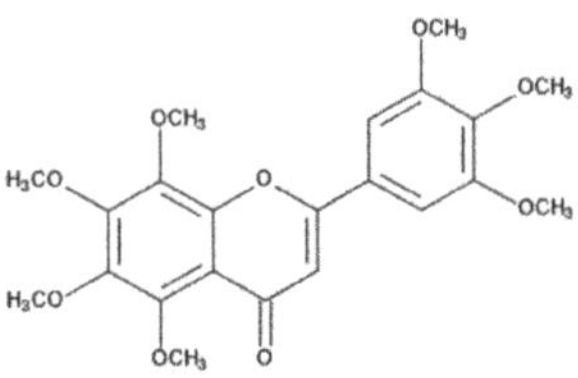

5′-Methoxynobiletin

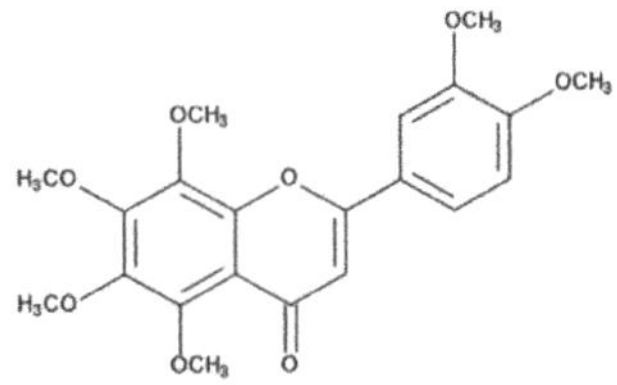

Nobiletin

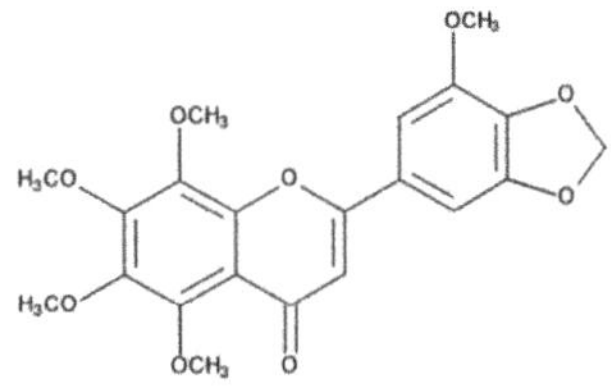

Eupalestin

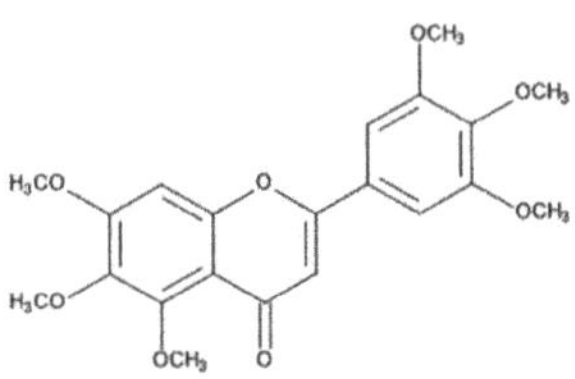

5,6,7,3′,4′,5′-Hexamethoxyflavone

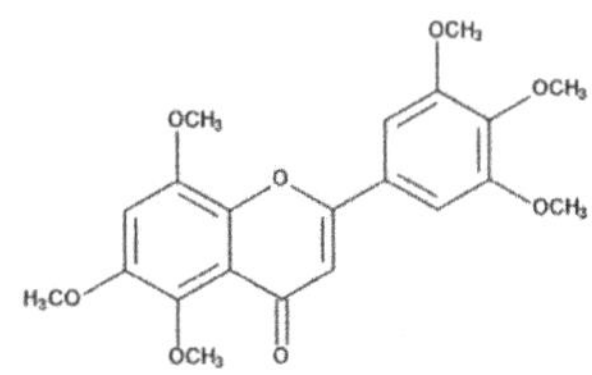

5,6,8,3,4′,5′-Hexamethoxyflavone

Figure 4. The compounds involved in the fungicidal activity of *Ageratum conyzoides*.

The intercropping of *Ageratum conyzoides* in citrus orchards decreased the populations of the soil-pathogenic fungi *Phytophthora citrophthora*, *Pythium aphanidermatum*, and *Fusarium solani*. Precocenes I and II and three flavonoids, 5′-methoxynobiletin (5,6,7,8,3,4′,5′-heptamethoxyflavone), 5,6,7,3′,4′,5′-hexamethoxyflavone, and 5,6,8,3,4′,5′-hexamethoxyflavone, were found in the soil where *Ageratum conyzoides* was intercropped. These compounds inhibited the spore germination of these pathogenic fungi [92]. These observations suggest that *Ageratum conyzoides* possesses antifungal activity and precocenes I and II, as well as the mentioned flavonoids, may be involved in this activity.

Precocenes I and II were reported to inhibit the production of trichothecene mycotoxin in a pathogenic fungus, *Fusarium graminearum*. The inhibitory activity of precocene II was much greater than that of precocene I [93,94]. Trichothecene is synthesized from farnesyl pyrophosphate, which is produced through the mevalonate pathway, and its synthesis is regulated by the TRI6 (trichothecene biosynthesis positive transcription factor) protein encoded by *Tri6* genes [95,96]. Precocenes II binds to a mitochondrial outer membrane protein and elevates the mitochondrial superoxide levels. The high levels of superoxide in mitochondria decrease the *Tri6* gene levels and TRI6 protein, resulting in the suppression of trichothecene production [95–97]. In addition, the insect juvenile hormone is also synthesized from farnesyl pyrophosphate in the corpus allatum cells of insects [98]. As described in Section 2, precocene II was reported to interrupt mitochondrial function [72] and to inhibit the biosynthesis of the juvenile hormone [70]. Therefore, precocene II may bind to the mitochondrial membrane proteins of the corpus allatum cells and interrupt juvenile hormone biosynthesis.

These observations suggest that precocenes I and II and these flavonoids may work as defense molecules against fungal pathogen attacks and help the invasion of *Ageratum conyzoides* into the introduced ranges.

5. Inhibitors for Symbiosis

When the whole plant residues of *Ageratum conyzoides* were mixed with soil, the soil suppressed the growth and nodulation of a leguminous plant chickpea (*Cicer arietinum*) [99]. Leguminous plants generally coexist with symbiotic rhizobia [100–102]. Rhizobium nodulation enhances the host plant's performance through the supply of nitrogen and ammonium to the host plant [103,104]. *Ageratum conyzoides* may possess certain compounds that degrade the nodulation of nearby legume plants. A reduction in rhizobium nodulation weakens the ability of these legumes to perform nitrogen and ammonium acquisition, which may cause the growth suppression of these plant species. Some other invasive plant species were also reported to suppress the colonization of the rhizobia and arbuscular mycorrhiza of native plant species [105,106]. Certain flavonoids released from leguminous plant species are known to act as signals for the induction of the nodulation genes in rhizobia and the initiation of symbiosis [103,104]. The compounds in *Ageratum conyzoides* may reduce the rhizobium population and interfere with the flavonoid signals and/or nodulation, resulting in the interruption of the symbiosis between the legumes and rhizobia. However, there is no information available on the compounds involved in the interruption of this symbiosis. The identification of these compounds is necessary.

6. Defense Molecules against Neighboring Plants

Allelopathy is the plant-to-plant interaction in the local plant community, occurring through certain secondary metabolites defied as allelochemicals. The donor plant species produce and release allelochemicals into their neighboring environments, and these released allelochemicals suppress the germination, growth, development, and/or regeneration process of the receiver plant species. Subsequently, the donor plants gain a relatively large quantity of resources, such as light, water, and nutrients, in the local plant community [107–110]. The competitive ability of invasive plant species against indigenous plant species for resource acquisition is one of the most important factors for their success in the introduced ranges [19,20,111,112]. The allelopathic potential of invasive plant species against indigenous plant species is often reported to be high [113–115].

The inhibitory effects of certain allelochemicals in invasive plant species against competitive plant species are considered to be greater in the introduced ranges than in the native ranges of the invasive plant species. In their native ranges, the competitive plant species may have developed tolerance to these allelochemicals because of their coevolutionary history. However, in their introduced ranges, the competitive plant species may not have had an opportunity to acquire tolerance to these allelochemicals because they had not existed together before. Therefore, according to the novel weapons hypothesis, the allelochemicals released from invasive plant species are more effective on indigenous plant species in the introduced ranges and contribute to their invasiveness [36,111,112].

Allelochemicals are synthesized, stored in certain plant organs, and released into the neighboring environment through volatilization, root exudation, and the decomposition of plant residues in the rhizosphere soil [107–110]. Therefore, allelochemicals have been identified in the extracts of plant organs (leaves, stems, and roots), essential oils, volatiles, root exudates, and rhizosphere soil [116–118].

Aqueous extracts of *Ageratum conyzoides* leaves inhibited the germination and growth of *Parthenium hysterophorus* [119]. Acetone extracts of *Ageratum conyzoides* leaves and roots inhibited the germination and growth of *Oryza sativa* [120]. Acetone extracts of *Ageratum conyzoides* shoots (leaves and stems) inhibited the germination and growth of *Amaranthus caudatus*, *Digitaria sanguinalis*, and *Lactuca sativa* in an extract concentration-dependent manner [121]. Meanwhile, *n*-hexane and ethyl acetate extracts of *Ageratum conyzoides* leaves inhibited the growth of *Amaranthus spinosus*, and a major constituent in both extracts was precocene II [122,123]. These observations suggest that *Ageratum conyzoides* contains certain extractable allelochemicals, including precocene II.

The whole plant powder of *Ageratum conyzoides* incorporated into the soil inhibited the germination and growth of *Echinochloa crus-galli*, *Monochoria vaginalis*, and *Aeschynomene indica*. Coumalic acid, gallic acid, and benzoic acid were major constituents in the aqueous methanol extracts of *Ageratum conyzoides* whole plants [124]. When the root residues of *Ageratum conyzoides* were incorporated into soil, the soil suppressed the growth of *Oryza sativa* [125], and protocatechuic acid, *p*-coumaric acid, gallic acid, ferulic acid, and *p*-hydroxybenzoic acid were identified in the aqueous extracts of the soil as allelopathic agents [8]. The aqueous extracts of soil previously infested by *Ageratum conyzoides* inhibited the growth of *Triticum aestivum* [126]. The root exudates of *Ageratum conyzoides* suppressed the germination and growth of *Abelmoschus esculentus*, *Solanum lycopersicum*, *Phaseolus vulgaris*, *Zea mays*, *Cicer arietinum*, and *Cucumis sativus* [127]. These observations suggest that *Ageratum conyzoides* may contain certain allelochemicals, which are released into the rhizosphere soil through the root exudation and decomposition processes of plant residues. Protocatechuic acid, *p*-coumaric acid, gallic acid, ferulic acid, and *p*-hydroxybenzoic acid may be some of these allelochemicals.

The intact fresh leaves of *Ageratum conyzoides* and its essential oil inhibited the growth of *Cucumis sativus*, *Lolium ultiforum*, *Raphanus sativus*, *Phaseolus aureus*, *Triticum aestivum*, and *Lycapesicon* spp. in sealed bottles. Precocenes I and II and β-caryophyllene were found as active compounds [128]. This observation suggests that certain allelochemicals, including precocenes I and II and β-caryophyllene, may be released into the air through volatilization from *Ageratum conyzoides*.

Precocenes I and II elevate the mitochondrial superoxide levels in the cells of insects and fungi, leading to insecticidal activity and fungicidal activity, as described in Section 4. High levels of superoxide were also reported to cause allelopathic activity, such as germination and growth inhibition against several plant and alga species [129–131]. Therefore, the allelopathic activity of precocenes I and II may also be caused by the elevation of the superoxide levels in plant cells. Three sesquiterpenes, β-caryophyllene, β-bisabolene, and β-farnesene, emitted from *Ageratum conyzoides* showed allelopathic activity [132]. In addition, β-caryophyllene was identified in another invasive plant species, *Mikania micrantha* [133], and was considered to act as a allelochemical due to the elevation of the superoxide levels in the cells of the receiver plant species [134–136]. Therefore, these sesquiterpenes emitted from *Ageratum conyzoides* may induce allelopathic activity due to the elevation of the superoxide levels in the cells of the receiver plant species.

Soil samples obtained from *Ageratum conyzoides*-intercropped citrus orchards suppressed the growth of *Bidens pilosa*, *Digitaria sanguinalis*, and *Cyperus difformis*. Precocene II and three flavonoids, 5′-methozynobiletin, 5,6,7,3′,4′,5′-heptamethoxyflavone, and 5,6,8,3,4′, 5-hexamethoxyflavone, were identified in citrus orchard soil as allelopathic agents [92] (Figure 4). Flavonoids are polyphenolic secondary metabolites synthesized from phenylalanine through chalcone. Many flavonoids are reported to have anti-fungal, anti-herbivore, anti-bacterial, and allelopathic activity [137–140]. *Ageratum conyzoides* is rich in polyoxygenated flavonoids [141]. Therefore, some of these identified flavonoids and precocene II in *Ageratum conyzoides* may be released into the rhizosphere soil through the decomposition of plant residues and act as allelopathic agents. However, the molecular targets of the flavonoids in plant cells are unknown.

Benzoic acid and cinnamic acid derivatives, such as protocatechuic acid, gallic acid, *p*-coumaric acid, *p*-hydroxybenzoic acid, and ferulic acid, were identified in extracts of the roots, leaves, and stems of *Ageratum conyzoides* and/or in soil mixed with its root residues [8,124,125]. Cinnamic acid and its derivatives are synthesized via the shikimic acid pathway from phenylalanine [142,143]. These compounds have been identified in a wide range of plant extracts, plant residues, and plant rhizosphere soil. The involvement of benzoic acid and cinnamic acid derivatives in allelopathy and the mechanisms of their allelopathic action have been investigated in other plant species [144–146]. These compounds cause structural alterations in the plasma membrane lipids and proteins of plant cells and reduce the transmembrane electrochemical potential, which causes the depolarization of the membranes. The depolarization of the membranes induces the nonspecific efflux of both cations and anions, including phosphate, potassium, magnesium, and nitrate ions, and affects the water balance in the cells. These compounds also interrupt the activity of various enzymes involved in several types of metabolism, such as photosynthesis, respiration, phytohormone synthesis, protein synthesis, and the synthesis of other secondary metabolites, and they affect plant cell division, growth, and development [144–147]. Therefore, benzoic acid, protocatechuic acid, gallic acid, *p*-coumaric acid, *p*-hydroxybenzoic acid, and ferulic acid may affect the plasma membrane structure and certain enzymes' activity and act as allelopathic agents (Figure 5).

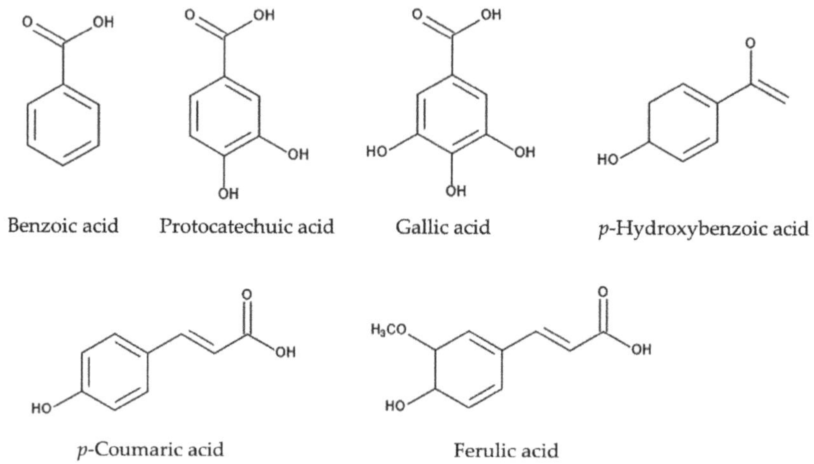

Figure 5. The compounds involved in the allelopathy of *Ageratum conyzoides*.

These allelochemicals identified in *Ageratum conyzoides* may contribute to the suppression of the germination and growth of indigenous plant species and increase the competitive ability of *Ageratum conyzoides* for the acquisition of nutrients, water, and light in the introduced ranges.

7. Contributions of Defense Molecules to Invasive Traits of *Ageratum conyzoides*

Ageratum conyzoides produces several defense molecules against insects, nematodes, fungal pathogens, and competitive neighboring plant species. Among them, precocenes I and II showed insecticidal activity through the inhibition of insect juvenile hormone biosynthesis [70]. Precocenes I and II also have fungicidal activity [92], and they exhibit inhibitory activity regarding trichothecene mycotoxin biosynthesis through the elevation of the mitochondrial superoxide levels [93,94]. Both compounds have shown allelopathic activity and suppressed the germination and growth of several plant species [122,123,128]. In addition, a mixture of volatiles, including precocenes I and II and three sesquiterpenes, namely β-caryophyllene, β-bisabolene, and β-farnesene, emitted from *Ageratum conyzoides*, may work as HIPVs involved in the indirect defense function against herbivore insects [67] (Figure 6).

Pyrrolizidine alkaloids, such as lycopsamine and echinatine, are highly toxic and possess insecticidal activity through the interruption of metabolism in insect cells, resulting in protection from herbivore insect attacks. These compounds may also work as defense agents and be involved in nematicidal activity. Flavonoids, such as nobiletin, 5′-methoxynobiletin, eupalestin, 5,6,7,3′,4′,5′-hexamethoxyflavone, and 5,6,8,3,4′,5′-hexamethoxyflavone, found in *Ageratum conyzoides* were reported to show inhibitory activity regarding the spore germination of pathogenic fungi [91,92]. Benzoic acid, protocatechuic acid, gallic acid, *p*-coumaric acid, *p*-hydroxybenzoic acid, and ferulic acid may act as allelopathic agents, causing the inhibition of the germination and growth of other plant species [124–126]. The sesquiterpene β-caryophyllene and the flavonoids found in *Ageratum conyzoides* may also act as allelopathic agents [128] (Figure 6).

Pharmacological and phytochemical investigations have shown that *Ageratum conyzoides* contains many other secondary metabolites in several chemical classes, such as monoterpenes, sesquiterpenes, flavonoids, and sterols. Some of these compounds are related to pharmacological activity, such as anti-pyretic, anti-inflammatory, cardiovascular, and analgesic activity, which is exploited in medicinal treatment, and anti-microbial activity, which benefits food security [94,148–153]. Although the identified compounds have not yet been related to the invasiveness of *Ageratum conyzoides*, some of them may act as defense molecules for unknown functions.

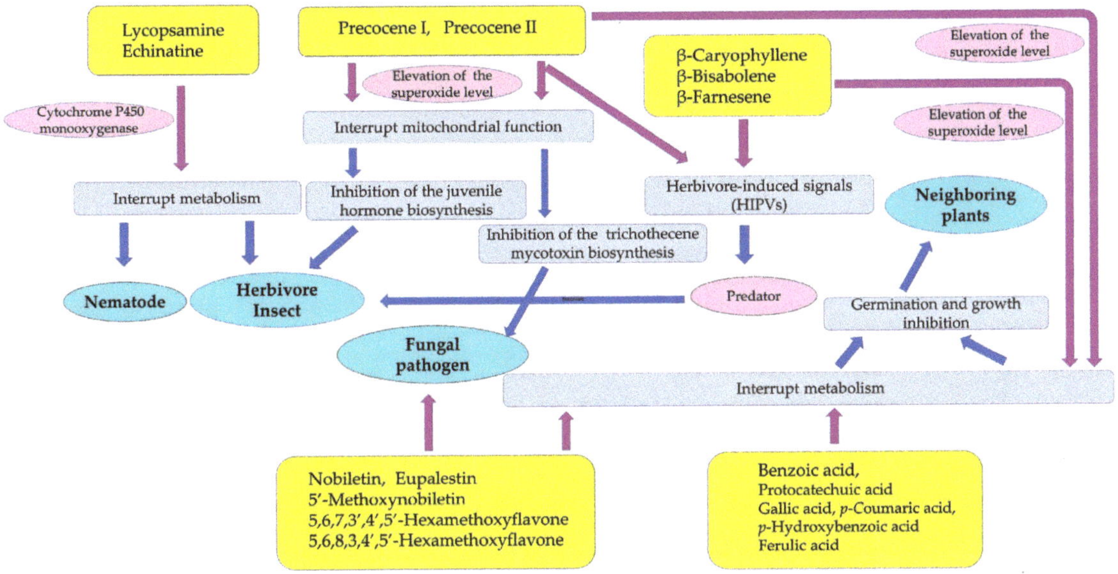

Figure 6. Defense molecules involved in the invasive abilities of *Ageratum conyzoides*. These compounds act as nematicidal, insecticidal, fungicidal, and allelopathic agents of *Ageratum conyzoides*. Purple arrow: direct action; blue arrow: secondary and tertiary action.

In conclusion, the defense responses of invasive plants to their natural enemies, such as herbivores and pathogens, is one of the essential functions for their naturalization and population expansion in their introduced ranges. The allelopathy of invasive plants against indigenous plant species is also one of these functions. As described above, *Ageratum conyzoides* produces several compounds that act as defense molecules against its natural enemies, such as herbivore insects, parasitic nematodes, and fungal pathogens, and act as allelochemicals against neighboring plant species. Therefore, these compounds may contribute to the naturalization and expanding population of *Ageratum conyzoides* in new habitats as an invasive plant species. These compounds may be used in the development of insecticides, fungicides, and/or herbicides.

Funding: This research received no external funding.

Institutional Review Board Statement: Not applicable.

Informed Consent Statement: Not applicable.

Data Availability Statement: Not applicable.

Conflicts of Interest: The authors declare no conflicts of interest.

References

1. Ming, L.C. *Ageratum conyzoides*: A tropical source of medicinal and agricultural products. In *Perspectives on New Crops and New Uses*; Janick, J., Ed.; ASHS Press: Alexandria, VA, USA, 1999; pp. 469–473.
2. Global Invasive Species Database. Species Profile: *Ageratum conyzoides*. Available online: https://www.iucngisd.org/gisd/species.php?sc=1493 (accessed on 12 August 2024).
3. Royal Botanical Gardens, Kew, *Ageratum conyzoides*. Available online: https://powo.science.kew.org/taxon/urn:lsid:ipni.org:names:7086-2 (accessed on 12 August 2024).
4. CABI Copmpendium. *Ageratum conyzoides* (Billy Goat Weed). Available online: https://www.cabidigitallibrary.org/doi/10.1079/cabicompendium.3572 (accessed on 12 August 2024).

5. Kaur, A.; Kaur, S.; Singh, H.P.; Datta, A.; Chauhan, B.S.; Ullah, H.; Kohli, R.K.; Batish, D.R. Ecology, biology, environmental impacts, and management of an agro-environmental weed *Ageratum conyzoides*. *Plants* **2023**, *12*, 2329. [CrossRef] [PubMed]
6. Paraseth, P.; Banerjee, K. Goat weed (*Ageratum conyzoides* L.): A biological threat to plant diversity in Eastern Ghats of India. *J. Biosci.* **2024**, *49*, 72. [CrossRef]
7. Manandhar, S.; Shrestha, B.B.; Lekhak, H.D. Weeds of paddy field at Kirtipur, Kathmandu. *Sci. World* **2007**, *5*, 100–106. [CrossRef]
8. Batish, D.R.; Kaur, S.; Singh, H.P.; Kohli, R.K. Role of root-mediated interactions in phytotoxic interference of *Ageratum conyzoides* with rice (*Oryza sativa*). *Flora* **2009**, *204*, 388–395. [CrossRef]
9. Devi, C.; Khwairakpam, M. Feasibility of vermicomposting for the management of terrestrial weed *Ageratum conyzoides* using earthworm species *Eisenia fetida*. *Environ. Technol. Innov.* **2020**, *18*, 100696. [CrossRef]
10. Gharde, Y.; Singh, P.K.; Dubey, R.P.; Gupta, P.K. Assessment of yield and economic losses in agriculture due to weeds in India. *Crop Prot.* **2018**, *107*, 12–18. [CrossRef]
11. Anwar, I.; Bukhari, H.A.; Nahid, N.; Rashid, K.; Amin, I.; Shaheen, S.; Hussain, K.; Mansoor, S. Association of cotton leaf curl *Multan betasatellite* and *Ageratum conyzoides* symptomless alphasatellite with tomato leaf curl New Delhi virus in *Luffa cylindrica* in Pakistan. *Australas. Plant Pathol.* **2020**, *49*, 25–29. [CrossRef]
12. Sharman, M.; Thomas, J.E.; Tree, D.; Persley, D.M. Natural host range and thrips transmission of capsicum chlorosis virus in Australia. *Australas. Plant Pathol.* **2020**, *49*, 45–51. [CrossRef]
13. Serfraz, S.; Amin, I.; Akhtar, K.P.; Mansoor, S. Recombination among Begomoviruses on Malvaceous plants leads to the evolution of okra enation leaf curl virus in Pakistan. *J. Phytopathol.* **2015**, *163*, 764–776. [CrossRef]
14. Martins, D.D.S.; Ventura, J.A.; Paula, R.D.C.A.L.; Fornazier, M.J.; Rezende, J.A.M.; Culik, M.P.; Ferreira, P.S.F.; Peronti, A.L.B.G.; de Carvalho, R.C.Z.; Sousa-Silva, C.R. Aphid vectors of Papaya ringspot virus and their weed hosts in orchards in the major papaya producing and exporting region of Brazil. *Crop Prot.* **2016**, *90*, 191–196. [CrossRef]
15. Kohli, R.K.; Batish, D.R.; Singh, H.P.; Dogra, K.S. Status, invasiveness and environmental threats of three tropical American invasive weeds (*Parthenium hysterophorus* L., *Ageratum conyzoides* L., *Lantana camara* L.) in India. *Biol. Invasions* **2006**, *8*, 1501–1510. [CrossRef]
16. Dogra, K.S.; Kohli, R.K.; Sood, S.K.; Dobhal, P.K. Impact of *Ageratum conyzoides* L. on the diversity and composition of vegetation in the Shivalik hills of Himachal Pradesh (Northwestern Himalaya), India. *Int. J. Biodivers. Conser.* **2009**, *1*, 135–145.
17. US Fish and Wildlife Service. 5-Year Review: Summary and Evaluation. In *Lsodendrion longifolium (aupaka)*; US Fish and Wildlife Service: Falls Church, VA, USA, 2011. Available online: http://ecos.fws.gov/docs/five_year_review/doc3809.pdf (accessed on 12 August 2024).
18. Thompson, J.D.; McNeilly, T.; Gray, A.J. Population variation in *Spartina anglica* C.E. Hubbard. I. Evidence from a common garden experiment. *New Phytol.* **1991**, *117*, 115–128. [CrossRef]
19. Mack, R.M. Predicting the identity and fate of plant invaders: Emergent and emerging approaches. *Biol. Conserv.* **1996**, *78*, 107–121. [CrossRef]
20. Chengxu, W.; Mingxing, Z.; Xuhui, C.; Bo, Q. Review on allelopathy of exotic invasive plants. *Procedia Engin.* **2011**, *18*, 240–246. [CrossRef]
21. Theoharides, K.A.; Dukes, J.S. Plant invasion across space and time: Factors affecting nonindigenous species success during four stages of invasion. *New Phytol.* **2007**, *176*, 256–273. [CrossRef]
22. Warren, R.J.; Matt Candeias, M.; Labatore, A.; Olejniczak, M.; Yang, L. Multiple mechanisms in woodland plant species invasion. *J. Plant Ecol.* **2019**, *12*, 201–209. [CrossRef]
23. Holm, L.G.; Plucknett, D.L.; Pancho, J.V.; Herberger, J.P. *The World's Worst Weeds. Distribution and Biology*; University Press of Hawaii: Honolulu, HI, USA, 1977; pp. 1–609.
24. Kaur, S.; Batish, D.R.; Kohli, R.K.; Singh, H.P. *Ageratum conyzoides*: An alien invasive weed in India. In *Invasive Alien Plants: An Ecological Appraisal for the Indian Subcontinent*; Bhatt, J.R., Singh, J.S., Singh, S.P., Tripathi, R.S., Kohli, R.K., Eds.; CABI: Wallingford, UK, 2012; pp. 57–76.
25. Horvitz, N.; Wang, R.; Wan, F.H.; Nathan, R. Pervasive human-mediated large-scale invasion: Analysis of spread patterns and their underlying mechanisms in 17 of China's worst invasive plants. *J. Ecol.* **2017**, *105*, 85–94. [CrossRef]
26. Marks, M.K.; Nwachuku, A.C. Seed-bank characteristics in a group of tropical weeds. *Weed Res.* **1986**, *26*, 151–157. [CrossRef]
27. Sauerborn, J.; Koch, W.; Krage, J. On the influence of light, temperature, depth of burial and water stress on the germination of selected weed species. *Z. Pflanzenkr. Pflanzenschutz Sonderh.* **1988**, *11*, 47–53.
28. PIER. Pacific Island Ecosystems at Risk, *Ageratum conyzoides*. Available online: http://www.hear.org/pier/species/ageratum_conyzoides.htm (accessed on 12 August 2024).
29. PROTA. PROTA4U Web Database. Plant Resources of Tropical Africa. 2018. Available online: https://www.prota4u.org/database/ (accessed on 12 August 2024).
30. Gupta, R.C. Meiotic abnormalities in *Ageratum conyzoides* from hot desert of India (Rajasthan). *Chromosome Bot.* **2015**, *10*, 67–74.
31. do Rosário, C.J.R.M.; Lima, A.S.; de Mendonça, C.; Soares, I.S.; Júnior, E.B.A.; Gomes, M.N.; Costa-Junior, L.M.; Maia, J.G.S.; da Rocha, C.Q. Essential oil *Ageratum conyzoides* chemotypes and anti-tick activities. *Vet. Parasitol.* **2023**, *319*, 109942. [CrossRef] [PubMed]
32. Dogra, K.S.; Kohli, R.K.; Sood, S.K. An assessment and impact of three invasive species in the Shivalik hills of Himachal Pradesh, India. *Int. J. Biodiv. Conserv.* **2009**, *1*, 4–10.
33. Chaudhary, N.; Narayan, R. The advancing dominance of *Ageratum conyzoides* L. and *Lantana camara* L. in dry tropical peri-urban vegetation in India. *Int. Res. J. Environ. Sci.* **2013**, *2*, 88–95.

34. Sengupta, R.; Dash, S.S. A comprehensive inventory of alien plants in the protected forest areas of Tripura and their ecological consequences. *Nelumbo* **2021**, *63*, 163–182. [CrossRef]
35. Semy, K.; Singh, M.R. Changes in plant diversity and community attributes of coal mine affected forest in relation to a community reserve forest of Nagaland, Northeast India. *Trop. Ecol.* **2024**, *65*, 16–25. [CrossRef]
36. Callaway, R.M.; Aschehoug, E.T. Invasive plants versus their new and old neighbors: A mechanism for exotic invasion. *Science* **2000**, *290*, 521–523. [CrossRef]
37. Meiners, S.J.; Kong, C.H.; Ladwig, L.M.; Pisula, N.L.; Lang, K.A. Developing an ecological context for allelopathy. *Plant Ecol.* **2012**, *213*, 1861–1867. [CrossRef]
38. Kato-Noguchi, H. Involvement of allelopathy in the invasive potential of *Tithonia diversifolia*. *Plants* **2020**, *9*, 766. [CrossRef]
39. Kato-Noguchi, H.; Kurniadie, D. Allelopathy and allelochemicals of *Leucaena leucocephala* as an invasive plant species. *Plants* **2022**, *11*, 1672. [CrossRef]
40. Keane, R.M.; Crawley, M.L. Exotic plant invasions and the enemy release hypothesis. *Trend Ecol. Evol.* **2002**, *17*, 164–170. [CrossRef]
41. Blossey, B.; Notzold, R. Evolution of increased competitive ability in invasive nonindigenous plants—A hypothesis. *J. Ecol.* **1995**, *83*, 887–889. [CrossRef]
42. Muller-Scharer, H.; Schaffner, U.; Steinger, T. Evolution in invasive plants: Implications for biological control. *Trends Ecol. Evol.* **2004**, *19*, 417–422. [CrossRef] [PubMed]
43. Kato-Noguchi, H.; Kurniadie, D. Allelopathy of *Lantana camara* as an invasive plant. *Plants* **2021**, *10*, 1028. [CrossRef]
44. Kato-Noguchi, H. Defensive molecules momilactones A and B: Function, biosynthesis, induction and occurrence. *Toxins* **2023**, *15*, 241. [CrossRef]
45. Ingrid, D.T.; Akwanjoh, S.R.; Yacouba, M. Insecticidal activity of *Ageratum conyzoides* (Asteraceae) aqueous extracts against the grasshopper *Zonocerus variegatus* (Orthoptera: Pyrgomorphidae). *J. Agric. Ecol. Res. Int.* **2020**, *21*, 29–36. [CrossRef]
46. Moreira, M.D.; Picanco, M.C.; Barbosa, L.C.A.; Guedes, R.N.C.; Barros, E.C.; Campos, M.R. Compounds from *Ageratum conyzoides*: Isolation, structural elucidation and insecticidal activity. *Pest Manag. Sci.* **2007**, *63*, 615–621. [CrossRef]
47. Raja, S.S.; Singh, A.; Rao, S. Effect of *Ageratum conyzoides* on *Chilo partelus* swinhoe (Lepidoptera: Pyralidae). *J. Anim. Morphol. Physiol.* **1987**, *34*, 35–37.
48. Fagoonee, I.; Umrit, G. Antigonadotropic hormones from the goatweed, *Ageratum conyzoides*. *Insect Sci. Appl.* **1981**, *4*, 373–376.
49. Suwaiba, H.; Barde, A.A.; Mao, P.S.; Aliyu, O.A. Larvicidal activity of *Ageratum conyzoides* L. extracts on *Anopheles gambiae* complex. *GSC Biol. Pharm. Sci.* **2018**, *3*, 1–5.
50. Singh, P.J.; Prakash, B.; Dubey, N.K. Insecticidal activity of *Ageratum conyzoides* L., *Coleus aromaticus* Benth. and *Hyptis suaveolens* (L.) Poit essential oils as fumigant against storage grain insect *Tribolium castaneum* Herbst. *J. Food Sci. Technol.* **2014**, *51*, 2210–2215.
51. Gbolade, A.A.; Onayade, O.A.; Ayinde, B.A. Insecticidal activity of *Ageratum conyzoides* L. volatile oil against *Callosobruchus chinensis* F in seed treatment and fumigation laboratory tests. *Insect Sci. Appl.* **1999**, *19*, 237.
52. Wiedenfeld, H.; Roder, E. Pyrrozidine alkaloids form *Ageratum conyzoides*. *Planta Med.* **1991**, *57*, 578–579. [CrossRef] [PubMed]
53. Boppré, M. Lepidoptera and pyrrolizidine alkaloids. Exemplification of complexity in chemical ecology. *J. Chem. Ecol.* **1990**, *16*, 165–185. [CrossRef]
54. Ober, D.; Hartmann, T. Homospermidine synthase, the first pathway-specific enzyme of pyrrolizidine alkaloid biosynthesis, evolved from deoxyhypusine synthase. *Proc. Natl. Acad. Sci. USA* **1999**, *96*, 14777–14782. [CrossRef]
55. Schramm, S.; Köhler, N.; Rozhon, W. Pyrrolizidine alkaloids: Biosynthesis, biological activities and occurrence in crop plants. *Molecules* **2019**, *24*, 498. [CrossRef]
56. van Dam, N.M.; Vuister, L.W.; Bergshoeff, C.; de Vos, H.; van der Meijden, E.D. The "Raison D'être" of pyrrolizidine alkaloids in *Cynoglossum officinale*: Deterrent effects against generalist herbivores. *J. Chem. Ecol.* **1995**, *21*, 507–523. [CrossRef]
57. Joshi, J.; Vrieling, K. The enemy release and EICA hypothesis revisited: Incorporating the fundamental difference between specialist and generalist herbivores. *Ecol. Lett.* **2005**, *8*, 704–714. [CrossRef]
58. Gardner, D.R.; Thorne, M.S.; Molyneux, R.J.; Pfister, J.A.; Seawright, A.A. Pyrrolizidine alkaloids in *Senecio madagascariensis* from Australia and Hawaii and assessment of possible livestock poisoning. *Biochem. Syst. Ecol.* **2006**, *34*, 736–744. [CrossRef]
59. Stegelmeier, B.L.; Colegate, S.M.; Brown, A.W. Dehydropyrrolizidine alkaloid toxicity, cytotoxicity, and carcinogenicity. *Toxins* **2016**, *8*, 356. [CrossRef]
60. Gordon, G.J.; Coleman, W.B.; Grisham, J.W. Induction of cytochrome P450 enzymes in the livers of rats treated with the pyrrolizidine alkaloid retrorsine. *Exp. Mol. Pathol.* **2000**, *69*, 17–26. [CrossRef] [PubMed]
61. Xu, J.; Wang, W.; Yang, X.; Xiong, A.; Yang, L.; Wang, Z. Pyrrolizidine alkaloids: An update on their metabolism and hepatotoxicity mechanism. *Liver Res.* **2019**, *3*, 176–184. [CrossRef]
62. Cheeke, P.R. Toxicity and metabolism of pyrrolizidine alkaloids. *J. Anim. Sci.* **1988**, *66*, 2343–2350. [CrossRef] [PubMed]
63. Tamariz, J.; Burgueño-Tapia, E.; Vázquez, M.A.; Delgado, F. Pyrrolizidine Alkaloids. In *The Alkaloids: Chemistry and Biology*; Hans-Joachim Knölker, H.J., Ed.; Academic Press: Cambridge, UK, 2018; pp. 1–314.
64. Macel, M. Attract and deter: A dual role for pyrrolizidine alkaloids in plant-insect interactions. *Phytochem. Rev.* **2011**, *10*, 75–82. [CrossRef] [PubMed]
65. Livshultz, T.; Kaltenegger, E.; Straub, S.C.; Weitemier, K.; Hirsch, E.; Koval, K.; Mema, L.; Liston, A. Evolution of pyrrolizidine alkaloid biosynthesis in Apocynaceae: Revisiting the defense de-escalation hypothesis. *New Phytol.* **2018**, *218*, 762–773. [CrossRef]

66. Bowers, W.S.; Ohta, T.; Cleere, J.S.; Marsella, P.A. Discovery of insect anti-juvenile hormones in plants. *Science* **1976**, *193*, 542–547. [CrossRef]
67. Kong, C.H.; Hu, F.; Xu, X.H.; Zhang, M.X.; Liang, W.J. Volatile allelochemicals in the *Ageratum conyzoides* intercropped citrus orchard and their effects on mites *Amblyseius newsami* and *Panonychus citri*. *J. Chem. Ecol.* **2005**, *31*, 2193–2203. [CrossRef]
68. Mathai, S.; Nair, V.S.K. Effects of precocene II on last instar larvae of *Spodoptera mauritia* (Lepidoptera: Noctuidae). *Curr. Sci.* **1983**, *52*, 376–377.
69. Oi, C.A.; Ferreira, H.M.; da Silva, R.C.; Bienstman, A.; do Nascimento, F.S.; Wenseleers, T. Effects of juvenile hormone in fertility and fertility-signaling in workers of the common wasp *Vespula vulgaris*. *PLoS ONE* **2021**, *16*, e0250720. [CrossRef]
70. Amsalem, E.; Teal, P.; Grozinger, C.M.; Hefetz, A. Precocene-I inhibits juvenile hormone biosynthesis, ovarian activation, aggression and alters sterility signal production in bumble bee (*Bombus terrestris*) workers. *J. Exp. Biol.* **2014**, *217*, 3178–3185. [CrossRef]
71. Gupta, P.R.; Dogra, G.S. Bioactivity of Precocene II against the potato beetle *Epilachna vigintioctopunctata*. In *Presented in National Symposium on Problems and Prospects of Botanical Pesticides in Integrated Pest Management*; CTRI Press: Rajahmundry, India, 1990; pp. 21–22.
72. Hammond, A.H.; Garle, M.J.; Fry, J.R. Mechanism of toxicity of precocene II in rat hepatocyte cultures. *J. Biochem. Toxicol.* **1995**, *10*, 265–273. [CrossRef] [PubMed]
73. Liang, W.G.; Huang, M.D. Influence of citrus orchard ground cover plants on arthropod communities in China: A review. *Agric. Ecosyst. Environ.* **1994**, *50*, 29–37. [CrossRef]
74. Dicke, M.; Baldwin, I.T. The evolutionary context for herbivore-induced plant volatiles: Beyond the 'cry for help'. *Trends Plant Sci.* **2010**, *15*, 167–175. [CrossRef]
75. Aartsma, Y.; Bianchi, F.J.; van der Werf, W.; Poelman, E.H.; Dicke, M. Herbivore-induced plant volatiles and tritrophic interactions across spatial scales. *New Phytol.* **2017**, *216*, 1054–1063. [CrossRef] [PubMed]
76. Seid, A.; Fininsa, C.; Mekete, T.; Decraemer, W.; Wesemael, W.M. Tomato (*Solanum lycopersicum*) and root-knot nematodes (*Meloidogyne* spp.)—A century-old battle. *Nematology* **2015**, *17*, 995–1009. [CrossRef]
77. Sikandar, A.; Zhang, M.Y.; Wang, Y.Y.; Zhu, X.F.; Liu, X.Y.; Fan, H.Y.; Xuan, Y.H.; Chen, L.J.; Duan, Y.X. *Meloidogyne incognita* (root-knot nematode) a risk to agriculture. *Appl. Ecol. Environ. Res.* **2020**, *18*, 1679–1690. [CrossRef]
78. Lambert, K.; Bekal, S. Introduction to Plant-Parasitic Nematodes. The Plant Health Instructor. Available online: https://www.apsnet.org/edcenter/disandpath/nematode/intro/Pages/IntroNematodes.aspx (accessed on 12 August 2024).
79. den Akker, S.E. Plant–nematode interactions. *Curr. Opin. Plant Biol.* **2021**, *62*, 102035.
80. Pires, D.; Vicente, C.S.L.; Menéndez, E.; Faria, J.M.S.; Rusinque, L.; Camacho, M.J.; Inácio, M.L. The fight against plant-parasitic nematodes: Current status of bacterial and fungal biocontrol agents. *Pathogens* **2022**, *11*, 1178. [CrossRef]
81. Akhter, G.; Zafar, A.; Khan, W.; Jamshed, M. In vitro nemato-toxic potential of some leaf extracts on juvenile mortality of *Meloidogyne incognita* race-3. *Arch. Phytopathol. Plant Prot.* **2018**, *51*, 399–407. [CrossRef]
82. Mamman, A. Nematicidal activity of *Ageratum conyzoides* leaf extract against root-knot nematode (*Meloidogyne javanica*) on eggplant in Jalingo, Nigeria. *Niger. Dutse J. Pure Appl. Sci.* **2023**, *9*, 120–128. [CrossRef]
83. Pavaraj, M.; Karthikairaj, K.; Rajan, M.K. Effect of leaf extract of *Ageratum conyzoides* on the biochemical profile of blackgram *Vigna mungo* infected by root-knot nematode, *Meloidogyne incognita*. *J. Biopest.* **2010**, *3*, 313–316.
84. Levine, J.M.; Adler, P.B.; Yelenik, S.G. A meta-analysis of biotic resistance to exotic plant invasions. *Ecol. Lett.* **2004**, *7*, 975–989. [CrossRef]
85. Reinhart, K.O.; Callaway, R.M. Soil biota and invasive plants. *New Phytol.* **2006**, *170*, 445–457. [CrossRef] [PubMed]
86. Ehrenfeld, J.G. Ecosystem consequences of biological invasions. *Ann. Rev. Ecol. Evol. Syst.* **2010**, *41*, 59–80. [CrossRef]
87. Desmond, O.J.; Manners, J.M.; Stephens, A.E.; Maclean, D.J.; Schenk, P.M.; Gardiner, D.M.; Munn, A.L.; Kazan, K. The *Fusarium* mycotoxin deoxynivalenol elicits hydrogen peroxide production, programmed cell death and defense responses in wheat. *Mol. Plant Pathol.* **2008**, *9*, 435–445. [CrossRef] [PubMed]
88. Ma, L.J.; Geiser, D.M.; Proctor, R.H.; Rooney, A.P.; O'Donnell, K.; Trail, F.; Gardiner, D.M.; Manners, J.M.; Kazan, K. *Fusarium* Pathogenomics. *Annu. Rev. Microbiol.* **2013**, *67*, 399–416. [CrossRef]
89. Javed, S.; Basir, U. Antifungal activity of different extracts of *Ageratum conyzoides* for the management of *Fusarium solani*. *Afr. J. Biotechnol.* **2012**, *11*, 11022–11029.
90. Hazirah, M.F.; Hamizah, O.; Natasya, W.A.W. Antifungal activity of *Ageratum conyzoides* extract against *Fusarium oxysporum* in *Musa* spp. *IOP Conf. Ser. Earth Environ. Sci.* **2023**, *1182*, 012074. [CrossRef]
91. Nguyen, C.C.; Nguyen, T.Q.C.; Kanaori, K.; Binh, T.D.; Dao, X.H.T.; Vang, L.V.; Kamei, K. Antifungal activities of *Ageratum conyzoides* L. extract against rice pathogens *Pyricularia oryzae* Cavara and *Rhizoctonia solani* Kühn. *Agriculture* **2021**, *11*, 1169. [CrossRef]
92. Kong, C.H.; Liang, W.J.; Hu, F.; Xu, X.H.; Wang, P.; Jiang, Y. Allelochemicals and their transformations in *A. conyzoides* intercropped citrus orchard soil. *Plant Soil* **2004**, *264*, 149–157. [CrossRef]
93. Yaguchi, A.; Yoshinari, T.; Tsuyuki, R.; Takahashi, H.; Nakajima, T.; Sugita-Konishi, Y. Isolation and identification of precocenes and piperitone from essential oils as specific inhibitors of trichothecene production by *Fusarium graminearum*. *J. Agric. Food. Chem.* **2009**, *57*, 846–851. [CrossRef] [PubMed]

94. Chahal, R.; Nanda, A.; Akkol, E.K.; Sobarzo-Sánchez, E.; Arya, A.; Kaushik, D.; Dutt, R.; Bhardwaj, R.; Rahman, M.H.; Mittal, V. *Ageratum conyzoides* L. and its secondary metabolites in the management of different fungal pathogens. *Molecules* **2021**, *26*, 2933. [CrossRef] [PubMed]
95. Nasmith, C.G.; Walkowiak, S.; Wang, L.; Leung, W.Y.Y.; Gong, Y.; Johnston, A.; Harris, L.J.; Guttman, D.S.; Subramaniamet, R. Tri6 is a global transcription regulator in the phytopathogen *Fusarium graminearum*. *PLoS Pathog.* **2011**, *7*, e1002266. [CrossRef] [PubMed]
96. Sakuda, S.; Yoshinari, T.; Furukawa, T.; Jermnak, U.; Takagi, K.; Kimura, M.; Yamamoto, T.; Suzuki, M.; Nagasawa, H. Search for aflatoxin and trichothecene production inhibitors and analysis of their modes of action. *Biosci. Biotech. Biochem.* **2016**, *80*, 43–54. [CrossRef]
97. Furukawa, T.; Sakamoto, N.; Suzuki, M.; Kimura, M.; Nagasawa, H.; Sakuda, S. Precocene II, a trichothecene production inhibitor, binds to voltage-dependent anion channel and increases the superoxide level in mitochondria of *Fusarium graminearum*. *PLoS ONE* **2015**, *10*, e0135031. [CrossRef]
98. Noriega, F.G. Juvenile hormone biosynthesis in insects: What is new, what do we know, and what questions remain? *Int. Sch. Res. Notices* **2014**, *1*, 967361. [CrossRef]
99. Batish, D.R.; Singh, H.P.; Kaur, S.; Kohli, R.K. Phytotoxicity of *Ageratum conyzoides* residues towards growth and nodulation of *Cicer arietinum*. *Agric. Ecosyst. Environ.* **2006**, *113*, 399–401. [CrossRef]
100. Barrett, C.F.; Parker, M.A. Coexistence of *Burkholderia*, *Cupriavidus* and *Rhizobium* sp. nodule bacteria on two *Mimosa* species in Costa Rica. *Appl. Environ. Microbiol.* **2006**, *72*, 1198–1206. [CrossRef]
101. Chen, W.M.; James, E.K.; Coenye, T.; Chou, J.H.; Barrios, E.; de Faria, S.M.; Ellio, N.; Sheu, S.Y.; Sprent, J.I.; Vandamme, P. *Burkholderia mimosarum* sp. nov., isolated from root nodules of *Mimosa* spp. from Taiwan and South America. *Int. J. Syst. Evol. Microbiol.* **2006**, *56*, 1847–1851. [CrossRef]
102. Elliott, G.N.; Chou, J.H.; Chen, W.M.; Bloemberg, G.V.; Bontemps, C.; Martínez-Romero, E.; Velázquez, E.; Young, J.P.W.; Sprent, J.I.; James, E.K. *Burkholderia* spp. are the most competitive symbionts of *Mimosa*, particularly under N-limited conditions. *Environ. Microbiol.* **2009**, *11*, 762–778. [CrossRef]
103. Tsyganova, A.V.; Brewin, N.J.; Tsyganov, V.E. Structure and development of the legume-rhizobial symbiotic interface in infection threads. *Cells* **2021**, *10*, 1050. [CrossRef] [PubMed]
104. Mathesius, U. Are legumes different? Origins and consequences of evolving nitrogen fixing symbioses. *J. Plant Physiol.* **2022**, *276*, 153765. [CrossRef] [PubMed]
105. Kato-Noguchi, H. Allelopathy of knotweeds as invasive plants. *Plants* **2022**, *11*, 3. [CrossRef] [PubMed]
106. Kato-Noguchi, H. Allelopathy and allelochemicals of *Imperata cylindrica* as an invasive plant species. *Plants* **2022**, *11*, 2551. [CrossRef] [PubMed]
107. Rice, E.L. *Allelopathy*, 2nd ed.; Academic Press: Orlando, FL, USA, 1984; pp. 1–422.
108. Bais, H.P.; Weir, T.L.; Perry, L.G.; Gilroy, S.; Vivanco, J.M. The role of root exudates in rhizosphere interactions with plants and other organisms. *Annu. Rev. Plant Biol.* **2006**, *57*, 233–266. [CrossRef]
109. Bonanomi, G.; Sicurezza, M.G.; Caporaso, S.; Esposito, A.; Mazzoleni, S. Phytotoxicity dynamics of decaying plant materials. *New Phytol.* **2006**, *169*, 571–578. [CrossRef]
110. Belz, R.G. Allelopathy in crop/weed interactions—An update. *Pest. Manag. Sci.* **2007**, *63*, 308–326. [CrossRef]
111. Cappuccino, N.; Arnason, J.T. Novel chemistry of invasive exotic plants. *Biol. Lett.* **2006**, *2*, 189–193. [CrossRef]
112. Callaway, R.M.; Ridenour, W.M. Novel weapons: Invasive success and the evolution of increased competitive ability. *Front. Ecol. Environ.* **2004**, *2*, 419–426. [CrossRef]
113. Kato-Noguchi, H. The impact and invasive mechanisms of *Pueraria montana* var. *lobata*, one of the world's worst alien species. *Plants* **2023**, *12*, 3066. [CrossRef]
114. Kato-Noguchi, H.; Kato, M. Evolution of the secondary metabolites in invasive plant species *Chromolaena odorata* for the defense and allelopathic functions. *Plants* **2023**, *12*, 521. [CrossRef] [PubMed]
115. Kato-Noguchi, H. Isolation and identification of allelochemicals and their activities and functions. *J. Pesti. Sci.* **2024**, *49*, 1–14. [CrossRef] [PubMed]
116. Kato-Noguchi, H.; Kato, M. Allelopathy and allelochemicals of *Solidago canadensis* L. and *S. altissima* L. for their naturalization. *Plants* **2022**, *11*, 3235. [CrossRef] [PubMed]
117. Kato-Noguchi, H. Invasive mechanisms of one of the world's worst alien plant species *Mimosa pigra* and its management. *Plants* **2023**, *12*, 1960. [CrossRef] [PubMed]
118. Kato-Noguchi, H.; Kurniadie, D. The invasive mechanisms of the noxious alien plant species *Bidens pilosa*. *Plants* **2024**, *13*, 356. [CrossRef]
119. Javaid, N.; Shah, M.H.; Khan, I.H.; Javaid, A.; Waleed, S.M. Herbicidal activity of *Ageratum conyzoides* against *Parthenium*. *Pak. J. Weed Sci. Res.* **2020**, *26*, 137–146. [CrossRef]
120. Negi, B.; Bargali, S.S.; Bargali, K.; Khatri, K. Allelopathic interference of *Ageratum conyzoides* L. against rice varieties. *Curr. Agric. Res. J.* **2020**, *8*, 69–76. [CrossRef]
121. Kato-Noguchi, H. Assessment of the allelopathic potential of *Ageratum conyzoides*. *Biol. Plant.* **2001**, *44*, 309–311. [CrossRef]

122. Erida, G.; Saidi, N.; Hasanuddin, H.; Sampietro, D.A.; Amist, N. Herbicidal effects of *n*-hexane, ethyl acetate and methanol extracts of billygoat weed (*Ageratum conyzoides* L.) leaves on *Amaranthus spinosus* L. growth. *Allelopath. J.* **2021**, *54*, 211–220. [CrossRef]
123. Erida, G.; Saidi, N.; Hasanuddin, H.; Syafruddin, S. Herbicidal effects of ethyl acetate extracts of billygoat weed (*Ageratum conyzoides* L.) on spiny amaranth (*Amaranthus spinosus* L.) growth. *Agronomy* **2021**, *11*, 1991. [CrossRef]
124. Xuan, T.D.; Shinkichi, T.; Hong, N.H.; Khanh, T.D.; Min, C.I. Assessment of phytotoxic action of *Ageratum conyzoides* L. (Billy goat weed) on weeds. *Crop Prot.* **2004**, *23*, 915–922. [CrossRef]
125. Batish, D.R.; Harminder, P.S.; Shalinder, K.; Kohli, R.K. Nature of interference potential of leaf debris of *Ageratum conyzoides* L. *Plant Grow Regul.* **2008**, *57*, 137–144. [CrossRef]
126. Singh, H.P.; Batish, D.R.; Kaur, S.; Kohli, R.K. Phytotoxic interference of *Ageratum conyzoides* with wheat (*Triticum aestivum*). *J. Agron. Crop Sci.* **2003**, *189*, 341–346. [CrossRef]
127. Akter, P.; Begum, R. Allelopathic effects of *Ageratum conyzoides* root exudates on germinability of selected crops: A comparative analysis. *Middle East Res. J. Biol. Sci.* **2024**, *4*, 22–29. [CrossRef]
128. Kong, C.; Hu, F.; Xu, T.; Lu, Y. Allelopathic potential and chemical constituents of volatile oil from *Ageratum conyzoides*. *Allelopath. J.* **1999**, *25*, 2347–2356.
129. Zheng, H.; Wei, N.; Wang, L.; He, P. Effects of *Lantana camara* leaf extract on the activity of superoxide dismutase and accumulation of H_2O_2 in water hyacinth leaf. *J. Plant Physiol. Mol. Biol.* **2006**, *32*, 189.
130. Li, C.; Yang, X.; Tian, Y.; Yu, M.; Shi, S.; Qiao, B.; Zhao, C.; Mao, L. The effects of fig tree (*Ficus carica* L.) leaf aqueous extract on seed germination and seedling growth of three medicinal plants. *Agronomy* **2021**, *11*, 2564. [CrossRef]
131. Mao, X.T.; Xu, R.X.; Gao, Y.; Li, H.Y.; Liu, J.S.; Yang, W.D. Allelopathy of *Alexandrium pacificum* on *Thalassiosira pseudonana* in laboratory cultures. *Ecotoxicol. Environ. Saf.* **2021**, *215*, 112123. [CrossRef] [PubMed]
132. Kong, C.; Fei, F.; Wenju, L.; Weng, P.; Yong, J. Allelopathic potential of *Ageratum conyzoides* at various growth stages in different habitats. *Allelopath. J.* **2004**, *13*, 233–240.
133. Wang, R.; Peng, S.L.; Zeng, R.S.; Ding, L.W.; Xu, Z.F. Cloning, expression and wounding induction of β-caryophyllene synthase gene from *Mikania micrantha* HBK and allelopathic potential of β-caryophyllene. *Allelopathy J.* **2009**, *24*, 35–44.
134. Richter, A.; Seidl-Adams, I.; Köllner, T.G.; Schaff, C.; Tumlinson, J.H.; Degenhardt, J. A small, differentially regulated family of farnesyl diphosphate synthases in maize (*Zea mays*) provides farnesyl diphosphate for the biosynthesis of herbivore-induced sesquiterpenes. *Planta* **2015**, *241*, 1351–1361. [CrossRef] [PubMed]
135. Balasubramani, S.; Kumari, B.D.R.; Moola, A.K.; Sathish, D.; Kumar, G.P.; Srimurali, S.; Rajendran, R.B. Enhanced production of β-caryophyllene by farnesyl diphosphate precursor-treated callus and hairy root cultures of *Artemisia vulgaris* L. *Front. Plant Sci.* **2021**, *12*, 634178. [CrossRef] [PubMed]
136. Wang, H.; Zong, C.; Bai, A.; Yuan, S.; Li, Y.; Yu, Z.; Tian, R.; Liu, T.; Hou, X.; Li, Y. Transcriptome sequencing and gas chromatography-mass spectrometry analyses provide insights into β-caryophyllene biosynthesis in Brassica campestris. *Food Chem. Mol. Sci.* **2022**, *5*, 100129. [CrossRef] [PubMed]
137. Treutter, D. Significance of flavonoids in plant resistance: A review. *Environ. Chem. Lett.* **2006**, *4*, 147. [CrossRef]
138. Weston, L.A.; Mathesius, U. Flavonoids: Their structure, biosynthesis and role in the rhizosphere, including allelopathy. *J. Chem. Ecol.* **2013**, *39*, 283–297. [CrossRef]
139. Mierziak, J.; Kostyn, K.; Kulma, A. Flavonoids as important molecules of plant interactions with the environment. *Molecules* **2014**, *19*, 16240–16265. [CrossRef]
140. Fernández-Aparicio, M.; Masi, M.; Cimmino, A.; Vilariño, S.; Evidente, A. Allelopathic effect of quercetin, a flavonoid from *Fagopyrum esculentum* roots in the radicle growth of *Phelipanche ramosa*: Quercetin natural and semisynthetic analogues were used for a structure-activity relationship investigation. *Plants* **2021**, *10*, 543. [CrossRef]
141. Okunade, A.L. *Ageratum conyzoides* L. (asteraceae). *Fitoterapia* **2002**, *73*, 1–16. [CrossRef]
142. Li, Z.H.; Wang, Q.; Ruan, X.; Pan, C.D.; Jiang, D.A. Phenolics and plant allelopathy. *Molecules* **2010**, *15*, 8933–8952. [CrossRef]
143. Widhalm, J.R.; Dudareva, N. A familiar ring to it: Biosynthesis of plant benzoic acids. *Mol. Plant* **2015**, *8*, 83–97. [CrossRef]
144. Dalton, B.R. The occurrence and behavior of plant phenolic acids in soil environments and their potential involvement in allelochemical interference interactions: Methodological limitations in establishing conclusive proof of allelopathy. In *Principals and Practices in Plant Ecology: Allelochemical Interactions*; Inderjit, Dakshini, K.M.M., Foy, C.L., Eds.; CRC Press: Boca Raton, FL, USA, 1999; pp. 57–74.
145. Inderjit. Plant phenolics in allelopathy. *Bot. Rev.* **1996**, *62*, 186–202. [CrossRef]
146. Einhellig, F.A. Mode of action of allelochemical action of phenolic compounds. In *Chemistry and Mode of Action of Allelochemicals*; Macías, F.A., Galindo, J.C.G., Molino, J.M.G., Cutler, H.G., Eds.; CRC Press: Boca Raton, FL, USA; London, UK; New York, NY, USA; Washington, DC, USA, 2004; pp. 217–238.
147. Šoln, K.; Koce, J.D. Allelopathic root inhibition and its mechanisms. *Allelopath. J.* **2021**, *52*, 181–198. [CrossRef]
148. Paul, S.; Datta, B.K.; Ratnaparkhe, M.B.; Dholakia, B.B. Turning waste into beneficial resource: Implication of *Ageratum conyzoides* L. in sustainable agriculture, environment and biopharma sectors. *Mol. Biotechnol.* **2022**, *64*, 221–244. [CrossRef] [PubMed]
149. Sundufu, A.J.; Shoushan, H. Chemical composition of the essential oils of *Ageratum conyzoides* L. occurring in South China. *Flavour Fragr. J.* **2004**, *19*, 6–8. [CrossRef]

150. Kamboj, A.; Saluja, A.K. *Ageratum conyzoides* L.: A review on its phytochemical and pharmacological profile. *Int. J. Green Pharm.* **2008**, *2*, 59–68. [CrossRef]
151. Singh, S.B.; Devi, W.R.; Marina, A.; Devi, W.I.; Swapana, N.; Singh, C.B. Ethnobotany, phytochemistry and pharmacology of *Ageratum conyzoides* Linn (Asteraceae). *J. Med. Plants Res.* **2013**, *7*, 371–385.
152. Rioba, N.B.; Stevenson, P.C. *Ageratum conyzoides* L. for the management of pests and diseases by small holder farmers. *Ind. Crop Prod.* **2017**, *110*, 22–29. [CrossRef]
153. Yadav, N.; Ganie, S.A.; Singh, B.; Chhillar, A.K.; Yadav, S.S. Phytochemical constituents and ethnopharmacological properties of *Ageratum conyzoides* L. *Phytother. Res.* **2019**, *33*, 2163–2178. [CrossRef]

molecules

MDPI

Communication

Investigation of Trimethylenemethane Cyclopentyl-Annulations as a Strategy to Obtain a Functionalized Angular Triquinane Skeleton †

S. Mason Webber and Wade A. Russu *

Department of Pharmaceutical Sciences, Thomas J. Long School of Pharmacy, University of the Pacific, Stockton, CA 95211, USA; m_webber@u.pacific.edu

* Correspondence: wrussu@pacific.edu

† Dedicated to Professor R. Daniel Little.

Abstract: The angular triquinane carbocyclic ring system is a component of many natural products found in numerous terrestrial and marine plants. A strategy for the synthesis of functionalized angular triquinanes utilizing two trimethylenemethane (TMM)-based [3+2] cycloaddition reactions is presented. This synthetic strategy employs the intermolecular dyil-trapping reaction to give eventual access to the bicyclo[3.3.0]oct-1-en-3-one system. A subsequent [3+2] cycloaddition with a TMM equivalent provides the angular triquinane carbocyclic framework.

Keywords: angular triquinane; trimethylenemethane; TMM; diradical; bicyclo[3.3.0]octenones

1. Introduction

Triquinanes, or polycarbocyclic ring systems composed of three five-membered rings, occur in numerous terrestrial and marine plants. These naturally occurring quinanes have been the subject of synthetic and biological investigations for many decades [1,2]. The five-membered rings can be adjoined in a linear, angular, or propellane pattern. These triquinane molecules possess biological and medicinal value [3–5]. The family of angular triquinanes is characterized by three five-membered rings fused in an angular pattern so that all three rings share a common quaternary carbon in an all-cis-fused fashion. Subfamilies of angular triquinanes are characterized by the position of the methyl groups on the carbocyclic skeleton. Specific angular triquinanes are characterized by their specific structure, including their stereochemistry, such as silphinene, pentalenene, and subergorgic acid. Natural angular triquinanes also serve as biosynthetic precursors to pentalenolactone antibiotics [6]. We are interested in angular triquinanes because we believe that synthetic access to unique derivatives has the potential to deliver new drug lead molecules. This belief leads us not toward the total synthesis of a particular natural product but to the development of a general synthetic methodology to angular triquinane-bearing functional groups readily usable for analog synthesis.

We envisioned a relatively quick access to the angular triquinane ring system, with each ring bearing a synthetically useful functionalization, by the direct [3+2] cycloaddition of a trimethylenemethane (TMM) unit with a functionalized bicyclo[3.3.0]oct-1-en-3-one. This ring system can be accessed by the [3+2] addition of a TMM-based diradical with an olefin (Scheme 1) [7–9]. Reports in the literature of the direct cyclopentyl-annulation of bicyclo[3.3.0]oct-1-en-3-ones toward angular triquinanes are limited to two-step annulations using conjugate-addition reactions with sulfinylallyl anions or bifunctional cuprates, sometimes as one-pot reactions [10–13]. The drawbacks of using bifunctional reagents are additional synthetic reactions, the use of organotin reagents, and potentially sensitive transmetallation steps. There are also examples of Danheiser annulation with similar substrates having been successful in giving access to angular tetra- and triquinanes [14–16]. The drawback of employing this approach is the use of a strong Lewis acid that may not be tolerated by some functional groups. There are no examples of the direct cyclopentyl-annulation of bicyclo[3.3.0]oct-1-en-3-one with a TMM equivalent. We are aware of one other TMM-based diradical strategy toward angular triquinanes that involves the intramolecular [3+2] cycloaddition of a diazene-derived TMM in route to the total synthesis of crinipellin A [17–19]. Our motivation for investigating this synthetic route is the production of a useful intermediate for elaboration into non-natural angular triquinane analogs for the eventual identification of new antimicrobial and anticancer drug lead molecules.

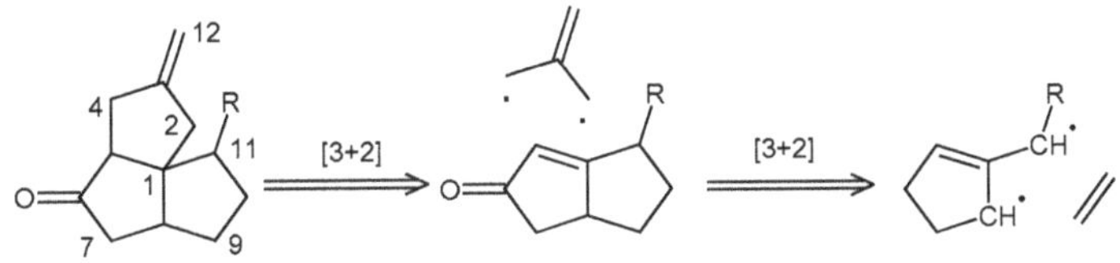

1 2 3

Scheme 1. Retrosynthetic scheme depicting the TMM-based [3+2] cycloaddition strategy to access functionalized angular triquinanes.

2. Results and Discussion

To test our proposed route to the creation of functionalized angular triquinanes, we used diazene **4** (Scheme 2) [20,21]. This compound provides the functionalization of one of the rings of the product in the form of a tether that could be used for the future attachment of various labeling moieties. Heating **4** in degassed acetonitrile to generate the corresponding TMM diyl, in the presence of phenylvinylsulfone as the diylophile, resulted in the formation of **5** as a mixture of isomers. Phenylvinylsulfone was chosen as the diylophile because of its ability to serve as an ethylene and a ketene equivalent [22–24]. The phenylsulfone group was removed under reducing conditions with sodium amalgam to provide compound **6** and reveal relative stereoselectivity in the diyl-trapping reaction. Purification by column chromatography provided the major isomer contaminated with a small amount of the minor isomer. The nuclear magnetic resonance (NMR) spectra (^{1}H, ^{13}C, TOCSY, HMQC, NOSEY) were consistent with the syn-relative stereochemistry of the predominant isomer. The vinyl and ring juncture methine ^{1}H chemical shifts in the major isomer of **6** appeared downfield of the same resonances for the minor isomer. Additionally, the ^{13}C resonances of the ring juncture methine carbon and the ring juncture vinyl were downfield in the case of the major isomer, and the methinyl vinyl carbon was upfield compared to the minor isomer (Figures S4–S6). This type of stereoselectivity in the intermolecular diyl-trapping reaction has previously been observed [25–28]. Attempts at the allylic oxidation of TBDMS-protected **6** in order to access **9** using SeO_2 or chromium oxide were unsuccessful. A multistep procedure through epoxide **7** and allylic alcohol **8** provided the desired enone. The epoxidation of **6** with *m*-chloroperbenzoic acid (mCPBA) exhibited a low facial selectivity and provided a mixture of diastereomers, presumably due to steric hinderance or hydrogen bonding effects of the tether moiety. The integration of the two epoxide methine proton resonances, present in the product ^{1}H NMR spectra, indicated a 4:1 ratio of isomers. This result is consistent with the formation of both cis- and trans-fused products resulting from the epoxidation of similar systems [29]. Attempts to open the epoxide with a strong base to obtain allylic alcohol **8** were unsuccessful, but the phenylselenide ion facilitated nucleophilic opening of the epoxide, followed by oxidative elimination, producing allylic alcohol **8** [30,31]. Finally, oxidation of the allylic alcohols using pyridinum chlorochromate (PCC) provided the desired enone, **9** [32].

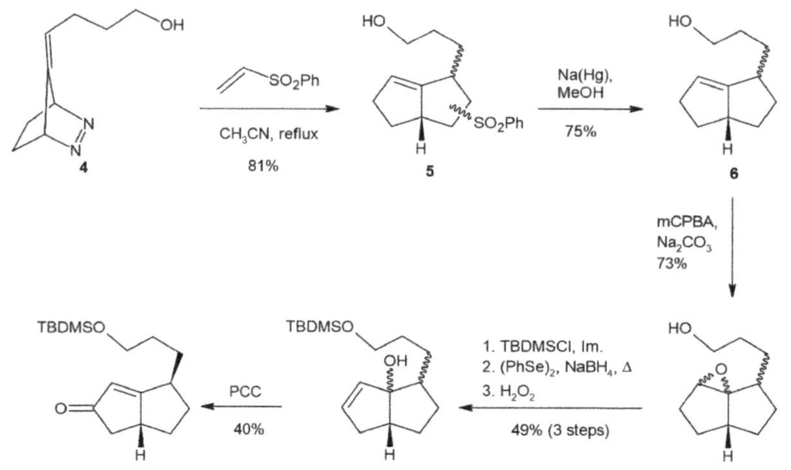

Scheme 2. Synthesis of bicyclo[3.3.0]octeneone **9**.

Enone **9** was subjected to [3+2] cycloaddition with Trost's TMM precursor (Figure 1(1)) [33–37]. To our disappointment, a mixture of isomers was observed as the product. The expectation that the reaction of the bicyclo[3.3.0]oct-1-en-3-one system should exhibit facial selectivity to produce the thermodynamically more stable all-cis-fused angular triquinane product was not realized. The mixture of isomers consisting of the expected all-cis-fused product and the mixed cis–trans-fused product was not readily separable. Mass spectrometry confirmed the presence of **10**. The ^{1}H NMR of the product mixture showed two distinct pairs of methylene vinyl peaks in a 60:40 ratio, estimated by integration (Figure S17). This result is consistent with our initial assignment of the relative stereochemistry of a major isomer of **6** and its subsequent epoxidation result. We believe that the tether present in the allylic position of molecule **9** presents a significant steric effect to the approach of the palladium–TMM complex.

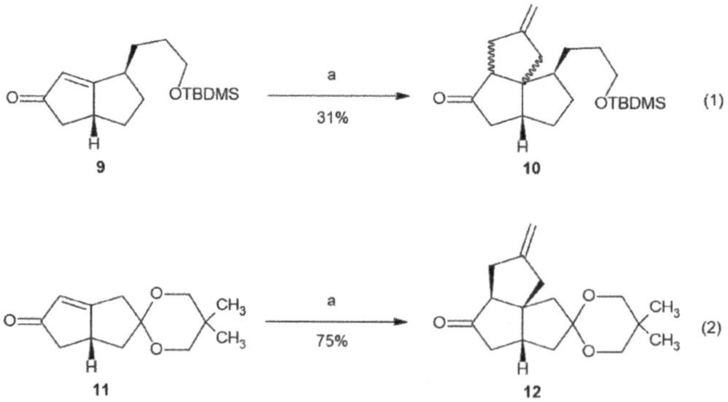

Figure 1. The [3+2] cycloaddition of **9** and **11**. Conditions: a—$TMSCH_2C(CH_2)CH_2OAc$, $Pd(Ph_3P)_4$, dppe, THF, and reflux.

To test whether the tether present in the allylic position was the cause of the creation of the isomeric mixture in the [3+2] cycloaddition reaction, we subjected enone **11** to the same reaction conditions. Only one major isomer, **12**, was isolated from the reaction (Figure 1(2)). It is likely that another isomer was also formed. The NMR (^{1}H, ^{13}C, TOCSY, NOESY) data support product **12** as the all-cis-fused angular triquinane. The NMR chemical shifts were consistent with similar angular triquinanes [13,38]. Notable nuclear Overhauser effects

(NOEs) were observed between C2Hβ and C8H and between the ketal methylene protons and both C2Hα and C5H (Figure 2). It should be noted here that **12** possesses a carbonyl or carbonyl equivalent in each of the cyclopentane rings, thus having the synthetic potential to further functionalize all but the quaternary carbon atom.

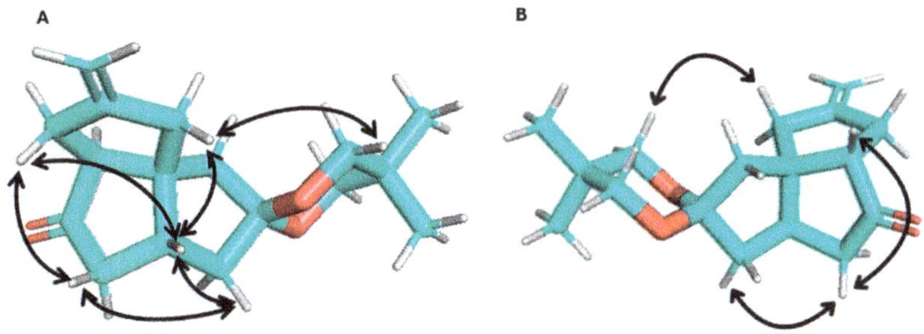

Figure 2. Observed NOEs for compound **12**: (**A**) β-face and (**B**) α-face views.

3. Conclusions

In conclusion, we have demonstrated that the intermolecular trapping of a diazene-derived TMM-based diyl may be used in route, via [3+2] cycloaddition with an olefin, to the bicyclo[3.3.0]oct-1-en-3-one system. The subsequent [3+2] cyclopentyl annulation of this ring system with a TMM equivalent can give access to the angular triquinane carbocyclic framework. The synthesis of **9** was plagued by the persistence of a minor isomer and low facial selectivity in the epoxidation step. Low facial selectivity was again observed in the [3+2] cycloaddition of **9** to give a mixture of two major isomers. To test the hypothesis that the allylic substituent in **9** was the cause of the formation of significant amounts of the undesired isomer, **11** was subjected to the reaction conditions. The reaction formed one major isomer of **12**, and this result supports the hypothesis. The advantage of using this TMM equivalent strategy is that the TMM precursor is commercially available and provides a masked carbonyl in the product. The route presented here complements previous approaches but possesses the drawback of sensitivity to allylic substitution in the bicyclo[3.3.0]oct-1-en-3-one substrate, which reduces facial selectivity, resulting in the formation of significant amounts of undesired isomers.

Supplementary Materials: The following supporting information can be downloaded at: https://www.mdpi.com/article/10.3390/molecules29225358/s1, Experimental procedures and compound characterization data.

Author Contributions: Conceptualization and manuscript preparation, W.A.R.; experiment execution and compound characterization, S.M.W. All authors have read and agreed to the published version of the manuscript.

Funding: This research received no external funding.

Institutional Review Board Statement: Not applicable.

Informed Consent Statement: Not applicable.

Data Availability Statement: No new data were created or analyzed in this study. Data sharing is not applicable to this article.

Acknowledgments: The authors acknowledge the support of the FRC at the University of the Pacific in the form of an SAAG grant. The authors also thank Andreas Franze for recording the 2D NMR data and extend their sincere gratitude to the reviewers and editors for their comments and suggestions, which have improved this manuscript.

Conflicts of Interest: The authors declare no conflicts of interest.

References

1. Qiu, Y.; Lan, H.-J.; Chen, L.-P. Linear Triquinane Sesquiterpenoids: Their Isolation, Structures, Biological Activities, and Chemical Synthesis. *Molecules* **2018**, *23*, 2095. [CrossRef] [PubMed]
2. Mehta, G.; Srikrishna, A. Synthesis of Polyquinane Natural Products: An Update. *Chem. Rev.* **1997**, *97*, 671–719. [CrossRef] [PubMed]
3. Hudlicky, T.; Price, J.D. Anionic Approaches to the Construction of Cyclopentanoids. *Chem. Rev.* **1989**, *89*, 1467–1486. [CrossRef]
4. Jeon, H.; Winkler, J.D. Synthesis of Cyclohexane-Angularly-Fused Triquinanes. *Synthesis* **2021**, *53*, 475–488. [CrossRef] [PubMed]
5. González-Coloma, A.; Gutiérrez, C.; Cabrera, R.; Reina, M. Silphinene Derivatives: Their Effects and Modes of Action on Colorado Potato Beetle. *J. Agric. Food Chem.* **1997**, *45*, 946–950. [CrossRef]
6. Li, H.; Li, H.; Chen, S.; Wu, W.; Sun, P. Isolation and Identification of Pentalenolactone Analogs from *Steptomyces* sp. NRRL S-4. *Molecules* **2021**, *26*, 7377. [CrossRef]
7. Dowd, P. Trimethylenemethane. *J. Am. Chem. Soc.* **1966**, *88*, 2587–2589. [CrossRef]
8. Corwin, L.R.; McDaniel, D.M.; Bushby, R.J.; Berson, J.A. Dimerization and cycloaddition reactions of a trimethylenemethane derivative, 2-isoprpylidenecyclopenta-1,3-diyl. Mechanistic separation of triplet and singlet reactions. *J. Am. Chem. Soc.* **1980**, *102*, 276–287. [CrossRef]
9. Little, R.D. Diyl Trapping and Electroreductive Cyclization Reactions. *Chem. Rev.* **1996**, *96*, 93–114. [CrossRef]
10. Hua, D.H. Asymmetric Total Synthesis of (+)-Pentalenene via Chiral Sulfinylallyl Anions. Hydrolytic Ring Closure of Enol Thioether Ketones. *J. Am. Chem. Soc.* **1986**, *108*, 3835–3837. [CrossRef]
11. Piers, E.; Karunaratne, V. 4-Chloro-2-lithio-1-butene, a Novel Donor-Acceptor Conjunctive Reagent. *J. Org. Chem.* **1983**, *48*, 1774–1776. [CrossRef]
12. Piers, E.; Karunaratne, V. Organotin-based reagents: 4-Chloro-2-lithio-1-butene and related sustances. Methylenecyclopentane annulations. Total synthesis of (±)-$\delta^{9(12)}$-capnellene. *Tetrahedron* **1989**, *45*, 1089–1104. [CrossRef]
13. Dragojlovic, V. Synthesis of a Highly Functionalized Triquinane: Studies Towards a Total Synthesis of Subergorgic Acid and Its Analogues. *Molecules* **2000**, *5*, 674–698. [CrossRef]
14. Schmidt, A.W.; Olpp, T.; Baum, E.; Stiffle, T.; Knölker, H.-J. Organosilicon-Mediated Total Synthesis of the Triquinane Sesquiterpenes (±)-β-Isocomene and (±)-Isocomene. *Org. Biomol. Chem.* **2010**, *8*, 4562. [CrossRef] [PubMed]
15. Danheiser, R.L.; Carini, D.J.; Basak, A. (Trimethylsilyl)cyclopentene Annulation: A Regiocontrolled Approach to the Synthesis of Five-Membered Rings. *J. Am. Chem. Soc.* **1981**, *103*, 1604–1606. [CrossRef]
16. Xu, B.; Xun, W.; Su, S.; Zhai, H. Total Synthesis of (−)-Conidiogenone B, (−)-Conidiogenone, and (−)-Conidiogenol. *Angew. Chem.* **2020**, *132*, 16617–16621. [CrossRef]
17. Lee, H.-Y.; Jung, Y.; Yoon, Y.; Kim, B.G.; Kim, Y. Angularly Fused Triquinanes from Linear Substrates through Trimethylenemethane Diyl [2+3] Cycloaddition Reaction. *Org. Lett.* **2010**, *12*, 2672–2674. [CrossRef]
18. Kang, T.; Kim, W.-Y.; Yoon, Y.; Kim, B.G.; Lee, H.-Y. Tandem Cycloaddition Reactions of Allenyl Diazo Compounds Forming Triquinanes via Trimethylenemethane Diyls. *J. Am. Chem. Soc.* **2011**, *133*, 18050–18053. [CrossRef]
19. Kang, T.; Song, S.B.; Kim, W.-Y.; Kim, B.G.; Lee, H.-Y. Total Synthesi of (−)-Crinipellin A. *J. Am. Chem. Soc.* **2014**, *136*, 10274–10276. [CrossRef]
20. Campopiano, O.; Little, R.D.; Petersen, J.L. Evidence for Hydrogen Atom Abstraction and Loss of Diylophile Stereochemistry in an Intramolecular 1,3-Diyl Trapping Reaction. *J. Am. Chem. Soc.* **1985**, *107*, 3721–3722. [CrossRef]
21. Masjedizadeh, M.R.; Fite, C.; Little, R.D. Direct observation of intermediates involved in the intramolecular diyl trapping reaction. *Tetrahedron Lett.* **1990**, *31*, 1229. [CrossRef]
22. Carr, R.V.C.; Paquette, L.A. An Ethylene and Terminal Olefin Equivalent in [4+2] π Cycloadditions. General Synthetic Application of Phenyl Vinyl Sulfone to the Construction of Functionalized Six-Membered Rings. *J. Am. Chem. Soc.* **1980**, *102*, 853–855. [CrossRef]
23. Little, R.D.; Brown, L. Facile Construction of C10 Modified Prostaglandin Precursors. Diyl Trapping Reactions Using Phenyl Vinyl Sulfoxide and Phenyl Vinyl Sulfone. *Tetrahedron Lett.* **1980**, *21*, 2303–2304. [CrossRef]
24. Little, R.D.; Myong, S.O. Oxidative desulfonylation. Phenyl vinyl sulfone as a ketene synthetic equivalent. *Tetrahedron Lett.* **1980**, *21*, 3339–3342. [CrossRef]
25. Little, R.D.; Bukhari, A.; Venegas, M.G. A new route to linearly fused tricyclopentanoids. Diyl trapping reactions in organic synthesis. *Tetrahedron Lett.* **1979**, *20*, 305–308. [CrossRef]
26. Venegas, M.G.; Little, R.D. Carbon-13 chemical shifts in tricyclo[6.3.0.0^{3,7}] undecanes (linearly fused tricyclopentanoids). *Tetrahedron Lett.* **1979**, *20*, 309–312. [CrossRef]
27. Little, R.D.; Carroll, G.L. Elecrochemical Generation of the Azo Linkage. Synthesis of Bicyclic Azo Compounds, Precursors of 1,3-Diyls. *J. Org. Chem.* **1979**, *44*, 4720–4722. [CrossRef]
28. Whitesell, J.K.; Matthews, R.S. Carbon-13 Chemical Shifts in Bicyclo[3.3.0]octanes. *J. Org. Chem.* **1977**, *24*, 3878–3882. [CrossRef]
29. Van Hijfte, L.; Little, R.D.; Petersen, J.L.; Moeller, K.D. Intramolecular 1,3-Diyl Trapping Reactions. Total Synthesis of (±)-Hypnophilin and (±)-Coriolin. Formation of the Trans-Fused Bicyclo[3.3.0]octane Ring System. *J. Org. Chem.* **1987**, *52*, 4647–4661. [CrossRef]
30. Kissel, C.L.; Rickborn, B. The Base-Induced Rearrangement of Epoxides. IV. Reaction of Cyclohexene Oxide wih Various Lithium Alkylamides. *J. Org. Chem.* **1972**, *37*, 2060–2063. [CrossRef]

31. Sharpless, K.B.; Lauer, R.F. A Mild Method for the Conversion of Epoxides to Allylic Alcohols. The First Organoselenium Reagent. *J. Am. Chem. Soc.* **1973**, *95*, 2697–2699. [CrossRef]
32. Dauben, W.G.; Michno, D.M. Direct oxidation of tertiary allylic alcohols. A simple and effective method for alkylative carbonyl transposition. *J. Org. Chem.* **1977**, *42*, 682–685. [CrossRef]
33. Trost, B.M.; Chan, D.M.T. Regiochemistry of the Cycloaddition of a Substituted Trimethylenemethanepalladium Complex. *J. Am. Chem. Soc.* **1981**, *103*, 5972–5974. [CrossRef]
34. Trost, B.M.; Chan, D.M.T. Intramolecular Carbocyclic [3+2] Cycloaddition via Organopalladium Intermediates. *J. Am. Chem. Soc.* **1982**, *104*, 3733–3735. [CrossRef]
35. Trost, B.M.; Chan, D.M.T. Palladium-Mediated Cycloaddition Approach to Cyclopentanoids. Introduction and Initial Studies. *J. Am. Chem. Soc.* **1983**, *105*, 2315–2325. [CrossRef]
36. Trost, B.M.; Chan, D.M.T. Palladium-Mediated Cycloaddition Approach to Cyclopentanoids. Mechanistic Studies. *J. Am. Chem. Soc.* **1983**, *105*, 2326–2335. [CrossRef]
37. Nanninga, T.N.; Trost, B.M. Palladium-Mediated Cycloaddition Approach to Loganin Aglucon. *J. Am. Chem. Soc.* **1985**, *107*, 1293–1299.
38. Rowley, E.G.; Schore, N.E. The Pauson-Khand Reaction in Triquinane Synthesis: Approaches to Pentalenene, Pentalenic Acid, and Silphinene. *J. Org. Chem.* **1992**, *57*, 6853–6861. [CrossRef]

molecules

MDPI

Article

Efficient Consecutive Synthesis of Fluorinated Isoflavone Analogs, X-Ray Structures, Hirshfeld Analysis, and Anticancer Activity Assessment

Mohammed Salah Ayoup [1,*], Malak Daqa [2], Yousef Salama [3], Rand Hazzam [2], Mohammed B. Hawsawi [4], Saied M. Soliman [5] and Nawaf Al-Maharik [2,*]

[1] Department of Chemistry, College of Science, King Faisal University, Al-Ahsa 31982, Saudi Arabia
[2] Department of Chemistry, Science College, An-Najah National University, P.O. Box 7, Nablus 00970, Palestine; malak.d@najah.edu (M.D.); rand.hazzam@najah.edu (R.H.)
[3] An-Najah Center for Cancer and Stem Cell Research, Faculty of Medicine and Health Sciences, An-Najah National University, P.O. Box 7, Nablus 00970, Palestine; yousef.ut@najah.edu
[4] Department of Chemistry, Faculty of Science, Umm Al-Qura University, Makkah 21955, Saudi Arabia; mbhawsawi@uqu.edu.sa
[5] Department of Chemistry, Faculty of Science, Alexandria University, Alexandria 21321, Egypt; saeed.soliman@alexu.edu.eg
* Correspondence: mayoup@kfu.edu.sa (M.S.A.); n.maharik@najah.edu (N.A.-M.)

Abstract: The synthesis of 7-*O*-carboxymethyl-4′-fluoroisoflavone **4** and 7-*O*-carboxymethyl-4′-fluoro-2-trifluormethylisoflavone **7** involved the cyclization of 2,4-dihydroxy-4′-fluoro deoxybenzoin **1**, followed by 7-*O*-alkylation with methyl bromoacetate and subsequent acid-catalyzed hydrolysis. The structures of the novel compounds were validated using a range of techniques, including XRD crystallography (^{1}H, ^{19}F, ^{13}C)-NMR, and IR. Only inter-halogen contacts were detected in **5**, while they were completely lacking in **2** and **4**, owing to the presence of crystalline ethanol in the crystal structure. The %F...F in **5** was 12.2% based on Hirshfeld calculations. The aromatic π-π stacking interactions were important only in **2** and **4** but not observed in **5**. Isoflavones **4**, **5**, and **7** displayed anticancer activity against MCF-7 cancer cells, with IC_{50} values of 13.66, 15.43, and 11.73 μM, respectively.

Keywords: 4′-fluoroisflavones; 7-*O*-carboxmethyl-4′-fluoroisoflavone; XRD crystallography; anticancer; MCF7 cancer cells

1. Introduction

Scientists and health enthusiasts have expressed significant interest in isoflavones owing to their fascinating properties and prospective health benefits. Isoflavones are the primary subgroup of a broader category of isoflavonoids, which collectively form a subset of flavonoids. Unlike other flavonoid subclasses, isoflavones demonstrate a restricted distribution throughout 20 plant families, attributable to the scarce presence of isoflavone synthase, which is a crucial enzyme involved in the synthesis of isoflavones [1–3]. Soybeans serve as the primary source of isoflavones, predominantly in glycosylated forms, including the following prominent isoflavone aglycones: genistein, daidzein, glycitein, and biochanin A (Figure 1).

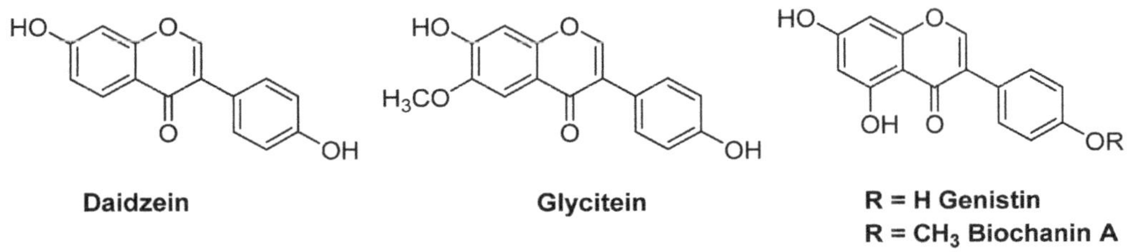

Figure 1. The predominant isoflavones found in soy.

Plant isoflavones can be classified into three categories: isoflavone glycosides, prenylated derivatives, and isoflavones of basic substitution patterns such as hydroxy, methoxy, methylenedioxy, hydroxymethyl, and acetyl patterns [3]. Furthermore, in whole-cell biotransformation, microbes such as fungi and actinomycetes have been used to synthesize non-plant-chlorinated isoflavones, as well as simple and complex isoflavones [3–5]. Isoflavones are well known for their high pharmacological activity and low toxicity, making them a focus of interest in medicinal research and development [5,6]. They play an important role in plant growth and development, as well as in the prevention of bacterial infections and illnesses [7–9]. Notably, they demonstrate a diverse range of biological capacities, encompassing antibacterial [10], antifungal [11], antiviral [12], anticancer [13–15], anti-inflammatory [16], antiplatelet [17], and antiaging [18] properties. Isoflavones have estrogenic effects as they share structural and functional similarities with 17β-estradiol, the primary form of estrogen in the human body. They predominantly bind to estrogen receptors (ERs), specifically ER-α and ER-β [19]. Epidemiological studies have revealed that Asian women have a reduced incidence of breast cancer, the most common malignant tumor among women, in contrast to their Western counterparts, which is a difference ascribed to their elevated consumption of phytoestrogens [20]. Thus, phytoestrogens may function as a viable strategy in the prevention and treatment of breast cancer via mechanisms such as estrogen receptor modulation and anti-angiogenesis [21].

Despite the potential of natural isoflavones for pharmaceutical development, their advancement in the drug discovery process is impeded by various issues, including inadequate solubility, bioavailability, and selectivity [22]. Various efforts have been made to improve the therapeutic effectiveness of isoflavones by including functional groups such as halogens, amino groups, and amino acids [22]. Fluorinated pharmaceuticals have considerable emphasis in pharmaceutical science, with around 20% of medications containing one or more fluorine atoms [23]. The diminutive atomic size and elevated electronegativity of fluorine significantly influence the characteristics of medicinal compounds. These characteristics encompass drug–target interactions, selectivity, metabolic stability, acidity or basicity, membrane permeability, and toxicity. The fluorine atom can function as a bioisostere for amino and hydroxyl groups, as well as hydrogen atoms, modifying the processes of pharmacological action and their impacts on biological systems [24]. The incorporation of fluorine into an aryl ring or other π-system enhances lipophilicity due to the resonance donation of fluorine's lone-pair electrons [25].

To further advance our endeavors in identifying potential therapeutic candidates, we introduced the synthesis of the novel fluorinated isoflavone-bearing carboxymethyl group at the 7-*O*-position. The anticancer potential of these compounds was subsequently assessed against the MCF-7, B16F10, and MEF-1 cell lines. An analysis of this unique chemical's structure was conducted utilizing IR, (^{1}H, ^{19}F, ^{13}C)-NMR, HR ESI-MS, and single-crystal XRD.

2. Results

Schemes 1 and 2 illustrate the synthetic procedures for the new fluorinated isoflavone **4** and **7** analogs, starting with 2,4-dihydroxy-4′-fluorodeoxybenzoin **1**. A highly efficient and pure synthesis of 4′-fluoro-7-hydroxyisoflavone **2** was achieved by formylating and cyclizing deoxybenzoin **1** using dry DMF in the presence of $BF_3.Et_2O$ and methanesulfonyl chloride (CH_3SO_2Cl) at a temperature of 70 °C [26]. Deprotonation of the 7-OH group of isoflavone **2** with non-nucleophilic potassium *tert*-butoxide (*t*-BuOK) at ambient temperature under an N_2 atmosphere generated the phenoxide. Subsequently, the phenoxide was treated with methyl bromoacetate to produce methyl 2-((3-(4-fluorophenyl)-4-oxo-4*H*-chromen-7-yl)oxy)acetate **3** in excellent yields. The desired acid **4** was obtained in high yield and purity by subjecting ester **3** to *p*-toluenesulfonic acid-catalyzed hydrolysis in formic acid at 75 °C.

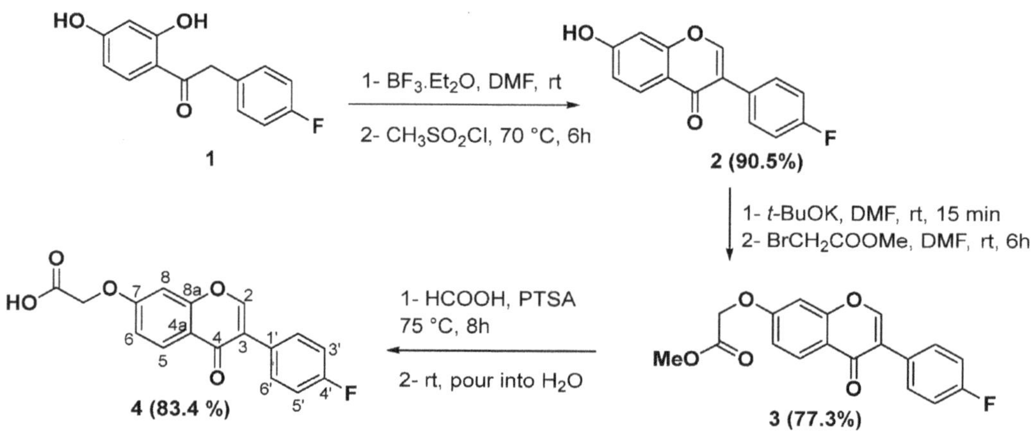

Scheme 1. Total synthetic pathway of 2-((3-(4-fluorophenyl)-4-oxo-4*H*-chromen-7-yl)oxy)acetic acid **4**.

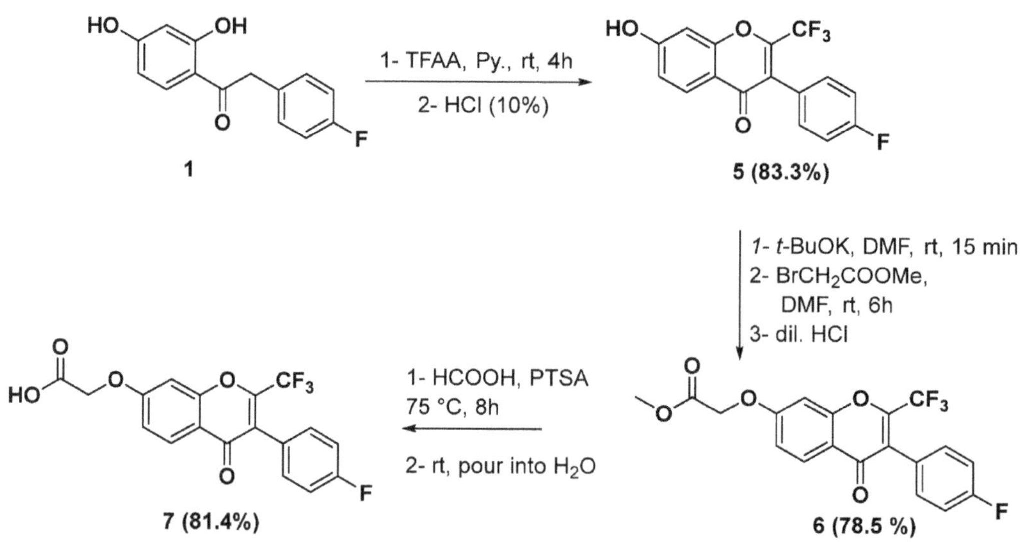

Scheme 2. Total synthetic pathway of 2-((3-(4-fluorophenyl)-4-oxo-2-(trifluoromethyl)-4H-chromen-7-yl)oxy)acetic acid **7**.

Hydroxyl groups were acylated in deoxybenzoin **1** with an excess of trifluoroacetic anhydride (TFAA) in dry pyridine under cooling, followed by the Baker–Venkataraman rearrangement and Allan–Robinson reaction, which afforded 3-(4-fluorophenyl)-7-hydroxy-2-(trifluoromethyl)-4*H*-chromen-4-one **5** in high yield (Scheme 2). After being treated with *t*-BuOK, the latter chemical **5** was subjected to 7-*O*-alkylation with methyl bromoacetate, resulting in the formation of methyl 2-((3-(4-fluorophenyl)-4-oxo-2-(trifluoromethyl)-4*H*-chromen-7-yl)oxy)acetate **6**. Upon treatment with a catalytic quantity of *p*-toluenesulfonic acid in formic acid at 75 °C, this compound produced the intended acid with a high yield and purity. The structures of the synthesized compounds were confirmed using IR, ^{1}H NMR, ^{13}C NMR (DEPTQ), HRMS and ^{19}F NMR spectroscopy. IR spectra exhibited a broad band in the range of 3262–3204 cm^{-1}, indicating the presence of phenolic OH groups for compounds **2** and **5**; additionally, the C=O group manifested as a sharp band in the region of 1763–1624 cm^{-1} for compounds **2**–**7**.

The structures of the synthesized compounds were confirmed using IR, ^{1}H NMR, ^{13}C NMR (DEPTQ), and ^{19}F NMR spectroscopy. IR spectra exhibited a broad band in the range of 3262–3204 cm^{-1}, indicating the presence of phenolic OH groups for compounds **2** and **5**; additionally, the C=O group manifested as a sharp band in the region of 1763–1624 cm^{-1} for compounds **2**–**7**. The ^{1}H NMR spectra of the final product **4** exhibited six resonances corresponding to eight aromatic protons and one peak for methylene protons at 4.91 ppm. A singlet at 8.49 ppm was assigned to H-2. A doublet of doublets for two protons (H-2′,6′) at 7.63 ppm, with $^{3}J_{H2'\text{-}H3'}$ = 8.7 Hz and $^{4}J_{H2'\text{-}F}$ = 5.6 Hz, and another doublet of doublets appearing as a triplet for two protons (H-3′,5′) at 7.14 ppm, with $^{3}J_{H2'\text{-}H3'}$ = 8.7 Hz and $^{3}J_{H2'\text{-}F}$ = 8.7 Hz, were designated. The DEPTQ spectra displayed fifteen peaks, and the positioning of the F atom at the 4-position was validated by the $^{1}J_{C4',F}$ value of 244 Hz, in conjunction with the $^{2}J_{C,F}$, $^{3}J_{C,F}$, and $^{4}J_{C,F}$ values of 21.2, 8.2, and 3.1 Hz, respectively, which corresponded with the expected values. The ^{1}H NMR of isoflavone **7** was distinguished by the absence of the H-2 proton. The DEPTQ spectra for compound 7 indicated the positioning of the CF_3 group at the C-2 site, corroborated by a quartet between 119.3 and 147.0 ppm (C-2), with $^{1}J_{C,F}$ = 275 Hz and $^{2}J_{C,F}$ = 35.5 Hz. Finally, the FNMR of compounds 4 and 7 showed a singlet signal at δ_F -114.22 (s, F) and two different signals at δ_F −62.77 (CF_3), −113.38 (1F) for compounds **4** and **7**, respectively.

3. Crystal Structure Description

The X-ray structure of compounds **2**, **4**, and **5**, showing the atom numbering for the heavy atoms, is presented in Figure 2. The crystal parameters and some important bond distances and angles are depicted in Tables 1 and 2, respectively. The structure of the three compounds comprised a planar 4*H*-chromen-4-one moiety with the *p-fluorophenyl* group as a substituent at C3. The 4*H*-chromen-4-one and fluorophenyl moieties were not in the same plane, whereas the mean planes between the two moieties showed different degrees of twists in the three compounds. The twist angles were 41.43, 32.30, and 62.22° for **2**, **4**, and **5**, respectively. The values of the twist angles were close to one another for both **2** and **4**, while it was significantly higher in **5**, which could be attributed to the presence of the trifluoromethyl substituent at C2. Hence, the presence of two bulky substituents in the neighborhood increased the twist angle between the 4H-chromen-4-one and fluorophenyl moieties due to the steric–electronic factors. Another interesting difference between the three compounds was the presence of a crystal solvent (methanol) in the case of compounds **2** and **4** but not in **5**, which had a significant impact on the molecular packing of the studied compounds.

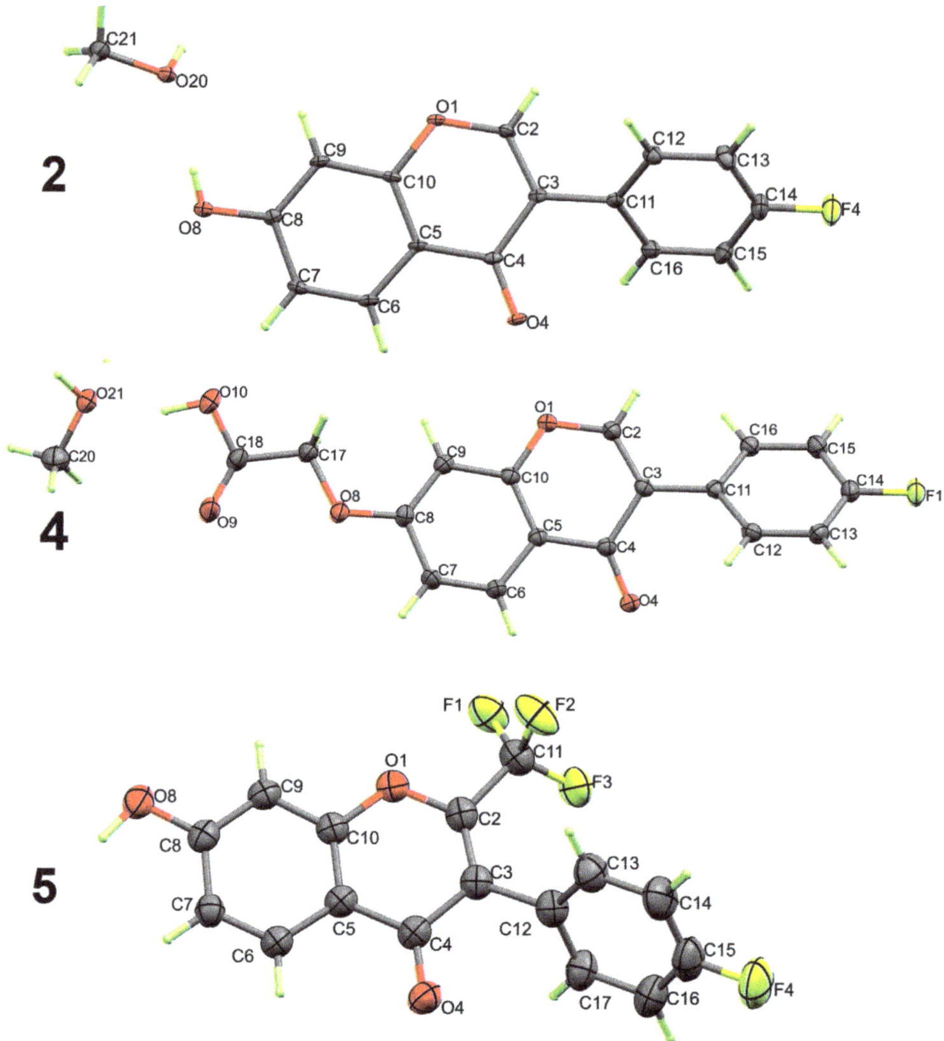

Figure 2. Structure with atom numbering for **2**, **4**, and **5**.

The molecular packing of the three compounds was controlled by the O-H. . .O hydrogen bonds shown in Figure 3. For **5**, the O-H, which is the hydrogen bond donor, makes with carbonyl oxygen (O4), which is the hydrogen acceptor for the significantly strong O8-H8. . .O4 hydrogen bond, where the hydrogen-to-acceptor (A) distance is only 1.70(2) Å, and the donor (D)-to-acceptor (A) distance is 2.664(3) Å. In addition, there is another relatively longer C7-H7. . .O4 interaction where the D. . .A distance is 3.092(3) Å. The presence of the methanol molecule as a crystal solvent in the case of **2** increases the number of O. . .H interactions. The O8-H8. . .O20 and O20-H20. . .O4 hydrogen bonds, which have H. . .A distances of 1.91(4) and 1.91(3) Å, respectively, in addition to the C2-H2. . .O4 interaction with the D. . .A distance of 3.121(4) Å are the important O. . .H contacts. Moreover, compound **4** not only has a methanol molecule as a crystal solvent but also has the polar COOH in its structure, which maximizes the hydrogen bonding interaction in this case (Table 3).

Table 1. Crystal data for the studied compounds.

Compound	2	5	4
CCDC	2382565	2382566	2382567
Empirical formula	$C_{16}H_{13}FO_4$	$C_{16}H_8O_3F_4$	$C_{18}H_{15}FO_6$
Formula weight	288.26	324.22	346.3
Temperature/K	100	173	173
Crystal system	monoclinic	orthorhombic	triclinic
Space group	$P2_1/c$	*Pccn*	*P-1*
a/Å	6.3586(2)	26.4115(18)	9.2015(5)
b/Å	33.5685(13)	13.5418(11)	9.2999(5)
c/Å	6.7957(4)	7.7907(4)	9.8368(6)
α/°	90	90	89.288(5)
β/°	107.328(5)	90	71.493(5)
γ/°	90	90	86.818(5)
Volume/Å^3	1384.70(11)	2786.4(3)	796.99(8)
Z	4	8	2
ρ_{calc}g/cm^3	1.383	1.546	1.443
μ/mm^{-1}	0.108	1.248	0.991
F(000)	600	1312	360
Crystal size/mm^3	0.2 × 0.04 × 0.02	0.14 × 0.08 × 0.015	0.14 × 0.06 × 0.04
Radiation	Mo Kα (λ = 0.71073)	Cu Kα (λ = 1.54184)	Cu Kα (λ = 1.54184)
2Θ range for data collection/°	4.854 to 58.114	6.694 to 163.266	9.482 to 133.29
Index ranges	$-8 \le h \le 8, -43 \le k \le 45, -9 \le l \le 9$	$-30 \le h \le 32, -16 \le k \le 16, -9 \le l \le 9$	$-10 \le h \le 9, -9 \le k \le 11, -11 \le l \le 11$
Reflections collected	27,429	25,327	14,066
Independent reflections	3374 [R_{int} = 0.0848, R_{sigma} = 0.0681]	2911 [R_{int} = 0.0847, R_{sigma} = 0.0312]	2774 [R_{int} = 0.0258, R_{sigma} = 0.0183]
Data/restraints/parameters	3374/0/193	2911/1/212	2774/2/235
Goodness-of-fit on F^2	1.218	1.07	1.039
Final R indexes [I ≥ 2σ (I)]	R_1 = 0.1001, wR_2 = 0.1961	R_1 = 0.0596, wR_2 = 0.1810	R_1 = 0.0350, wR_2 = 0.0981
Final R indexes [all data]	R_1 = 0.1396, wR_2 = 0.2092	R_1 = 0.0785, wR_2 = 0.2073	R_1 = 0.0371, wR_2 = 0.1002
Largest diff. peak/hole/e Å^{-3}	0.42/−0.31	0.28/−0.33	0.27/−0.23

Table 2. Bond lengths (Å) and angles (°) for **2**, **4**, and **5**.

Bond	Length/Å	Bond	Length/Å	Bond	Length/Å
2		**4**		**5**	
F4-C14	1.365(4)	F1-C11	1.328(3)	C7-C8	1.409(3)
O1-C2	1.346(4)	F2-C11	1.324(3)	C8-C9	1.381(3)
O1-C10	1.375(4)	F3-C11	1.327(3)	O1-C2	1.360(3)
O4-C4	1.251(4)	F4-C15	1.357(5)	O1-C10	1.379(3)
O8-C8	1.343(4)	O8-C8	1.356(3)	O4-C4	1.234(3)
Bond	**Length/Å**	**Bonds**	**Angle/°**	**Bonds**	**Angle/°**
C2-O1-C10	118.9(2)	C2-O1-C10	118.93(18)	F3-C11-C2	112.3(2)
C8-O8-H8	109.5(11)	C8-O8-H8	106.0(16)	F1-C11-F3	106.50(19)
O1-C2-C3	125.7(3)	O1-C2-C11	108.1(2)	C3-C12-C17	121.2(2)
C2-C3-C11	119.7(3)	C3-C2-C11	126.4(2)	C13-C12-C17	119.4(3)
C2-O1-C10	118.9(2)	C2-O1-C10	118.93(18)	F3-C11-C2	112.3(2)

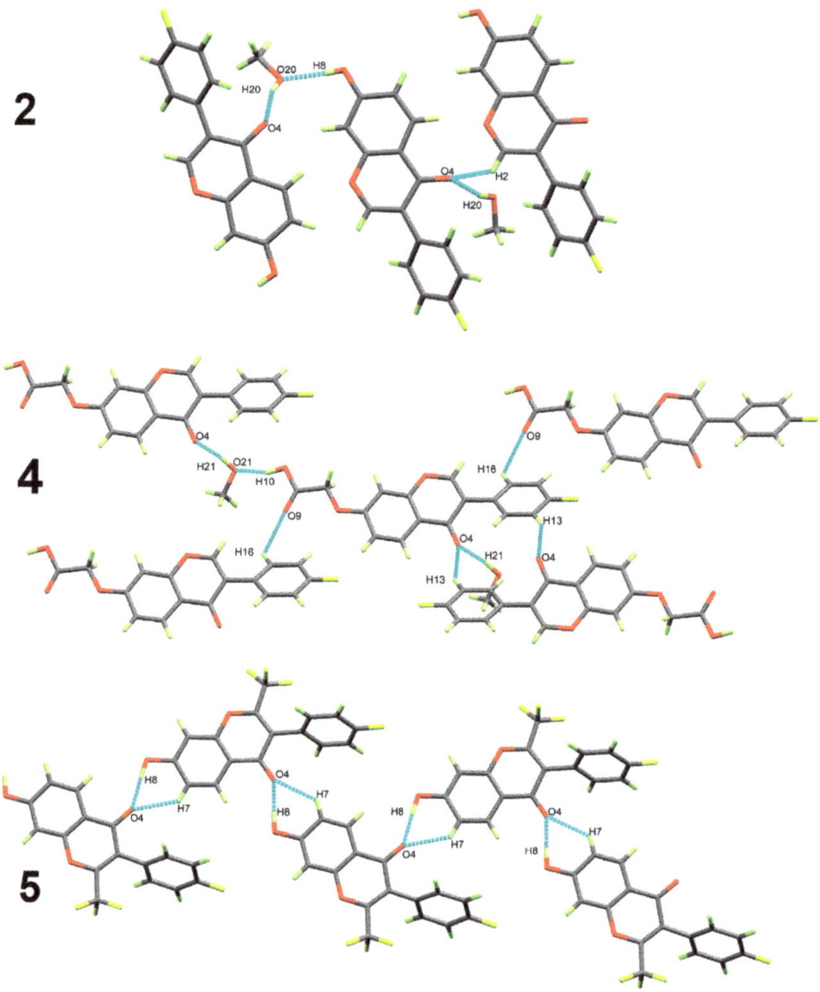

Figure 3. The hydrogen bond packing views for **2**, **4**, and **5**.

Table 3. Hydrogen bonds for **2**, **4**, and **5** [Å and °].

D-H...A	d(D-H)	d(H...A)	d(D...A)	<(DHA)	Symm. Code
2					
O8-H8...O20	0.75(4)	1.91(4)	2.664(4)	175.7(16)	
O20-H20...O4	0.81(4)	1.91(3)	2.690(4)	162(2)	−1 + x,1/2 − y, −1/2 + z
C2-H2...O4	0.95	2.57	3.121(4)	117	−1 + x, y, z
4					
O10-H10...O21	0.960(19)	1.667(19)	2.5945(18)	161.2(18)	
O21-H21...O4	0.969(18)	1.704(18)	2.6674(14)	171.8(17)	1 + x, −1 + y, −1 + z
C13-H13...O4	0.95	2.46	3.3157(16)	150	−x, 1 − y, 2 − z
C16-H16...O9	0.95	2.59	3.2019(18)	123	−1 + x, 1 + y, z
5					
O8-H8...O4	0.97(2)	1.70(2)	2.664(3)	176.1(18)	−x, −1/2 + y, −1/2 − z
C7-H7...O4	0.95	2.38	3.092(3)	131	−x, −1/2 + y, −1/2 − z

In addition, the molecular packing of the studied compounds showed a number of π-π stacking interactions. The shortest π-π contacts in **2**, **4**, and **5** were the C7. . .C4 (3.408(5) Å), C8. . .C16 (3.280(2) Å), and C4. . .C9 (3.418(3) Å) interactions (Table 4). Many of these short aromatic–aromatic separations are shown in Figure 4, which support the supramolecular structure of the studied systems.

Table 4. The important π-π contacts and their distances in **2**, **4**, and **5**.

2			4			5		
C10. . .C10	3.432(5)	x, 1/2 − y, −1/2 + z	**C16. . .C2**	3.384(2)	−x, 1 − y, 1 − z	**C4. . .C9**	3.418(3)	x, 1/2 − y, −1/2 + z
C6. . .C6	3.430(5)	x, 1/2 − y, −1/2 + z	**C2. . .C15**	3.328(2)	−x, 1 − y, 1 − z	**C5. . .C10**	3.464(3)	x, 1/2 − y, −1/2 + z
C8. . .C4	3.498(5)	x, 1/2 − y, −1/2 + z	**C8. . .C8**	3.430(2)	1 − x, −y, 1 − z	**C6. . .C10**	3.421(3)	x, 1/2 − y, −1/2 + z
C7. . .C4	3.408(5)	x, 1/2 − y, −1/2 + z	**C10. . .C4**	3.490(2)	1 − x, 1 − y, 1 − z	**C15. . .C16**	3.464(5)	x, 1.5 − y, −1/2 + z
			C8. . .C16	3.280(2)	1 − x, 1 − y, 1 − z			

2

4

5

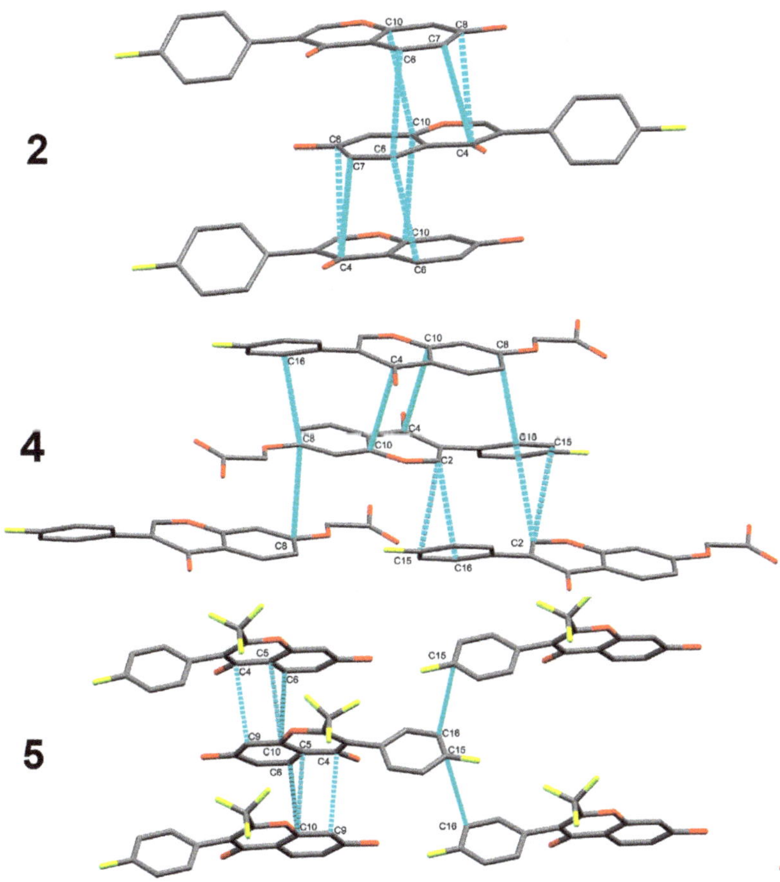

Figure 4. The π-π stacking interactions in **2**, **4**, and **5**.

It is worth noting that compound **5** is the only one that showed an interhalogen interaction (Figure 5). In this case, there was a short interhalogen F1. . .F2 interaction (2.837(2) Å) observed in **5**, which might be attributed to the absence of a solvent in the crystal structure. The presence of a methanol molecule as a crystal solvent could make further separation between the molecules in the crystals possible, which would decrease the possibility of interhalogen interactions, as found in **2** and **4**.

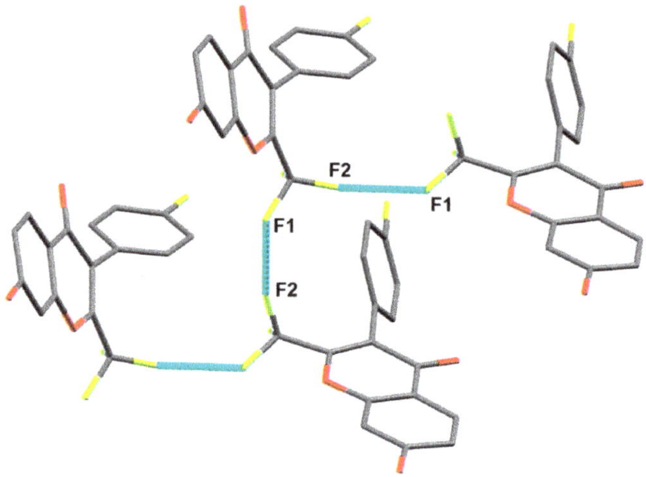

Figure 5. The interhalogen interaction in **5**.

4. Topology Analysis

Topology analysis, with the aid of Hirshfeld calculations, provides a full picture of all possible intermolecular interactions in the crystal structure and plays an important role in crystal stability. Even contacts that contribute a small amount to the molecular packing could be analyzed using this tool [27,28]

The analysis of molecular packing was performed using Hirshfeld topology calculations. The red spots in the d_{norm} map are related to short significant contacts in the studied systems (Figure 6). In **5**, the O...H and the interhalogen F...F interactions were the most important, while in both **2** and **4**, the important contacts were the O...H and F...H interactions. Additionally, there are many important C...C interactions in **4** that are related to the π-π interactions, where the C2...C15 (3.328 Å) and C8...C16 (3.280 Å) interactions are the shortest (Table 5). In addition, O20...H8 (1.684 Å), O4...H21 (1.691 Å), and O4...H8 (1.683 Å) are the most important O...H contacts in **2, 4,** and **5**, respectively. F4...H15 (2.481 Å) in **2** is slightly shorter than F1...H7 (2.489 Å) in **4**.

Table 5. Interaction distances for the short contacts in the compounds studied.

Contact	Distance	Contact	Distance	Contact	Distance
2		**4**		**5**	
O4...H2	2.511	O8...H15	2.575	O4...H7	2.299
O1...H6	2.56	O9...H16	2.517	O4...H8	1.683
O20...H8	1.684	O4...H13	2.345	F1...F2	2.837
O20...H7	2.541	O4...H21	1.691		
O4...H20	1.745	O4...H13	2.345		
F4...H15	2.481	F1...H7	2.489		
		C2...C15	3.280		
		C2...C16	3.384		
		C8...C16	3.280		

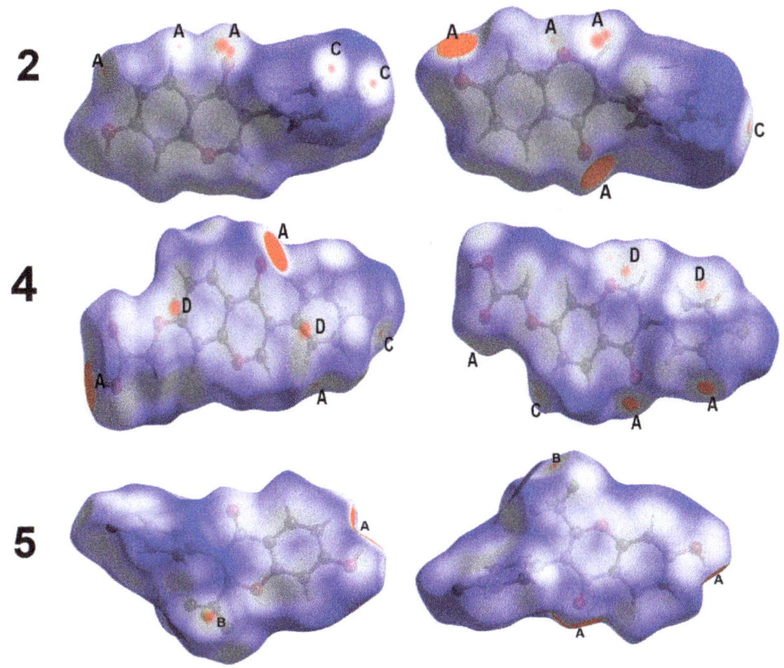

Figure 6. Hirshfeld d_{norm} maps showing important contacts in the studied compounds: O. . .H (A), F. . .F (B), F. . .H (C), and C. . .C (D).

In addition, the fingerprint plots for the important contacts are presented in Figure 7. The fingerprint plot further indicated the importance of the contacts presented in Figure 6. Also, the area of the fingerprint plot gave the percentage of each contact. The %O. . .H contacts in compounds **2**, **4**, and **5** were 23.2, 26.4, and 15.3%, respectively, while %F. . .H contacts were 10.0 and 9.8% for **2** and **4**, respectively. For **5**, the %F. . .F contact was 12.2%, while for **4**, the %C. . .C contact was 7.9%.

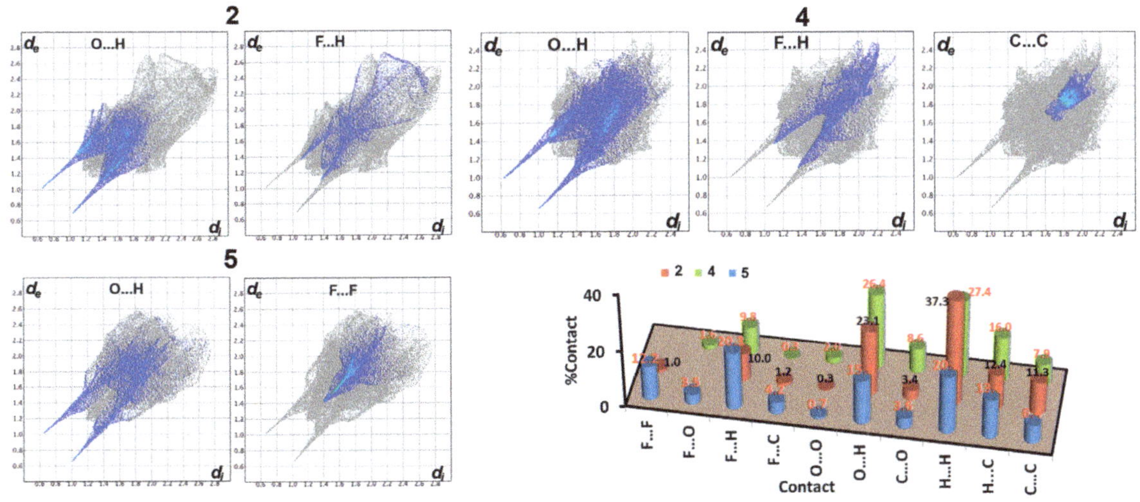

Figure 7. Fingerprint plots for the important contacts and %contacts in the studied compounds.

In Figure 8, the shape index maps of the studied compounds are presented. No red/blue triangles are observed in the shape index map of **5,** while the opposite is true for **2** and **4**. Hence, the π-π stacking interactions were important only in compounds **2** and **4**. It is worth noting that the C. . .C contacts are relatively longer in **2** than those found in **4**. In the former, the shortest C. . .C contact distance is 3.408 Å.

2 **4** **5**

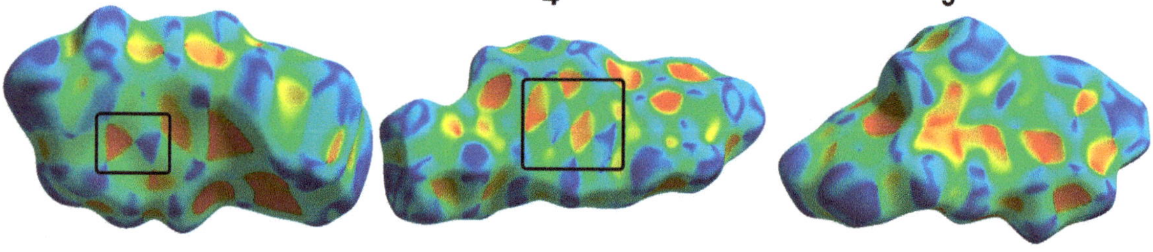

Figure 8. Shape index maps for the studied compounds.

5. Anticancer Activity

Breast cancer is the most prevalent cancer among women and the second most common disease globally [29,30]. The MCF-7 cell line is a typical model for human breast cancer that is dependent on estrogen [31]. MCF-7 cells, which are part of the luminal A molecular subtype, not only express progesterone receptors but also lack HER2/neu overexpression [32,33]. Upon exposure to the main isoflavones, genistein, and daidzein, which share structural and functional similarities with 17-estradiol, it was observed that the binding affinity of genistein to estrogen receptors of alpha (ERα) and beta (ERβ) was one to three orders of magnitude lower than that of 17-estradiol [34–36]. Studies were conducted to evaluate the impact of varying doses of isoflavones **7**, **4**, **5** and daidzein on cell proliferation in the highly metastatic murine B16F10 and human amelanotic MCF-7 breast cancer cell lines, as depicted in Figure 9A–C. The proliferation of MCF-7 cells was selectively suppressed by isoflavones, whereas B16F10 cells were not, in a concentration-dependent manner following 24 h of in vitro treatment. Conversely, the carrier treatment (DMSO) had no effect on cell proliferation (0 μM; Figure 9A–C).

For MCF-7 cells, the doses of isoflavones **7**, **4**, **5,** and daidzein that caused a 50% growth inhibition (IC_{50}) were 11.23, 13.66, 15.43, and 11.87 μM, respectively, as shown in Figure 9B, C and Table 6. Daidzein and the three fluoroisoflavones studied showed significant activity against the MCF-7 cell line, activating the apoptotic pathway and inducing cell death in a dose-dependent manner. Our findings indicate that substituting 4′-OH with F and replacing the H-atom with the CF_3 group did not influence the anticancer efficacy of daidzein. Moreover, we also investigated the impact of the isoflavones presented to MCF-7 cells on B16F10 melanoma cells. Following 24 h of exposure to isoflavones **7**, **4**, **5**, and daidzein at the indicated concentration, as shown in Figure 10A–C, it was confirmed that isoflavones have little impact on B16F10 cells when administered at high doses. Unlike B16F10 melanoma cells, breast cancer (BC) and other hormone-sensitive malignancies rely on estrogen receptor (ER) signaling as a crucial control mechanism for cell division, population growth, and survival. Our results corroborate with previous research indicating that isoflavones, by virtue of their structural and functional resemblance to 17-estradiol, suppress the growth and cell migration of breast cancer cells [36]. Our findings support other studies which state that isoflavones inhibit the proliferation and migration of breast cancer cells [36]. It is interesting that our study showed isoflavones to have less of an effect on B16F10 melanoma cell lines. The dose-limiting toxicity of anticancer drugs is called cytotoxicity. According to earlier studies [37], mouse embryonic fibroblasts (MEF-1) can be used to evaluate the toxicity of non-malignant cells. When 25 μM of isoflavones was introduced, MEF-1 did not decrease proliferation (Figure 10D). These findings support the idea that isoflavones improve anti-proliferative effects on cancer cells, lowering cytotoxicity and requiring less medication.

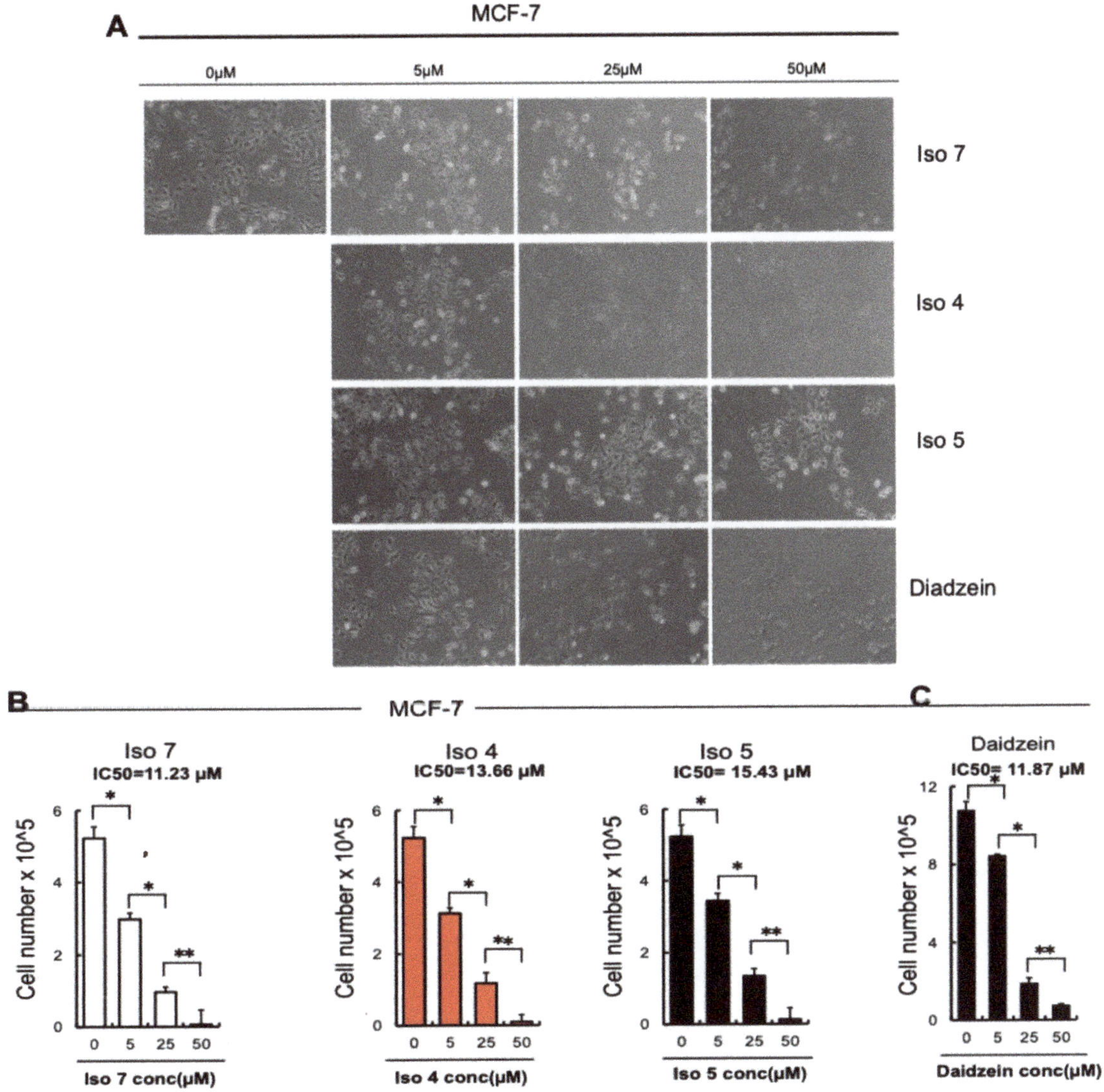

Figure 9. The synthetic isoflavones **4**, **5**, **7**, and daidzein were added in varying concentrations to MCF-7 cells. (**A**) Macroscopic images of MCF-7 cells under an inverted microscope after 24 h of treatment with **4**, **5**, **7**, and daidzein or DMSO as a control (n = 3 groups). (magnification 20×). (**B**,**C**). Isoflavones at the indicated concentrations were applied to human MCF-7 cells. After 24 h, viable cells (n = 3/group) were counted using Trypan blue. Data are expressed as mean ± SEM (unpaired Student's t-test or one-way ANOVA * $p < 0.05$, ** $p < 0.01$). The linear regression curve was used to obtain the IC_{50} value, which is as follows: $Y = a * X + b$, $IC_{50} = (0.5 - b)/a$.

Table 6. Anticancer activity of isoflavones.

Compounds #	IC50 (μM)/MCF-7	IC50 (μM)/MEF-1	SI (μM)
7	11.23	71.6	6.4
4	13.66	75.2	5.5
5	15.43	81.3	5.3
Daidzein	11.87	77.1	6.5

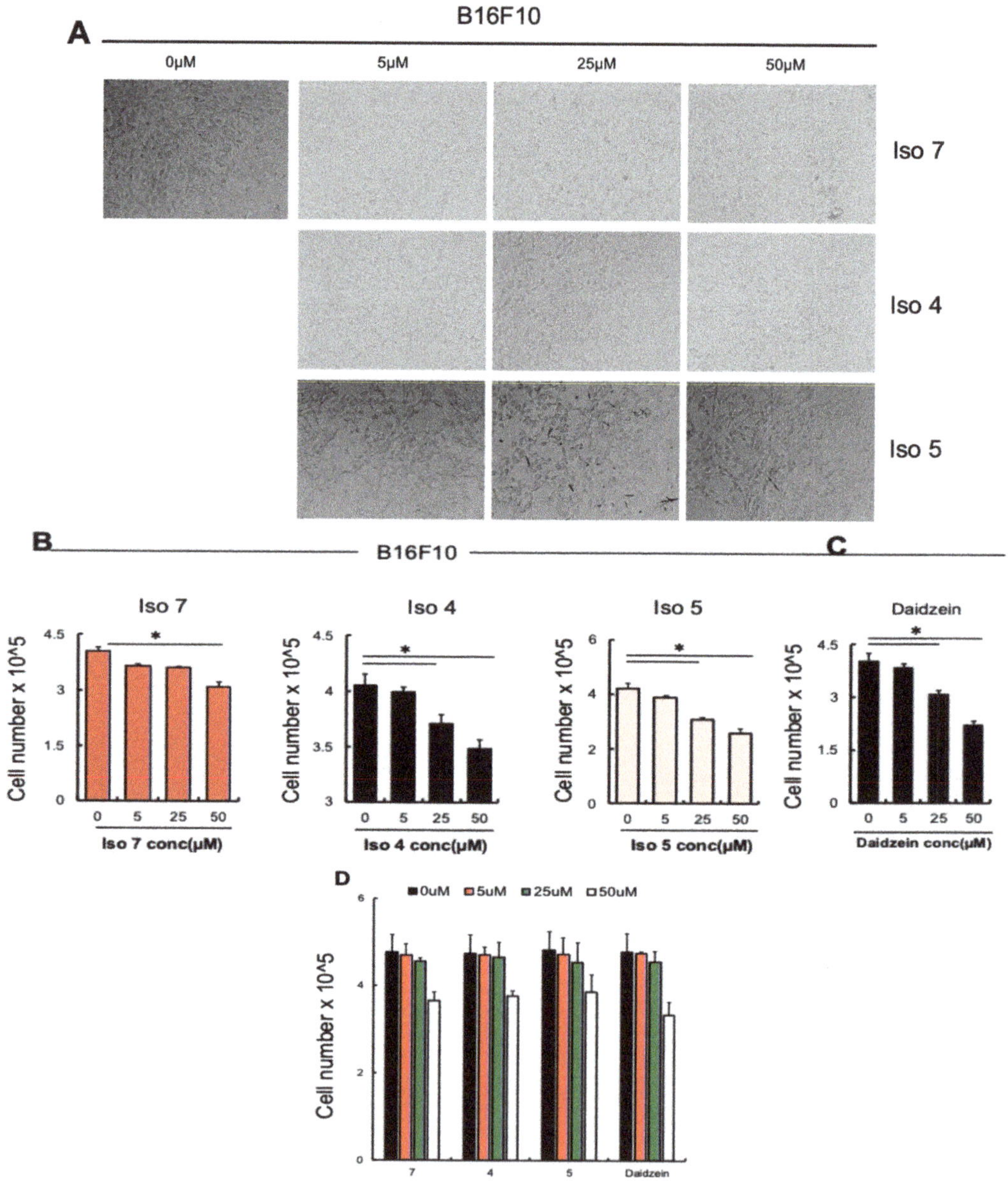

Figure 10. Various synthetic isoflavones, **4**, **5**, **7**, and daidzein, were added at varying concentrations to B16F10 cells. (**A**) Macroscopic images of B16F10 cells under an inverted microscope after treatment

with different isoflavones (magnification 20×). (**B**,**C**). Isoflavones at the indicated concentrations were applied to human B16F10 cells. (**D**). The mouse embryonic fibroblast-1 (MEF-1) cell line was treated with the indicated concentrations of isoflavones **4**, **5**, **7**, and daidzein; after 24 h, viable cells (n = 3/group) were counted using Trypan blue. Data are expressed as mean ± SEM (unpaired Student's *t*-test or one-way ANOVA * $p < 0.05$).

IC_{50} values for the normal cell line MEF-1 and the cancer cell line MCF-7 are shown following 24 h of exposure to the specified isoflavones (Table 6). Half-maximal inhibitory concentration (IC_{50}) values from three separate tests conducted in triplicate were used to display the data. Selectivity index: IC_{50} on normal cells/IC_{50} on cancer cells.

6. Experimental Section

6.1. Material and Measurement Details Are Reported in the Supplementary Information

All solvents and reagents were procured from [Sigma-Aldrich, St Louis, USA] and used without additional purification. ^{1}H-, ^{19}F-, and ^{13}C-NMR (DEPTQ) were recorded in $CDCl_3$ and DMSO-d_6 or CD_3OD on a 400 and 500 MHz Bruker AV III spectrometer (Billerica, Massachusetts, USA). Chemical shifts are represented by the value δ (ppm), whereas coupling constants (*J*) are expressed in Hertz (Hz). The flash column chromatography employed Merck silica gel 60 with a particle size of 0.040–0.063 mm

6.2. Chemistry

6.2.1. 4′-Fluoro7-hydroxyisoflavone (2)

$BF_3.Et_2O$ (7.43 mL, 0.06 mol) was added to a solution of 1-(2,4-dihydroxyphenyl)-2-(4-fluorophenyl)ethan-1-one (**1**) (4.92 g, 0.02 mol) in DMF (30 mL) under N_2. After 15 min, stirring at room temperature, a solution of methanesulfonyl chloride (4.67 mL, 0.06 mol) in DMF (10 mL) was added dropwise. After heating at 70 °C for 6 h, the reaction mixture was cooled to room temperature and poured into ice-cold aqueous sodium acetate (12 g/100 mL). The solid precipitate was filtered off and recrystallized from aqueous ethanol to produce the title compound **2** as a pale yellow solid (4.64 g, 0.0181 mol, 90.5%); Mp = 245–246 °C; FTIR (ν_{max}/cm^{-1}) 3262 br (OH), 1624, 1572, 1514, 1267, 1242; ^{1}H NMR (500 MHz, DMSO-d_6) δ_H 10.87 (br s, 1H, 7-OH), 8.41 (s, 1H, H-2), 7.98 (d, *J* = 8.8 Hz, 1H, H-5), 7.62 (dd, *J* = 8.9, 5.4 Hz, 2H, H-2′,6′), 7.27 (dd, *J* = 8.9, 8.8 Hz, 2H, H-3′,5′), 6.96 (dd, *J* = 8.8, 2.2 Hz, 1H, H-6), 6.89 (d, *J* = 2.2 Hz, 1H, H-8). ^{19}F NMR (471 MHz, DMSO-d_6) δ_C −114.37 (dt, *J* = 15.3, 5.7 Hz). ^{13}C NMR (126 MHz, DMSO-d_6) δ 174.8, 163.2, 162.6 (d, *J* = 245 Hz), 158.0, 154.4, 131.4 (d, *J* = 8.0 Hz), 128.9 (d, *J* = 3.7 Hz), 127.8, 123.0, 117.0, 115.8, 115.4 (d, *J* = 8.0 Hz), 102.7. HRMS calculated $C_{15}H_9O_3FNa$ (M + Na$^+$) 279.0433, found 279.0421.

6.2.2. Methyl 2-((3-(4-fluorophenyl)-4-oxo-4H-chromen-7-yl)oxy)acetate (3)

A solution of 4′-fluoro-7-hydroxyisoflavone (**2**) (0.4 g, 1.56 mmol) and potassium *tert*-butoxide (0.21 g, 1.87 mmol) in dry DMF (15 mL) was stirred at room temperature for 15 min under a nitrogen atmosphere. Thereafter, methyl bromoacetate (0.177 mL, 1.87 mmol) was added, and the mixture was stirred at room temperature for 6 h. The mixture was poured into ice water, neutralized with diluted HCl, and the yellow precipitate was filtered. The solid was subjected to flash chromatography to obtain the title compound **3** as a white solid (0.396 g, 0.00121 mol, 77.3%); Mp = 156–158 °C. FTIR (ν_{max}/cm^{-1}) ν_{max}/cm^{-1} 1764, 1631, 1509, 1438, 1218, 1197. ^{1}H NMR (400 MHz, $CDCl_3$) δ_H 8.24 (dd, *J* = 8.9, 0.9 Hz, 1H, H-5), 7.92 (s, 1H, H-2), 7.53 (dd, *J* = 8.9, 5.4 Hz, 2H, H-2′,6′), 7.12 (t, *J* = 8.8 Hz, 2H, H-3′,5′), 7.04 (dd, *J* = 8.9, 2.4 Hz, 1H, H-6), 6.84 (d, *J* = 2.4 Hz, 1H, H-8), 4.74 (s, 2H, -CH_2-), 3.83 (s, 3H, CH_3). ^{19}F NMR (377 MHz, $CDCl_3$) δ_F −113.7 (s, 1F). ^{13}C NMR (101 MHz, $CDCl_3$) δc 175.4, 168.3, 162.7 (d, *J* = 245 Hz), 162.0, 157.7, 152.1, 130.7 (d, *J* = 8.3 Hz), 128.2, 127.7 (d,

J = 8.3 Hz), 124.5, 119.1, 115.4 (d, *J* = 21.5 Hz), 114.5, 101.4, 65.3, 51.5. HRMS calculated $C_{18}H_{13}O_5FNa$ (M + Na$^+$) 351.0645, found 351.0641.

6.2.3. 2-((3-(4-Fluorophenyl)-4-oxo-4H-chromen-7-yl)oxy)acetic Acid **4**

The 4′-fluoro-7-O-(methoxycarbonylmethyl)isoflavone (**3**) (150 mg, 0.457 mmol) was dissolved in formic acid (5 mL), and a catalytic amount of *p*-toluenesulphonic acid (10 mg, 0.058 mmol) was added to the solution under a nitrogen atmosphere. The solution was stirred at 75 °C for 8 h. The completion of the reaction was monitored by TLC. After the disappearance of the starting material, the mixture was cooled to room temperature and diluted with distilled water. The white precipitate was collected, washed with water, and recrystallized from methanol to furnish **4** as a white solid (121 mg, 0.46 mmol, 83.4%), Mp = 244–245 °C. FTIR (ν_{max}/cm^{-1}) 2993 br (COOH), 1743, 1643, 1609, 1572, 1517, 1443, 1244, 1190. ^{1}H NMR (400 MHz, DMSO-d_6) δ_H 8.49 (s, 1H, H-2), 8.05 (dd, *J* = 8.9, 2,4 Hz, 1H, H-5), 7.63 (dd, *J* = 8.7, 5.6 Hz, 2H, H-2′,6′), 7.28 (t, *J* = 8.7 Hz, 2H, H-3′,5′), 7.18 (d, *J* = 2.4 Hz, 1H, H-8), 7.14 (dd, *J* = 8.9, 2.4 Hz, 1H, H-6), 4.91 (s, 2H, -CH$_2$-). ^{19}F NMR (377 MHz, DMSO-d_6) δ_F −114.22 (s, F). ^{13}C NMR (101 MHz, DMSO-d_6) δ_C 174.4, 169.5, 163.09, 162.3, 161.9 (d, *J* = 244 Hz), 157.3, 154.29, 131.0 (d, *J* = 8.2 Hz), 128.2 (d, *J* = 3.1 Hz), 127.1, 122.8, 117.92, 115.1, 115.0 2 (d, *J* = 7.5 Hz), 101.3, 65.0. HRMS calculated $C_{17}H_{11}O_5FNa$ (M + Na$^+$) 337.0488, found 337.0485.

6.2.4. 7-Hydroxy-3-(4-fluorophenyl)-2-(trifluoromethyl)-4H-chromen-4-one (**5**)

Trifluoroacetic anhydride (8.25 mL, 0.06 mol) was slowly added under a nitrogen atmosphere to a solution of 1-(2,4-dihydroxyphenyl)-2-(4-fluorophenyl)ethan-1-one (**1**) (4.92 g, 0.02 mol) in dry pyridine (15 mL). The mixture was stirred for 4 h, after which it was poured into a 10% HCl solution (100 mL). The mixture was stirred at 50 °C for 3 h. The precipitate was filtered and recrystallized from 70% ethanol to obtain the title compound **5** as a pale yellow solid (5.40 g, 0.0167 mol, 83.3%), Mp = 218–219 °C. FTIR (ν_{max}/cm^{-1}) 3204 br (OH), 1638, 1600, 1459, 1271, 1192, 1164, 1150; ^{1}H NMR (400 MHz, CD$_3$OD) δ_H 8.01 (d, *J* = 8.8 Hz, 1H, H-5), 7.30 (dd, *J* = 8.8, 5.4 Hz, 2H, H-2′,6′), 7.19 (dd, *J* = 8.8, 8.8 Hz, 2H, H-3′,5′), 7.01 (dd, *J* = 8.8, 2.2 Hz, 1H, H-6), 6.92 (d, *J* = 2.2 Hz, 1H, H-8). ^{19}F NMR (377 MHz, CD$_3$OD) δ_F −65.11 (3F), −115.24 (1F). ^{13}C NMR (101 MHz, CD$_3$OD) δ_C 176.5, 164.5, 163.1 (d, *J* = 247 Hz), 157.2, 148.1 (d, *J* = 36 Hz), 131.8 (d, *J* = 8.6 Hz), 127.8, 125.5 (d, *J* = 3.5 Hz), 124.2, 119.4 (d, *J* = 277 Hz), 116.9, 115.6, 114.6 (d, *J* = 22.3 Hz), 101.9. HRMS calculated $C_{16}H_8O_3F_4Na$ (M + Na$^+$) 347.0307, found 347.0310.

6.2.5. Methyl 2-((3-(4-fluorophenyl)-4-oxo-2-(trifluoromethyl)-4H-chromen-7-yl)oxy)acetate (**6**)

A solution of 4′-fluoro-7-hydroxy-2-trifluoromethylisoflavone (**5**) (0.35 g, 1.08 mmol) and potassium *tert*-butoxide (0.145 g, 1.29 mmol) in dry DMF (15 mL) was stirred at room temperature for 15 min under a nitrogen atmosphere. Thereafter, methyl bromoacetate (0.113 mL, 1.19 mmol) was added, and the mixture was stirred at room temperature for 6 h. The mixture was poured into ice water, neutralized with diluted HCl, and the yellow precipitate was filtered. The solid was subjected to flash chromatography to obtain the title compound **6** as a white solid (0.336 g, 0.85 mmol, 78.5%); Mp = 157–159 °C. FTIR (ν_{max}/cm^{-1}) 1750, 1661, 1617, 1508, 1448, 1203, 1200, 1136. ^{1}H NMR (500 MHz, CDCl$_3$) δ_H 8.16 (d, *J* = 8.9 Hz, 1H, H-5), 7.23 (d, *J* = 8.7, 5.4 Hz, 2H, H-2′,6′), 7.14 (t, *J* = 8.7 Hz, 2H, H-3′,5′), 7.10 (dd, *J* = 8.9, 2.4 Hz, 1H, H-6), 6.91 (d, *J* = 2.4 Hz, 1H, H-8), 4.78 (s, 2H, -CH$_2$-), 3.85 (s, 3H, CH$_3$). ^{19}F NMR (471 MHz, CDCl$_3$) δ_F −63.53, −112.66. ^{13}C NMR (126 MHz, CDCl$_3$) δ_C 175.9, 168.0, 163.1 (d, *J* = 249 Hz), 163.0, 156.6, 148.3 (q, *J* = 36 Hz), 131.7 (d, *J* = 7.8 Hz), 128.2, 124.7 (q, *J* = 3.4 Hz), 124.7, 119.2 (q, *J* = 277 Hz), 117.8, 115.3, 115.4 (q, *J* = 22.1 Hz), 101.2, 65.3, 49.1. HRMS calculated $C_{19}H_{12}O_5F_4Na$ (M + Na$^+$) 419.0519, found 419.0508.

6.2.6. 2-((3-(4-Fluorophenyl)-4-oxo-2-(trifluoromethyl)-4H-chromen-7-yl)oxy)acetic Acid 7

Both **6** (150 mg, 0.378 mmol) and *p*-toluensulphonic acid (10 mg, 0.058 mmol) were added to formic acid 5 (mL) using the procedure described above for **4**, which afforded **7** as a white solid (118 mg, 0.38 mmol, 81.4%); Mp = 208–209 °C. FTIR (ν_{max}/cm^{-1}) 3466 br (COOH), 1708, 1648, 1611, 1435, 1253, 1208, 1166. ^{1}H NMR (400 MHz, DMSO-d_6) δ_H 8.01 (d, J = 8.9 Hz, 1H, H-5), 7.40–7.25 (m, 5H, H2′,6′,3′,5′, 8), 7.20 (dd, J = 8.9, 2.4 Hz, 1H, H-6), 4.96 (s, 2H, -CH_2-). ^{19}F NMR (377 MHz, DMSO-d_6) δ_F −62.77 (s, 3F), −113.38 (s, 1F). ^{13}C NMR (101 MHz, DMSO-d_6) δ_C 175.2, 169.4, 163.48, 163.3, 162.7 (d, J = 245 Hz), 156.3, 147.38, 147.0 (q, J = 35.5Hz), 132.08 (d, J = 8.3 Hz), 127.2, 125.7 (q, J = 3.5 Hz), 124.3, 119.3 (q, J = 275 Hz), 116.8, 116.3, 115.0 (q, J = 22.5 Hz), 101.6, 65.1. HRMS calculated $C_{18}H_{10}O_5F_4Na$ (M + Na^+) 405.0362 and found 405.0357.

6.3. Crystal Structure Determination

The crystallographic measurements for **2**, **5**, and **4** were accomplished as previously reported [38], where the CCDC in Table 6 represents crystal data and details of refinement. The crystallographic data were deposited with the Cambridge Crystallographic Data Centre as supplementary publication no. CCDC 2382565, 2382566, and 2382567, respectively. These data can be obtained free of charge from The Cambridge Crystallographic Data Centre via (www.ccdc.cam.ac.uk/structures).

6.4. Hirshfeld Surface Analysis

The topology analyses were performed using the Crystal Explorer 17.5 program [38].

The generation of Hirshfeld surfaces and 2D fingerprint plots around the primary molecule with all hydrates external was accomplished using Crystal Explorer 17.5.

6.5. Anticancer Activity and Statistical Analysis

The methods of anticancer assessments and statistical analysis are reported in the Supplementary Information.

7. Conclusions

The fluorinated isoflavones 7-*O*-carboxymethyl-4′-fluoroisoflavone **4** and 7-*O*-carboxy methyl-4′-fluoro-2-trifluormethylisoflavone **7** were prepared in high yields starting from the corresponding deoxybenzoin **1**. Single-crystal X-ray diffraction was used to prove the molecular and supramolecular structures of the studied compounds. Compounds **2** and **4** were found to contain the ethanol molecule as the crystal solvent, which has a significant impact on the intermolecular interactions observed in these crystalline materials. The O...H interactions are more important in **2** and **4** than in **5**. Also, no interhalogen (F...F) contacts were detected in **2** and **7**, while both showed π-π stacking interactions. The opposite was true for **5**. Our investigation indicates that the synthesized isoflavones demonstrate significant anticancer activity against the MCF-7 cell line, corroborating the current literature regarding their effectiveness in hormone-dependent malignancies. The diminished activity shown against B16F10 melanoma cells indicated a selective effect that may be advantageous for targeting particular cancer types. The specificity of isoflavones against estrogen receptors or their high-binding affinity with these receptors seen on MCF-7 cells can be used to explain their notable and targeted action against breast cancer cells, including MCF-7, which is positive for ER alpha [39]. However, a feature of melanoma is the fact that it is resistant to many chemotherapeutic treatments, particularly when it is in an advanced stage. This wider resistance profile may be mirrored by the observed decreased influence of isoflavones; more research is required to elucidate this. Developing a better understanding of resistance mechanisms, such as immune evasion or the overexpression of survival pathways like NF-κB, can help to improve treatment approaches. Also, certain receptors or signaling pathways necessary for isoflavone-induced cytotoxicity could be absent in them, as many reports have mentioned [40]. Also, the isoflavones used in our study showed similar effects on MCF-7 cells, as their influences appeared to be closely matched. Notably, these compounds exhibit almost similar IC_{50} values (Table 6), indicating the same potency in inhibiting cell growth. Additionally, the selectivity index for each isoflavone is closely matched, suggesting that they all have a comparable ability to target cancerous cells while minimizing their impact on normal cells. This consistency in their bioactivity highlights their potential as promising therapeutic agents for further investigation and development. Finally, conducting in vivo and pre-clinical investigations will be essential to validate our results and comprehend isoflavones' mechanisms of action and potential therapeutic applications. This research may substantially advance the field of cancer treatment.

Supplementary Materials: The supporting information can be downloaded at https://www.mdpi.com/article/10.3390/molecules30040795/s1. Figure S1. ^{1}HNMR of **2**, Figure S2. ^{13}CNMR of **2**, Figure S3. ^{1}HNMR of **3**, Figure S4. ^{19}FNMR of **3**, Figure S5. ^{13}CNMR of **3**, Figure S6. ^{1}HNMR of **4**, Figure S7. ^{19}FNMR of **4**, Figure S8. ^{13}CNMR of **4**, Figure S9. ^{1}HNMR of **5**, Figure S10. ^{19}FNMR of **5**, Figure S11. ^{13}CNMR of **5**, Figure S12. ^{1}HNMR of **6**, Figure S13. ^{19}FNMR of **6**, Figure S14. ^{13}CNMR of **6**, Figure S15. ^{1}HNMR of **7**, Figure S16. ^{19}FNMR of **7**, Figure S17. ^{13}CNMR of **7**. References [34–36,39] are cited in the supplementary materials.

Author Contributions: Conceptualization, N.A.-M. and M.D.; methodology, N.A.-M.; software, S.M.S.; validation, S.M.S., R.H. and Y.S.; formal analysis, M.S.A.; investigation, Y.S.; resources, N.A.-M.; software, S.M.S.; data curation, M.B.H. and N.A.-M.; software, S.M.S.; writing—original draft preparation, N.A.-M.; writing—review and editing, M.B.H. and N.A.-M.; visualization, M.D.; supervision, N.A.-M.; project administration, N.A.-M.; funding acquisition, M.S.A. All authors have read and agreed to the published version of the manuscript.

Funding: This work was supported by the Deanship of Scientific Research, Vice Presidency for Graduate Studies and Scientific Research, King Faisal University, Saudi Arabia (Project No. KFU250349).

Institutional Review Board Statement: Not applicable.

Informed Consent Statement: Not applicable.

Data Availability Statement: The data will be made available upon request.

Acknowledgments: We wish to express our gratitude to An Najah National University for its invaluable support. Also, MSA acknowledge the Deanship of Scientific Research, Vice Presidency for Graduate Studies and Scientific Research, King Faisal University, Saudi Arabia (Project No. KFU250349).

Conflicts of Interest: The authors declare no conflicts of interest.

References

1. Veitch, N.C. Isoflavonoids of the leguminosae. *Nat. Prod. Rep.* **2009**, *26*, 776–802. [CrossRef]
2. Veitch, N.C. Isoflavonoids of the leguminosae. *Nat. Prod. Rep.* **2013**, *30*, 988–1027. [CrossRef] [PubMed]
3. Al-Maharik, N. Isolation of naturally occurring novel isoflavonoids: An update. *Nat. Prod. Rep.* **2019**, *36*, 1156. [CrossRef] [PubMed]
4. Huang, R.; Ding, Z.G.; Long, Y.F.; Zhao, J.Y.; Li, M.G.; Cui, X.L.; Wen, M.L. A new isoflavone derivative from *Streptomyces* sp. YIM GS3536. *Chem. Nat. Compd.* **2013**, *48*, 966–969. [CrossRef]
5. Wang, J.F.; Liu, S.S.; Song, Z.Q.; Xu, T.C.; Liu, C.S.; Hou, Y.G.; Huang, R.; Wu, S.H. Naturally Occurring Flavonoids and Isoflavonoids and Their Microbial Transformation: A Review. *Molecules* **2020**, *25*, 5112. [CrossRef]
6. Kopustinskiene, D.M.; Jakstas, V.; Savickas, A.; Bernatoniene, J. Flavonoids as Anticancer Agents. *Nutrients* **2020**, *12*, 457. [CrossRef]
7. Dixon, R.A.; Steele, C.L. Flavonoids and isoflavonoids—A gold mine for metabolic engineering. *Trends Plant Sci.* **1999**, *4*, 394–400. [CrossRef] [PubMed]

8. Novelli, S.; Gismondi, A.; Di Marco, G.; Canuti, L.; Nanni, V.; Canini, A. Plant defense factors involved in *Olea europaea* resistance against *Xylella fastidiosa* infection. *J. Plant Res.* **2019**, *132*, 439–455. [CrossRef]
9. Sajid, M.; Stone, S.R.; Kaur, P. Recent Advances in Heterologous Synthesis Paving Way for Future Green-Modular Bioindustries: A Review With Special Reference to Isoflavonoids. *Front. Bioeng. Biotechnol.* **2021**, *9*, 673270. [CrossRef] [PubMed] [PubMed Central]
10. Mukne, A.P.; Viswanathan, V.; Phadatare, A.G. Structure pre-requisites for isoflavones as effective antibacterial agents. *Pharmacogn. Rev.* **2011**, *5*, 13–18. [CrossRef] [PubMed] [PubMed Central]
11. Aboody, M.S.A.; Mickymaray, S. Anti-Fungal Efficacy and Mechanisms of Flavonoids. *Antibiotics* **2020**, *9*, 45. [CrossRef] [PubMed] [PubMed Central]
12. Wang, L.; Song, J.; Liu, A.; Xiao, B.; Li, S.; Wen, Z.; Lu, Y.; Du, G. Research Progress of the Antiviral Bioactivities of Natural Flavonoids. *Nat. Prod. Bioprospect.* **2020**, *10*, 271–283. [CrossRef]
13. Bellou, S.; Karali, E.; Bagli, E.; Al-Maharik, N.; Morbidelli, L.; Ziche, M.; Adlercreutz, H.; Murphy, C.; Fotsis, T. The Isoflavone Metabolite 6-Methoxyequol Inhibits Angiogenesis and Suppresses Tumor Growth. *Mol. Cancer* **2012**, *11*, 35–46. [CrossRef] [PubMed]
14. Al-Maharik, N.; Jaradat, N.; Hedmi, A. Synthesis of nitro- and aminoisoflavone and their effects on the proliferation of endothelial cells. *J. Chem. Soc. Pak.* **2020**, *42*, 572–580.
15. Basu, P.; Maier, C. Phytoestrogens and breast cancer: In vitro anticancer activities of isoflavones, lignans, coumestans, stilbenes and their analogs and derivatives. *Biomed. Pharmacother.* **2018**, *107*, 1648–1666. [CrossRef]
16. Danciu, C.; Avram, S.; Pavel, I.Z.; Ghiulai, R.; Dehelean, C.A.; Ersilia, A.; Minda, D.; Petrescu, C.; Moaca, E.-A.; Soica, C. Main Isoflavones Found in Dietary Sources as Natural Anti-inflammatory Agents. *Curr. Drug Targets* **2018**, *19*, 841–853. [CrossRef] [PubMed]
17. Liu, M.; Wang, G.; Xu, R.; Shen, C.; Ni, H.; Lai, R. Soy Isoflavones Inhibit Both GPIb-IX Signaling and αIIbβ3 Outside-In Signaling via 14-3-3ζ in Platelet. *Molecules* **2021**, *26*, 4911. [CrossRef] [PubMed]
18. Rizzo, J.; Min, M.; Adnan, S.; Afzal, N.; Maloh, J.; Chambers, C.J.; Fam, V.; Sivamani, R.K. Soy Protein Containing Isoflavones Improves Facial Signs of Photoaging and Skin Hydration in Postmenopausal Women: Results of a Prospective Randomized Double-Blind Controlled Trial. *Nutrients* **2023**, *15*, 4113. [CrossRef]
19. Lecomte, S.; Demay, F.; Ferrière, F.; Pakdel, F. Phytochemicals Targeting Estrogen Receptors: Beneficial Rather Than Adverse Effects? *Int. J. Mol. Sci.* **2017**, *18*, 1381. [CrossRef] [PubMed]
20. Mense, S.M.; Hei, T.K.; Ganju, R.K.; Bhat, H.K. Phytoestrogens and breast cancer prevention: Possible mechanisms of action. *Environ. Health Perspect.* **2008**, *116*, 426–433. [CrossRef] [PubMed]
21. Bilal, I.; Chowdhury, A.; Davidson, J.; Whitehead, S. Phytoestrogens and prevention of breast cancer: The contentious debate. *World J. Clin. Oncol.* **2014**, *5*, 705–712. [CrossRef] [PubMed]
22. Selepe, M.A. Isoflavone Derivatives as Potential Anticancer Agents: Synthesis and Bioactivity Studies. *ChemMedChem* **2024**, *19*, e202400420. [CrossRef] [PubMed]
23. Inoue, M.; Sumii, Y.; Shibata, N. Contribution of Organofluorine Compounds to Pharmaceuticals. *ACS Omega* **2020**, *5*, 10633–10640. [CrossRef] [PubMed]
24. Meanwell, N.A. Fluorine and Fluorinated Motifs in the Design and Application of Bioisosteres for Drug Design. *J. Med. Chem.* **2018**, *61*, 5822–5880. Available online: https://pubs.acs.org/doi/10.1021/acs.jmedchem.7b01788 (accessed on 3 February 2025). [CrossRef] [PubMed]
25. Awad, L.F.; Ayoup, M.S. Fluorinated phenylalanines: Synthesis and pharmaceutical applications. *Beilstein J. Org. Chem.* **2020**, *16*, 1022–1050. [CrossRef] [PubMed]
26. Yadav, S.K. Process for the preparation of chromones, isoflavones and homoisoflavones using Vilsmeier reagent generated from phthaloyl dichloride and DMF. *Int. J. Org. Chem.* **2014**, *4*, 236–246. [CrossRef]
27. Spackman, M.A.; Jayatilaka, D. Hirshfeld surface analysis. *CrystEngComm* **2009**, *11*, 19–32. [CrossRef]
28. Spackman, M.A.; McKinnon, J.J.; Jayatilaka, D. Electrostatic potentials mapped on Hirshfeld surfaces provide direct insight into intermolecular interactions in crystals. *CrystEngComm* **2008**, *10*, 377–388. [CrossRef]
29. Wilkinson, L.; Gathani, T. Understanding breast cancer as a global health concern. *Br. J. Radiol.* **2022**, *95*, 20211033. [CrossRef] [PubMed]
30. Bray, F.; Ferlay, J.; Soerjomataram, I.; Siegel, R.L.; Torre, L.A.; Jemal, A. Global cancer statistics 2018: GLOBOCAN estimates of incidence and mortality worldwide for 36 cancers in 185 countries. *CA Cancer J. Clin.* **2018**, *68*, 394–424. [CrossRef]
31. Dai, X.; Cheng, H.; Bai, Z.; Li, J. Breast cancer cell line classification and its relevance with breast tumor subtyping. *J. Cancer* **2017**, *8*, 3131–3134. [CrossRef]
32. Lopes, C.; Piairo, P.; Chícharo, A.; Abalde-Cela, S.; Pires, L.R.; Corredeira, P.; Alves, P.; Muinelo-Romay, L.; Costa, L.; Diéguez, L. HER2 Expression in Circulating Tumour Cells Isolated from Metastatic Breast Cancer Patients Using a Size-Based Microfluidic Device. *Cancers* **2021**, *13*, 4446. [CrossRef] [PubMed]

33. Ilieș, M.; Uifălean, A.; Pașca, S.; Dhople, V.M.; Lalk, M.; Iuga, C.A.; Hammer, E. From Proteomics to Personalized Medicine: The Importance of Isoflavone Dose and Estrogen Receptor Status in Breast Cancer Cells. *J. Pers. Med.* **2020**, *10*, 292. [CrossRef] [PubMed]
34. Poschner, S.; Maier-Salamon, A.; Zehl, M.; Wackerlig, J.; Dobusch, D.; Pachmann, B.; Sterlini, K.L.; Jäger, W. The Impacts of Genistein and Daidzein on Estrogen Conjugations in Human Breast Cancer Cells: A Targeted Metabolomics Approach. *Front. Pharmacol.* **2017**, *8*, 699. [CrossRef]
35. Sotoca, A.M.; van den Berg, H.; Vervoort, J.; van der Saag, P.; Ström, A.; Gustafsson, J.A.; Rietjens, I.; Murk, A.J. Influence of cellular ERalpha/ERbeta ratio on the ERalpha-agonist induced proliferation of human T47D breast cancer cells. *Toxicol. Sci. Off. J. Soc. Toxicol.* **2008**, *105*, 303–311. [CrossRef]
36. Hatono, M.; Ikeda, H.; Suzuki, Y.; Kajiwara, Y.; Kawada, K.; Tsukioki, T.; Kochi, M.; Suzawa, K.; Iwamoto, T.; Yamamoto, H.; et al. Effect of isoflavones on breast cancer cell development and their impact on breast cancer treatments. *Breast Cancer Res. Treat.* **2021**, *185*, 307–316. [CrossRef] [PubMed]
37. Al-Maharik, N.; Salama, Y.; Al-Hajj, N.; Jaradat, N.; Jobran, N.T.; Warad, I.; Hamdan, L.; Alrob, M.A.; Sawafta, A.; Hidmi, A. Chemical composition, anticancer, antimicrobial activity of Aloysia citriodora Palau essential oils from four different locations in Palestine. *BMC Complement. Med. Ther.* **2024**, *24*, 94. [CrossRef] [PubMed]
38. Turner, M.J.; McKinnon, J.J.; Wolff, S.K.; Grimwood, D.J.; Spackman, P.R.; Jayatilaka, D.; Spackman, M.A. *Crystal Explorer17*; University of Western Australia: Crawley, WA, Australia, 2017; Available online: http://hirshfeldsurface.net (accessed on 3 November 2024).
39. Kumar, V.; Chauhan, S.S. Daidzein Induces Intrinsic Pathway of Apoptosis along with ER α/β Ratio Alteration and ROS Production. *Asian Pac. J. Cancer Prev. APJCP* **2021**, *22*, 603–610. [CrossRef] [PubMed]
40. Rajabi, P.; Bagheri, M.; Hani, M. Expression of Estrogen Receptor Alpha in Malignant Melanoma. *Adv. Biomed. Res.* **2017**, *6*, 14. [CrossRef]

molecules

MDPI

Article

Metabolomic Profiles and Differential Constituents of *Andrographis paniculata* (Burm. f.) in Different Growth Stages and Parts

Enming Hu [1,2,3], Rui Cheng [2], Annian Liu [2], Ya Wang [2], Huali Long [4], Jinjun Hou [4], Daoping Wang [1,3], Wanying Wu [4,*] and Xingdong Wu [1,2,4,*]

1 State Key Laboratory of Discovery and Utilization of Functional Components in Traditional Chinese Medicine, Guiyang 550014, China; 47780huhanqing@gmail.com (E.H.); wangdaoping@gmc.edu.cn (D.W.)
2 Guizhou Engineering Research Center of Industrial Key-Technology for Dendrobium Nobile, Joint International Research Laboratory of Ethnomedicine of Ministry of Education, Zunyi Medical University, Zunyi 563000, China; 18636703714@163.com (R.C.); liuan_0808@163.com (A.L.); 18275687211@163.com (Y.W.)
3 Natural Products Research Center of Guizhou Province, Guiyang 550014, China
4 National Engineering Research Center of TCM Standardization Technology, Shanghai Institute of Materia Medica, Chinese Academy of Sciences, Shanghai 201203, China; longhuali@simm.ac.cn (H.L.); jinjun_hou@simm.ac.cn (J.H.)
* Correspondence: wanyingwu@simm.ac.cn (W.W.); wuxingdong@zmu.edu.cn (X.W.)

Abstract: *Andrographis paniculata* (Burm. f.) and its products have a long history of medicinal use in Asia. *A. paniculata* products are mainly made from the root extraction of stems, leaves and parts, but there may be differences in the proportion of different parts and different harvest times, which ultimately leads to certain differences in product quality. In this study, the chemical components and non-targeted metabolomics were characterized, and the characteristic compounds in different parts of *A. paniculata* at various growth stages were analyzed. By utilizing polygonal mass defect filtering, precursor ion lists, and a self-built compound library, a total of 225 components were identified in *A. paniculata*. Notably, spermidine derivatives and phosphatidylcholines were reported for the first time in this plant species. In total, 41 differential components were identified in different parts of *A. paniculata*. These findings provide scientific evidence for the selection of quality markers in *A. paniculata* and its products.

Keywords: *Andrographis paniculata*; different plant parts; different growth stages; non-targeted metabolomics; quality markers

1. Introduction

Andrographis paniculata (Burm. f.), a member of the *genus I* in the Acanthaceae family, encompasses three species: *A. paniculata*, *A. laxiflora*, and *A.* var. *glomerulifera* [1]. It predominantly thrives in subtropical regions of China, India, Thailand, and other Asian countries [2,3]. *A. paniculata* is renowned for its abundance of diterpene lactones, flavonoids, and organic acids, and has been traditionally employed in Asian traditional medicine for the treatment of ailments such as cardiovascular diseases, snakebites, and malaria [2,4,5]. Its exceptional therapeutic efficacy has garnered recognition in major pharmacopoeias worldwide, including the Chinese Pharmacopoeia, United States Pharmacopeia, and European Pharmacopoeia. Presently, several *A. paniculata*-derived products have been developed, including tablets, capsules, and formulations based on the active diterpene lactones [6]. Andrographolide, dehydroandrographolide, 14-deoxyandrographolide, and neoandrographolide are the four major diterpene lactones commonly employed to assess the quality of *A. paniculata* and its related products [7]. However, our previous research conducted by our group involved a random examination of four diterpene lactones in *A. paniculata* tablets from ten different manufacturers in China, revealing significant variations in andrographolide content among the samples (Figure S1, Table S1). These variations may be attributed to differences in the proportion of roots and stems utilized as raw materials, as well as discrepancies in the harvesting seasons of the herbal ingredients [8]. Thus, relying solely on the four major diterpene lactones for the quality evaluation of *A. paniculata* and its formulations is insufficient. Consequently, it is imperative to systematically compare and analyze the chemical constituents of *A. paniculata* collected at different growth stages and from various plant parts to identify additional quality markers and determine the optimal harvesting period.

Plants exhibit remarkable plasticity in adapting to diverse growth stages and environmental conditions by producing a wide array of secondary metabolites, which play crucial roles in reproduction and self-protection [9,10]. Consequently, substantial variations in the chemical composition of plants are often observed across different growth stages and environmental contexts [11]. While previous studies have reported changes in the content of andrographolide, dehydroandrographolide, and neoandrographolide in *A. paniculata* at different growth stages, investigations into the differential chemical constituents among distinct growth stages and plant parts of *A. paniculata* remain scarce [12]. Non-targeted metabolomics, a comprehensive approach that encompasses the global analysis of metabolites, offers a valuable means to study the relative changes in metabolite types and quantities within biological systems under physiological and pathological conditions [13]. Notably, untargeted metabolomics has proven successful in identifying disease biomarkers and screening quality markers in the field of herbal medicine [14,15]. Moreover, the advent of high-resolution mass spectrometry has facilitated the high-throughput characterization of chemical constituents within complex systems, thanks to its exceptional precision, sensitivity, and resolution [16,17]. Consequently, a synergistic integration of high-resolution mass spectrometry and untargeted metabolomics can be employed to discern and compare the chemical composition of different parts of *A. paniculata* at various growth stages.

In this study, we aimed to comprehensively characterize the chemical constituents of *A. paniculata* based on samples collected from different growth stages and plant parts within the cultivation area. Firstly, we employed UHPLC-LTQ-Orbitrap-MS^n technology in conjunction with a self-built database for the systematic characterization of *A. paniculata*. Furthermore, untargeted metabolomics analysis was conducted to identify differential constituents among different growth stages and parts of *A. paniculata*. These analyses aimed to elucidate the composition of chemical constituents in *A. paniculata*, providing insights into the determination of optimal harvesting periods and contributing to the selection of quality markers for *A. paniculata* and its derived products.

2. Experiment

2.1. Reagents and Materials

A total of 22 chemical reference standards were used for the characterization of chemical constituents, including andrographidine A (R5)/B (R6)/E (R10), 5-hydroxy-7,8-dimethoxyflavanone (R4), 4′,5,7,8-tetramethoxyflavone (R7), moslosooflavone (R8), skullcapflavone I (R9), chlorogenic acid (R1), isochlorogenic acid B (R2), 3,5-di-O-caffeoylquinic acid (R3), andrographolide (R11), dehydroandrographolide (R18), 14-deoxyandrographolide (R14), neoandrographolide (R16), andrographoside (R12), andropanoside (R17), 14-Deoxy-11,12-didehydroandrographiside (R20), andrograpanin (R13), 14-deoxy-17-hydroxyandrographolide (R19), 14-deoxy-12-ethoxyl andrographolide (R15), and bisandrographolide A (R21)/C (R22). These reference standards were purchased from

Shanghai Natural-Standard Company (Shanghai, China), Sichuan Vikki Biotechnology Co., Ltd. (Chengdu, China), and BioBioPha Co., Ltd. (Kunming, China). The purity of these reference standards was more than 95% after detection by HPLC. These standards included seven flavonoids, three organic acids, and twelve diterpene lactones, and their chemical structures are shown in Figure 1. HPLC-grade and MS-grade acetonitrile were obtained from Merck (Darmstadt, Germany), and MS-grade formic acid was purchased from Roe Scientific Inc. (Newark, NJ, USA). All other reagents used in this study were of analytical grade. Ultra-pure water was prepared in the laboratory. *A. paniculata* samples at different growth stages and plant parts were provided by medicinal plant growers in Guigang, Guangxi province, China (Table S2) and authenticated as plants of *A. paniculata* in Lamiaceae family by Professor Guo Dean. Voucher specimens of *A. paniculata* were deposited in the Center for Modernization of Traditional Chinese Medicine, Shanghai Institute of Materia Medica, Chinese Academy of Sciences.

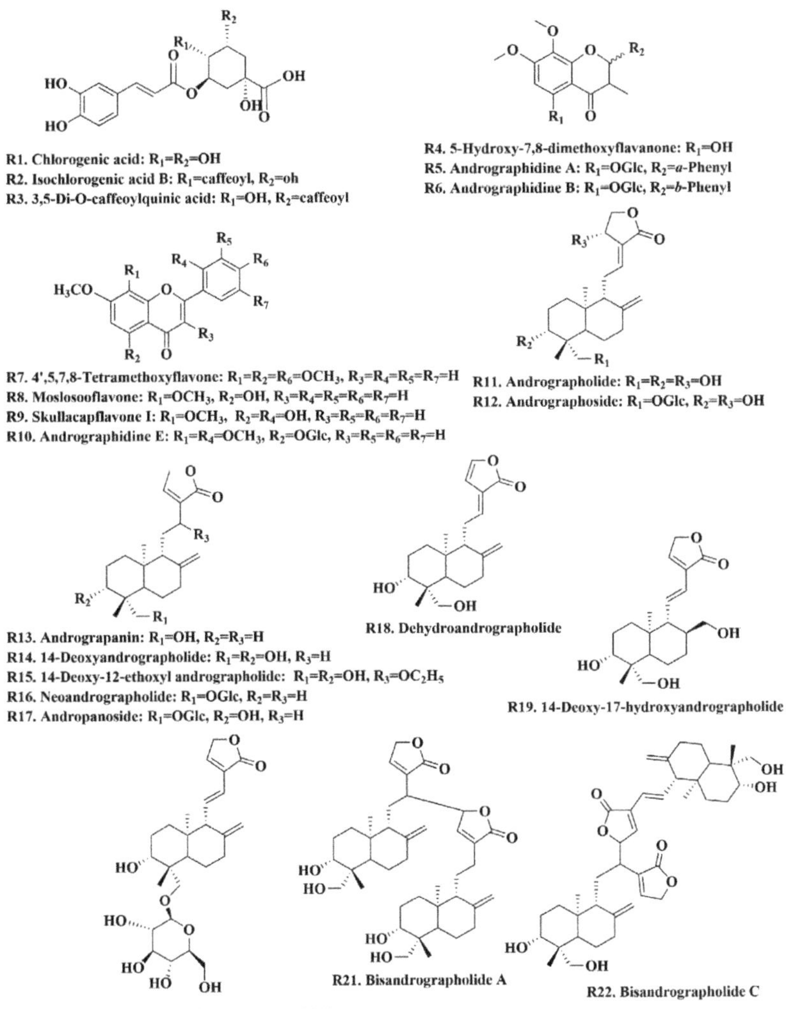

Figure 1. Chemical structure of 22 reference standards.

2.2. Preparation of Reference and Sample Solutions

Accurate amounts of the 22 reference standards were weighed. *A. paniculata* sample was ground to 60 mesh after drying under natural conditions, 0.5 g of each sample was accurately weighed, and sonicated with 25 mL of 75% methanol for 30 min (100 W, 35 kHz). After the extraction solution has cooled to room temperature, the lost weight is replenished with 75% methanol. After shaking, centrifuge at 12,000 rpm for 10 min and filter through a 50 μm Millipore filter. Weigh the appropriate amount of 12 diterpene lactones standard reference and diluted to 50 μg/mL. Different parts of *A. paniculata* at different harvest ages that including sixteen batches of stem, sixteen batches of leaf, fifteen batches of root, four batches of flower, and five batches of fruit were divided, respectively (Table S2) [18].

2.3. Chromatographic Conditions and Mass Spectrometry Parameters

The *A. paniculata* samples were analyzed using an Ultimate 3000 Standard Dual System (Thermo Fisher Scientific, San Jose, CA, USA) equipped with a binary solvent pump, an autosampler, and a diode-array detector. The samples were separated on an ACQUITY HSS T3 C18 column (2.1 100 mm, 1.7 μm, Waters, Milford, MA, USA). The mobile phase consisted of water containing 0.1% (*v*/*v*) formic acid (A) and acetonitrile (B); the flow rate was set to 0.3 mL/min. During the sample elution process, samples were eluted with an initial flow phase equilibrium for 2 min, a linear gradient increase in mobile phase B from 2% to 20% for 3 min, a linear gradient increase in mobile phase B from 20% to 55% for 20 min, a linear gradient increase in mobile phase B from 55% to 70% for 5 min, a linear gradient increase in mobile phase B from 70% to 100% for 5 min, a liner gradient decrease in mobile phase B from 100% to 0% for 5 min. The column temperature was maintained at 35 °C, and the injection volume of the test solution was 2 μL. In addition, the detection wavelength was 205 nm.

The experiments were performed at a spray voltage of 4600 V, a capillary temperature of 350 °C, an in-source CID of 20 V, a collision energy of 30 V, and source heater temperature of 300 °C. Nitrogen was applied as sheath gas and auxiliary gas, and their flow rate was 40 and 10 arb units, respectively. Data were acquired in positive ionization mode.

The chromatographic conditions and mass spectrometry parameters for untargeted metabolomics analysis of *A. paniculata* at different harvest periods and plant parts were consistent with the methods used in previous studies [18]. The UHPLC-LTQ-Orbitrap Velos Pro hybrid mass spectrometer (Thermo Fisher Scientific, San Jose, CA, USA) was employed for data acquisition, using different methods based on the compound types. Firstly, the collision-induced dissociation (CID) mode was selected to acquire the first-level mass spectrometry data for compounds with molecular weights ranging from 100 to 1200 Da, recorded as Event I. Event II recorded the fragmentation ions of the top three ions in Event I, while Event III captured the fragment ion information of the top three ions in Event II. Specifically, the data acquisition method for diterpene lactones in *A. paniculata* was consistent with our previous publication [18]. For flavonoid constituents, a polygonal mass defect filtering method was developed based on a literature survey of 66 compounds to screen potential flavonoid constituents in *A. paniculata*, and their multi-stage mass spectrometry information was acquired (Figure S2). As for caffeoylquinic acid constituents, a polygonal mass defect filtering method was devised based on a literature survey of six compounds to screen potential caffeoylquinic acid constituents in *A. paniculata* (Figure S3), and their multi-stage mass spectrometry information was obtained.

2.4. Chemical Characterization

A database was established by collecting information on 201 reported compounds of *A. paniculata*, including compound names, structural formulas, molecular formulas, and CAS numbers, from databases such as ScienceFinder^{n} (http://scifinder-n.cas.org/, accessed on 24 May 2023), PubMed (https://pubmed.ncbi.nlm.nih.gov/, accessed on 24 May 2023), Reaxys (https://www.reaxys.com/, accessed on 24 May 2023), and CNKI (https://c61.oversea.cnki.net/, accessed on 24 May 2023). The created compound database was imported into Compound Discoverer 3.3. Based on the characteristics of the constituents in *A. paniculata*, the following adduct ions were set in ESI^+ mode: $[M + H]^+$, $[2M + H]^+$, $[M + Na]^+$, $[2M + Na]^+$, $[M + H - H_2O]^+$, $[M + H - 2H_2O]^+$, and $[M + H - 3H_2O]^+$, with a mass error tolerance of 5 ppm, and potential known constituents in *A. paniculata* were searched. Finally, the mass spectra fragments of characterized compounds were compared with those of reference standards and literature data to further confirm the chemical constituents in *A. paniculata*.

2.5. Data Analysis

The raw data of *A. paniculata* collected from different growth stages and plant parts were imported into Progenesis QI 2.1 software for baseline correction, smoothing, peak extraction, and deconvolution. The processing parameters were set as follows: file type was selected as profile format, adduct ions were set as $[M + H]^+$, $[2M + H]^+$, $[M + Na]^+$, $[2M + Na]^+$, $[M + H - H_2O]^+$, $[M + H - 2H_2O]^+$, and $[M + H - 3H_2O]^+$; the minimum peak intensity was set to 2000, and the maximum peak width was set to 0.2 min. A data matrix containing retention time, m/z, and peak intensity information was obtained. Signal noise ions that did not meet the 30% and 80% rule and had high responses in the blank solvent were removed from the metabolomics data processing, resulting in the dataset used for metabolomics analysis. Multivariate statistical analysis and clustering analysis of the metabolomics data were performed using SIMCA-P 14.1 software (Umetrics, Umea, Sweden) and HemI software (CUCKOO Workgroup, Wuhan, China). Metabolites with VIP (Variable Importance in Projection) values greater than 3 were further subjected to t-tests to identify potential quality markers more accurately. The quantitative analysis results were plotted using Origin 2019b software (OriginLab, Northampton, MA, USA).

3. Results and Discussion

3.1. Optimization of Chromatographic Conditions and Mass Spectrometry Parameters

Due to the complexity and trace amounts of components in natural products, the chromatographic gradient directly affects the quality and quantity of compound data collected by mass spectrometry [19,20]. Therefore, it is necessary to optimize the chromatographic conditions before data acquisition. Similarly, the mass spectrometry parameters also affect the fragmentation pattern of compounds and thus influence their resolution [21]. In this study, the chromatographic conditions and mass spectrometry parameters used in metabolomics data acquisition were optimized, and the quantification of the four major diterpene lactones was performed using a method established in our laboratory for *A. paniculata* quality standard [18]. The total ion chromatogram of different plant parts of *A. paniculata* is shown in Figure 2A, and the chromatograms of different plant parts are shown in Figure 2B. In Figure 2A, it can be observed that there are significant differences in the constituents between the root of *A. paniculata* and other plant parts, while the stem, leaf, flower, and fruit show more similar profiles. The leaf of *A. paniculata* showed a higher concentration of constituents compared to the stem and leaf. Figure 2B shows that the four major diterpene lactones were not detected in the root of *A. paniculata*, while andrographolide, neoandrographolide, dehydroandrographolide, and 14-deoxyandrographolide were detected in the stem, leaf, flower, and fruit, with relatively higher levels in the leaf of *A. paniculata*.

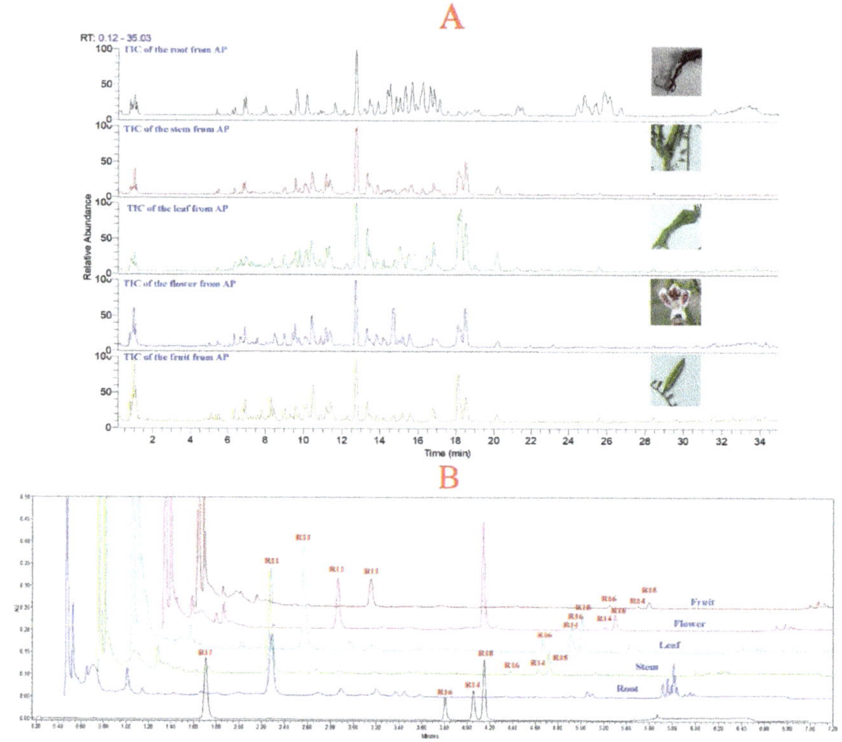

Figure 2. (**A**): Total ion chromatogram of different parts of *A. paniculata*; (**B**): chromatograms of different parts of *A. paniculata* (R11: andrographolide; R16: neoandrographolide; R14: 14-deoxyandrographolide; R18: dehydroandrographolide).

3.2. Identification of Chemical Constituents in Different Growth Stages and Plant Parts of A. paniculata

3.2.1. Analysis of Diterpene Lactones in *A. paniculata*

Diterpene lactones are the most abundant active components in *A. paniculata*, and their identification is of great significance [22]. However, the characterization of diterpene lactones in *A. paniculata* has been extensively reported in previous publications [18]. In this study, our focus was on the distribution of diterpene lactones in different plant parts of *A. paniculata*.

3.2.2. Analysis of Flavonoids in *A. paniculata*

Flavonoids belong to the natural polyphenolic compounds and are widely distributed in common foods such as vegetables, fruits, and tea [23]. Existing studies have shown that flavonoids possess various biological activities, including antioxidant, anti-inflammatory, antibacterial, and antiviral effects [24]. However, it has been reported that flavonoids account for 46.23% of the reported constituents in *A. paniculata*, including flavones, flavonols, and dihydroflavones [2]. Therefore, it is necessary to systematically characterize the flavonoid constituents.

Compounds **26** and **28** (Table S3) were positional isomers, both exhibiting molecular ion peaks at m/z 463.16 Da $[M + H]^+$ and $[M + Na]^+$ at m/z 485.14 Da in the protonated molecular ions. Furthermore, fragment ion peaks at m/z 301.11 Da, and 197.04 Da were detected in the MS^n analysis. The fragment ion at m/z 301.11 Da was the aglycone formed by the loss of one molecule of Glc. The fragment ion at m/z 197.04 Da represented the loss of one molecule of Glc and two molecules of CH_2 from compounds **26** and **28**. By comparing the retention time, m/z, and MS^n fragment patterns with reference standards, compounds **26** and **28** were identified as andrographidine A and andrographidine B, respectively, belonging to the dihydroflavone class. The mass spectrum and potential fragmentation pattern of compound **28** are shown in Figure 3A. Compound **36** exhibited a molecular ion peak at m/z 491.15 Da $[M + H]^+$ and an adduct ion peak $[M + Na]^+$ at m/z 513.14 Da in the MS. Fragment ion peaks at m/z 329.10, 314.08, 299.06, 183.03, and 165.02 Da were detected in the MS^n analysis. The fragment ion at m/z 329.10 Da mainly resulted from the loss of one molecule of Glc from the precursor ion, while the fragment ions at m/z 314.08 Da and 299.06 Da corresponded to the consecutive loss of two CH_3 groups from m/z 329.10 Da. The fragment ions at m/z 183.03 Da and 165.02 Da were generated by the RDA fragmentation of the parent nucleus of compound **36**. After comparing the retention time, m/z, and mass spectral fragments with reference standards, compound **36** was identified as andrographidine E. The potential fragmentation pattern of andrographidine E is shown in Figure 3B. Finally, a total of 72 flavonoid constituents (Table S3, 1–72) were characterized in *A. paniculata* based on the mass spectral fragments of reference compounds and literature data.

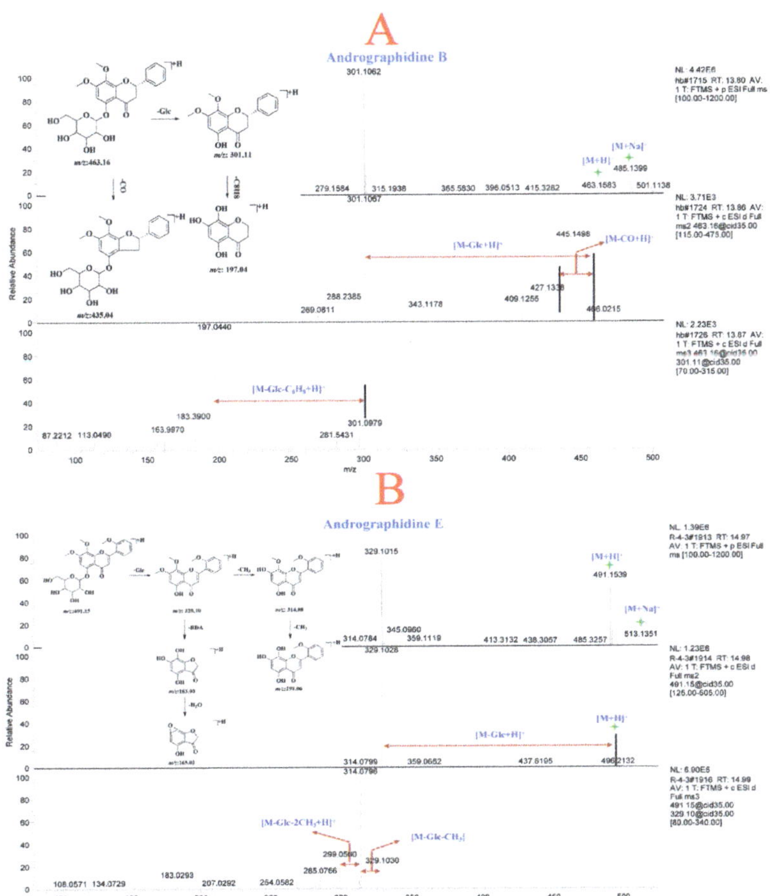

Figure 3. MS^n spectra and potential fragmentation patterns of andrographidine B (**A**) and andrographidine E (**B**).

3.2.3. Analysis of Organic Acids in *A. paniculata*

Organic acids are common constituents in plant species, and pharmacological studies have shown that these compounds possess various biological activities such as anti-inflammatory, antioxidant, and neuroprotective effects [25–28]. Thus, characterizing the organic acids in *A. paniculata* is of significance. In this study, based on the reported organic acids in *A. paniculata*, a polygonal mass defect window was established, and 190 potential organic acids were screened from the leaves of *A. paniculata*. Subsequently, the potential organic acids in *A. paniculata* were collected using a precursor ion list approach.

Compound **76** exhibited a $[M + H]^+$ ion peak at m/z 355.1014 Da and a $[M + Na]^+$ ion peak at m/z 377.083 Da in the MS spectrum. In the MS^2 spectrum, fragment ion peaks at m/z 337.09 Da and m/z 163.04 Da were observed, corresponding to the loss of one molecule of H_2O and $C_7H_{11}O_5$ from the precursor ion, respectively. In the MS^3 spectrum, fragment ion peaks at m/z 135.04 Da and m/z 117.03 Da were detected, which originated from the m/z 163.04 Da fragment with higher spectral intensity in the MS^2 spectrum. Through comparison with reference standards in terms of retention time and mass spectral fragmentation, compound **76** was identified as chlorogenic acid. The MS, MS^2 and MS^3 spectra and potential fragmentation patterns of compound **76** are shown in Figure 4. Finally, through comparison with reference standards and literature data, ten caffeoylquinic acid compounds (Table S3, 74–82) were characterized from different parts of *A. paniculata*.

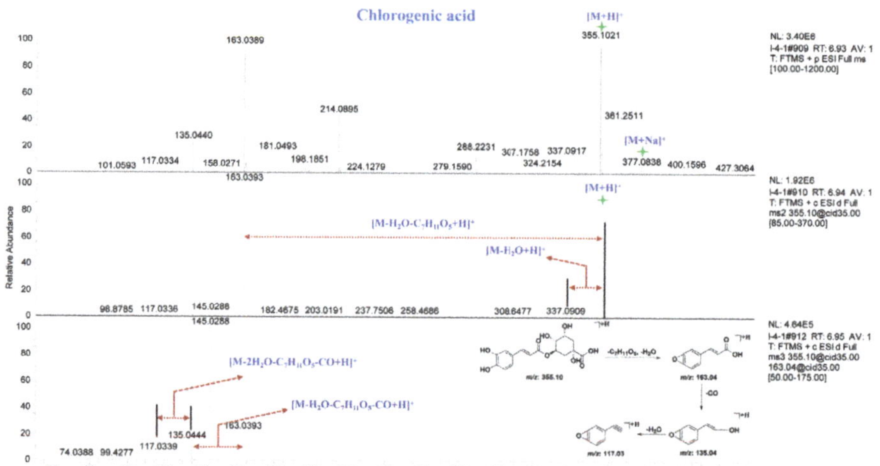

Figure 4. MS^n spectra and potential fragmentation patterns of chlorogenic acid.

3.2.4. Analysis of Other Components in *A. paniculata*

Previous reports have indicated that besides diterpene lactones, flavonoids, and organic acids, *A. paniculata* also contains other types of compounds such as triterpenoids and adenosine [3]. To systematically characterize other components in *A. paniculata*, the raw data obtained were imported into Compound Discoverer 3.3 software for local database identification and network database searching.

Compound **83** and **84** exhibited $[M + H]^+$ ion peaks at m/z 584.27 Da and $[M + Na]^+$ ion peaks at m/z 606.25 Da, indicating that compounds **83** and **84** are a pair of isomeric compounds. In the MS^n spectra, fragment ion peaks at m/z 438.24, 420.23, 292.20, 275.18, and 129.14 Da were detected. The fragment ions at m/z 438.24, 292.20, and 129.14 Da corresponded to the consecutive loss of three molecules of coumaroyl from the precursor ion. The fragment ions at m/z 420.23 Da and m/z 275.18 Da resulted from the loss of one molecule of coumaroyl, H_2O, and C_9H_7NO from the precursor ion, respectively. Through comparison with online mass spectral databases, compounds **83** and **84** were identified as tricoumaroyl spermidine or an isomer. The MS^n spectra and potential fragmentation patterns of compounds **83** and **84** are shown in Figure 5A [29]. The fragment ions at m/z 438.24, 420.23, 292.20, 275.18, and 129.14 Da could serve as diagnostic ions for spermidine derivatives in natural products.

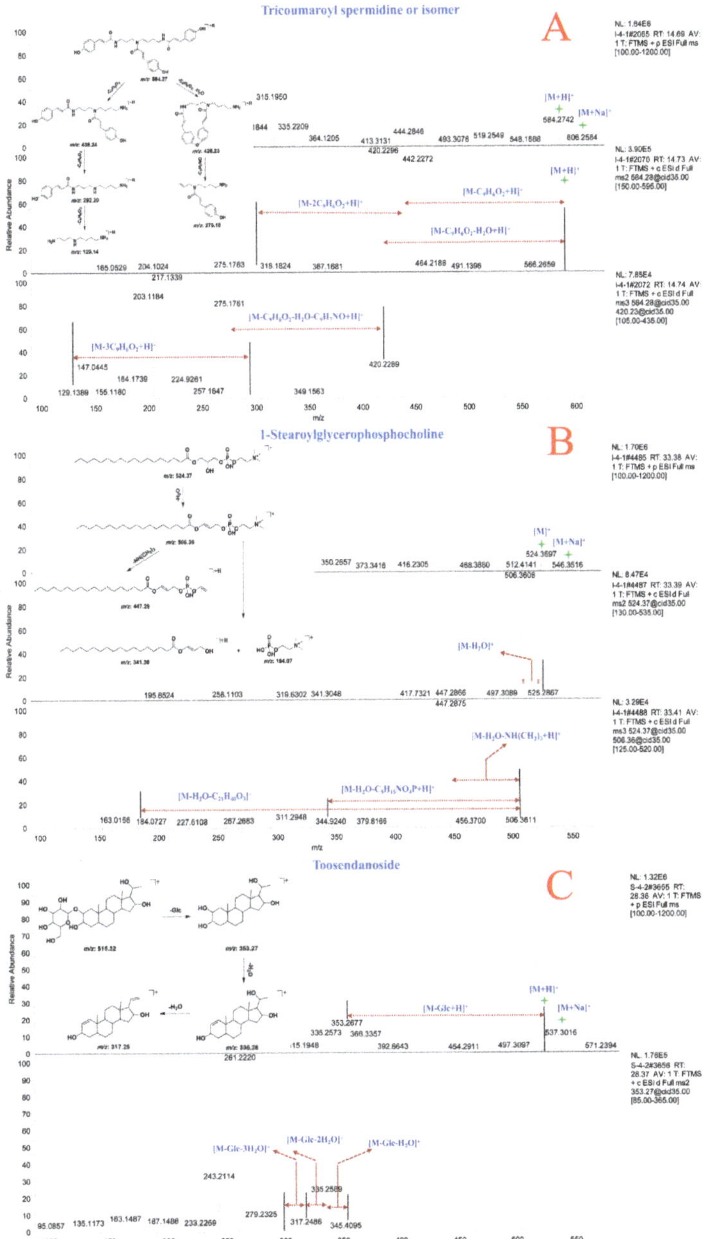

Figure 5. MS^n spectra and potential fragmentation patterns of tricoumaroyl spermidine or isomer (**A**), 1-stearoylglycerophosphocholine (**B**), and toosendanoside (**C**).

Compound **93** was identified as 1-stearoylglycerophosphocholine by comparing its MS^n data with the spectral information in the online spectral databases and preliminary research [30]. In the MS spectrum, compound **93** displayed $[M + H]^+$ ion peak at m/z 524.37 Da and $[M + Na]^+$ ion peak at m/z 546.35 Da. In the MS^2 and MS^3 spectra, fragment ions at m/z 506.36, 447.29, 341.30, and 184.07 Da were detected. The fragment ion at m/z 506.36 Da resulted from the loss of one molecule of H_2O from the precursor ion. Fragment ions at m/z 447.29, 341.30, and 184.07 Da were derived from the fragment ion at m/z 506.36 Da through subsequent losses of $NH(CH_3)_3$, $C_5H_{15}NO_4P$, and $C_{21}H_{40}O_3$, respectively. The MS^n spectrum and potential fragmentation patterns of compound **93** are shown in Figure 5B. Based on the characteristic fragment ions in the mass spectrum, compounds **86–93** were identified as phosphatidylcholines.

Compound **103** exhibited $[M + H]^+$ ion peak at m/z 515.32 Da and $[M + Na]^+$ ion peak at m/z 537.30 Da in MS spectrum. In the MS^n spectrum, fragment ion peaks at m/z 353.27, 335.26, 317.25, and 259.08 Da were detected, corresponding to consecutive loss of one molecule of Glc and two molecules of H_2O from the precursor ion at m/z 515.32 Da. Comparison with literature mass spectral data confirmed that compound **103** was toosendanoside [31]. The MS^n spectrum and potential fragmentation patterns of toosendanoside are shown in Figure 5C. Compared to compound **103**, compound **100** exhibited an m/z of 677.37 Da, indicating the presence of an additional molecule of Glc, and the glycone portion showed consistent fragmentation patterns. Based on the characteristic fragment ions in the mass spectrum, compounds **94–106** were identified as triterpenoids.

Consequently, through comparison with reference standards, the literature, and online mass spectral databases, a total of 126 compounds were characterized from *A. paniculata*, excluding diterpene lactones. The characterized compounds included 72 flavonoids, ten caffeoylquinic acid derivatives, three spermidine derivatives, eight phosphatidylcholines, 13 triterpenoids, and 20 other components. In the identified components, we identified 67, 42, 29, 30, and 20 flavonoids in the roots, stems, leaves, flowers, and fruits of *A. paniculata*, respectively. Additionally, we detected 9, 9, 9, 7, and 7 sphenylpropanoid in the roots, stems, leaves, flowers, and fruits, respectively. Spermidine derivatives and phosphatidylcholines were found to be present in all parts of *A. paniculata*. Furthermore, we identified 12, 12, 7, 5, and 5 triterpenoids in the roots, stems, leaves, flowers, and fruits, respectively. In addition, 15, 17, 16, 15, and 16 of other types of compounds were identified in the roots, stems, leaves, flowers, and fruits of *A. paniculata*, respectively.

3.3. Metabolite Analysis of A. paniculata at Different Growth Stages and Plant Parts

Previous studies have shown significant variations in the content of major diterpenoid lactones in *A. paniculata* leaves from different manufacturers and batches, which could be attributed to variations in harvesting time and inconsistent leaf-to-stem ratios [32,33]. To explore the differential metabolites in *A. paniculata* at different growth stages and plant parts, a non-targeted metabolomics approach was employed in this study. Raw data from 56 samples of *A. paniculata* roots, stems, leaves, and seven batches of quality control (QC) samples were imported into Progenesis QI 2.1 software for peak alignment and extraction, facilitating subsequent targeted. Finally, the exported data matrix is used for non-targeted metabolomics analyses.

3.3.1. Targeted Analysis of Major Compounds in *A. paniculata*

To investigate the distribution of diterpenoid lactones and flavonoids in different parts of *A. paniculata*, a polygonal mass defect filter was applied to screen potential diterpenoid lactones and flavonoids. In the roots of *A. paniculata*, 4342 ions were detected, and after the targeted metabolite screening using the polygonal mass defect filter, 556 potential diterpenoid lactones and 778 potential flavonoids were identified. Similarly, 4809 ions were detected in the stems of *A. paniculata*, and after the screening process, 868 potential diterpenoid lactones and 642 potential flavonoids were identified. In the leaves of *A. paniculata*, 4717 ions were detected, and the targeted analysis revealed 1550 potential diterpenoid lactones and 426 potential flavonoids. Due to the limited sample numbers of flowers and fruits, their data were combined for analysis. By applying the polygonal mass defect filter, 4385 ions were detected in the flowers and fruits of *A. paniculata*, including 886 potential diterpenoid lactones and 493 potential flavonoids. These results indicate that diterpenoid lactones were predominantly present in *A. paniculata* leaves, while flavonoids were relatively less diverse in this plant part. The roots exhibited a higher abundance of flavonoids compared to diterpenoid lactones, whereas the stems displayed the highest diversity of compounds, including a wide range of diterpenoid lactones and flavonoids. Flowers and fruits mainly contained diterpenoid lactones, with fewer flavonoid compounds.

3.3.2. Non-Targeted Metabolomics Analysis of Chemical Constituents in *A. paniculata*

To further explore differential metabolites in *A. paniculata* from different origins and medicinal plant parts, the raw data were processed using Progenesis QI 2.1 software, resulting in a data matrix containing 6192 variables, including retention time, m/z, and ion intensities. Subsequently, based on the "30% rule" and "80% rule" in metabolomics data analysis, 1969 data points that did not meet the criteria were excluded using Excel formulas, resulting in a final data matrix of 4223 variables. The processed data matrices (63 in total) were then imported into SIMCA-P 14.1 software for principal component analysis (PCA) and orthogonal partial least squares discriminant analysis (OPLS-DA). As shown in Figure 6, Figure 6A presents the PCA plot of the 63 datasets, with the seven QC samples tightly clustered, indicating good instrument precision and reproducibility for further analysis. Figure 6B shows the OPLS-DA results of different parts of *A. paniculata*, revealing clear differentiation among roots, stems, leaves, flowers, and fruits, indicating the presence of chemical composition variations across different plant parts. The loading plot in Figure 6C highlights andrographolide, dehydroandrographolide, and 14-deoxyandrographolide as the key differential compounds influencing the classification of *A. paniculata* plant parts. The OPLS-DA model exhibited good fitting (R2Y(cum) = 0.951) and predictive ability (Q2(cum) = 0.933), as validated through 200 permutations [i.e., R2 = (0.0, 0.157), Q2 = (0.0, −0.444)], indicating robustness and reliability. Subsequently, variables with VIP (Variable Importance in Projection) values greater than three were selected and further analyzed using *t*-tests in MetaboAnalyst 5.0 online platform. Variables with VIP values greater than 3 and *p*-values less than 0.05 were considered as differential compounds influencing the classification of *A. paniculata* plant parts (Table S4). A total of 41 compounds were selected as differentiating factors. To visually illustrate the impact of these 41 variables on the classification of *A. paniculata* plant parts, the mass spectrometry responses of these compounds in different plant parts were imported into HemI 2.0 software for cluster analysis. The cluster analysis included seven QC samples, 15 root samples, 16 stem and leaf samples, five fruit samples, and four flower samples, and employed the square Euclidean distance method. The results in Figure 6E demonstrate the classification of the 63 datasets into three main clusters, with distinct separation of roots from stems and leaves. Leaves and stems also exhibited good differentiation, while flowers and early-stage fruits showed similar profiles to leaves, with higher levels of diterpenoid lactones and lower levels of flavonoids. QC samples and later-stage fruits were more similar to stems, with higher levels of flavonoids compared to *A. paniculata* leaves. The identified differential compounds included andrographolide, andropanoside, dehydroandrographolide, 14-deoxyandrographolide, andrographidine A, and andrographidine

B, which could be served as characteristic markers for distinguishing different parts of *A. paniculata*. According to the heat map analysis, it can be seen that the content of the three main differential components in the third and fourth week of *A. paniculata* are more significant than those in other stages, and the proportion of roots and stems and yield are comprehensively analyzed, and the yield in the third week is less, so we believe that the collection time of the fourth week after planting is the best harvest time for *A. paniculata*.

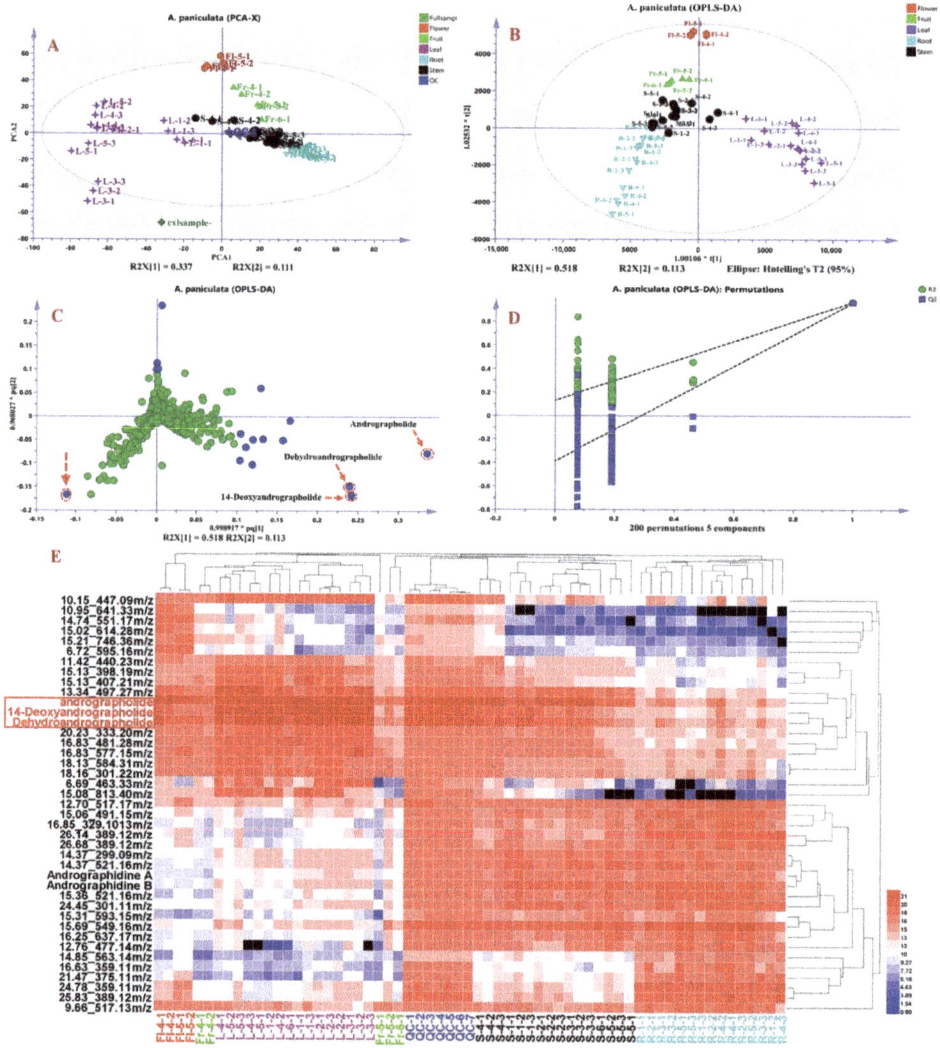

Figure 6. Principal component analysis (PCA) and cluster analysis results of different parts in *A. paniculata*. PCA plot (**A**), orthogonal partial least squares discriminant analysis (OPLS-DA) plot (**B**), OPLS-DA loading plot (**C**), OPLS-DA model validation results, *: $p < 0.05$ (**D**), and heatmap of differential metabolites (**E**).

4. Conclusions

In this study, a systematic characterization of chemical components in *A. paniculata* was performed, followed by the analysis of differential metabolites in different parts of the plant at various harvest periods using a non-targeted metabolomics approach. A total of 225 components were identified, including 99 diterpene lactones 18, 72 flavonoids, 10 caffeoylquinic acids, 3 spermidine derivatives, 8 phosphatidylcholines, 13 triterpenoids, and 20 other types of components. Notably, several component types, such as spermidine derivatives and phosphatidylcholines, were reported for the first time in *A. paniculata*. In addition to the four major diterpene lactones, 37 other components, including andrographidine A and andrographidine B, could serve as potential quality markers for the identification of raw materials in *A. paniculata* products. In addition to this, we also consider the fourth week after planting to be the best time to harvest *A. paniculata*. Our study provides important insights into the chemical composition and differential metabolites in different parts of *A. paniculata* and offers references for the selection of quality markers in *A. paniculata* herbal materials and related products.

Supplementary Materials: The following supporting information can be downloaded at: https://www.mdpi.com/article/10.3390/molecules30071490/s1, Figure S1: Determine results of four diterpene lactones in Chuanxinlian tablets from different manufacturers. Figure S2: Polygonal mass deficit map of flavonoids in *A. paniculata*. Figure S3: Polygonal mass deficit map of caffeoyl quinic acid components in *A. paniculata*. Table S1: Sample information of Chuanxinlian tablets from different manufacturers. Table S2: Collect information of samples from different parts of *A. paniculata* at different growth stages. Table S3: Detailed information about the characterized components in *A. paniculata*. Table S4: Components with VIP > 3 between different harvest periods and different plant parts of *A. paniculata* based on the OPLS-DA.

Author Contributions: Conceptualization, E.H.; methodology, E.H. and R.C.; software, A.L. and Y.W.; writing—original draft preparation, E.H. and R.C.; formal analysis, R.C. and A.L.; investigation, Y.W. validation, H.L., D.W. and J.H.; writing—review and editing, Y.W. and X.W.; visualization, D.W. and W.W.; supervision, W.W. and X.W.; funding acquisition, X.W. All authors have read and agreed to the published version of the manuscript.

Funding: The study was supported by the National Nature Science Foundation of China (82160812, 82304450), the Department of Science and Technology of Guizhou Province (QKHZC [2021]420, QKHPTRC-CXTD [2023]024), Guizhou Engineering Research Center of Industrial Key-technology for Dendrobium Nobile (QKJ [2022]048), Administration of Traditional Chinese Medicine of Guizhou Province (Grant no. 362 QZYY-2024-197).

Institutional Review Board Statement: Not applicable.

Informed Consent Statement: Not applicable.

Data Availability Statement: The original contributions presented in this study are included in the article/Supplementary Material. Further inquiries can be directed to the corresponding authors.

Conflicts of Interest: The authors have no conflicts of interest to declare.

References

1. Intharuksa, A.; Arunotayanun, W.; Yooin, W.; Sirisa-ard, P. A Comprehensive Review of *Andrographis paniculata* (Burm. f.) Nees and Its Constituents as Potential Lead Compounds for COVID-19 Drug Discovery. *Molecules* **2022**, *27*, 4479. [CrossRef] [PubMed]
2. Kumar, S.; Singh, B.; Bajpai, V. *Andrographis paniculata* (Burm.f.) Nees: Traditional uses, phytochemistry, pharmacological properties and quality control/quality assurance. *J. Ethnopharmacol.* **2021**, *275*, 114054. [PubMed]
3. Jiang, M.; Sheng, F.; Zhang, Z.; Ma, X.; Gao, T.; Fu, C.; Li, P. *Andrographis paniculata* (Burm.f.) Nees and its major constituent andrographolide as potential antiviral agents. *J. Ethnopharmacol.* **2021**, *272*, 113954. [PubMed]
4. Songvut, P.; Suriyo, T.; Panomvana, D.; Rangkadilok, N.; Satayavivad, J. A comprehensive review on disposition kinetics and dosage of oral administration of *Andrographis paniculata*, an alternative herbal medicine, in co-treatment of coronavirus disease. *Front. Pharmacol.* **2022**, *13*, 952660.
5. Rafi, M.; Karomah, A.H.; Heryanto, R.; Septaningsih, D.A.; Kusuma, W.A.; Amran, M.B.; Rohman, A.; Prajogo, B. Metabolite profiling of *Andrographis paniculata* leaves and stem extract using UHPLC-Orbitrap-MS/MS. *Nat. Prod. Res.* **2020**, *36*, 625–629.

6. Casamonti, M.; Risaliti, L.; Vanti, G.; Piazzini, V.; Bergonzi, M.C.; Bilia, A.R. Andrographolide Loaded in Micro- and Nano-Formulations: Improved Bioavailability, Target-Tissue Distribution, and Efficacy of the "King of Bitters". *Engineering* **2019**, *5*, 69–75.
7. *Pharmacopoeia of People's Republic of China*; Chinese Pharmacopoeia Commission, Ed.; China Medical Science Press: Beijing, China, 2020; Volume Part I, p. 280.
8. Dalawai, D.; Aware, C.; Jadhav, J.P.; Murthy, H.N. RP-HPLC analysis of diterpene lactones in leaves and stem of different species of Andrographis. *Nat. Prod. Res.* **2019**, *35*, 2239–2242.
9. Liang, X.; Ye, Y.; Zhu, Y.; Xiao, J.; Qiao, Y. Multivariate comparative analysis of chemical constituent changes and antioxidant properties of polysaccharides in ribes stenocarpum maxim. at different maturity stages on the Qinghai-Tibet Plateau. *Sci. Hortic.* **2023**, *308*, 111556.
10. Mahgoub, Y.A.; Shawky, E.; Ghareeb, D.A.; Darwish, F.A.; El Sebakhy, N.A.; El-Hawiet, A.M. UPLC-MS/MS multivariate data analysis reveals phenological growth stages affect silymarin bioactive components of the different organs of two Silybum marianum genotypes. *Microchem. J.* **2023**, *187*, 108436.
11. Yan, J.-K.; Chen, T.-T.; Wang, Z.-W.; Wang, C.; Liu, C.; Li, L. Comparison of physicochemical characteristics and biological activities of polysaccharides from barley (*Hordeum vulgare* L.) grass at different growth stages. *Food Chem.* **2022**, *389*, 133083.
12. Pholphana, N.; Rangkadilok, N.; Saehun, J.; Ritruechai, S.; Satayavivad, J. Changes in the contents of four active diterpenoids at different growth stages in *Andrographis paniculata* (Burm.f.) Nees (*Chuanxinlian*). *Chin. Med.* **2013**, *8*, 2. [CrossRef] [PubMed]
13. Waris, M.; Koçak, E.; Gonulalan, E.M.; Demirezer, L.O.; Kır, S.; Nemutlu, E. Metabolomics analysis insight into medicinal plant science. *Trends Anal. Chem.* **2022**, *157*, 116795. [CrossRef]
14. Wu, X.; Long, H.; Li, F.; Wu, W.; Zhou, J.; Liu, C.; Hou, J.; Wu, W.; Guo, D. Comprehensive feature-based molecular networking and metabolomics approaches to reveal the differences components in *Cinnamomum cassia* and *Cinnamomum verum*. *J. Sep. Sci.* **2021**, *44*, 3810–3821. [CrossRef]
15. Li, W.; Yang, X.; Chen, B.; Zhao, D.; Wang, H.; Sun, M.; Li, X.; Xu, X.; Liu, J.; Wang, S.; et al. Ultra-high performance liquid chromatography/ion mobility time-of-flight mass spectrometry-based untargeted metabolomics combined with quantitative assay unveiled the metabolic difference among the root, leaf, and flower bud of *Panax notoginseng*. *Arab. J. Chem.* **2021**, *14*, 103409. [CrossRef]
16. Wu, X.; Hou, J.; Zhang, Z.; Chen, L.; Ni, H.; Qian, Y.; Wu, W.; Long, H.; Zhang, L.; Li, F.; et al. In-depth exploration and comparison of chemical constituents from two *Lilium* species through offline two-dimensional liquid chromatography combined with multimode acquisition of high-resolution mass spectrometry. *J. Chromatogr. A* **2022**, *1670*, 462980. [CrossRef]
17. Qian, Y.; Li, W.; Wang, H.; Hu, W.; Wang, H.; Zhao, D.; Hu, Y.; Li, X.; Gao, X.; Yang, W. A four-dimensional separation approach by offline 2D-LC/IM-TOF-MS in combination with database-driven computational peak annotation facilitating the in-depth characterization of the multicomponents from Atractylodis Macrocephalae Rhizoma (*Atractylodes macrocephala*). *Arab. J. Chem.* **2021**, *14*, 102957.
18. Wu, X.; Ding, H.; Zhang, Z.; Zheng, M.; Ni, H.; Huang, Z.; Wu, W.; Long, H.; Zhou, Y.; Li, F.; et al. An improved strategy for identification and annotation of easily in-sourced dissociation diterpene lactones from plant natural products: Taking *Andrographis paniculata* (Burm. f.) as an example. *Rapid Commun. Mass Spectrom.* **2023**, *37*, e9483. [CrossRef]
19. Alvarez-Rivera, G.; Ballesteros-Vivas, D.; Parada-Alfonso, F.; Ibañez, E.; Cifuentes, A. Recent applications of high resolution mass spectrometry for the characterization of plant natural products. *Trends Anal. Chem.* **2019**, *112*, 87–101. [CrossRef]
20. Zuo, T.; Zhang, C.; Li, W.; Wang, H.; Hu, Y.; Yang, W.; Jia, L.; Wang, X.; Gao, X.; Guo, D. Offline two-dimensional liquid chromatography coupled with ion mobility-quadrupole time-of-flight mass spectrometry enabling four-dimensional separation and characterization of the multicomponents from white ginseng and red ginseng. *J. Pharm. Anal.* **2019**, *10*, 597–609. [CrossRef]
21. Ramabulana, A.-T.; Petras, D.; Madala, N.E.; Tugizimana, F. Mass spectrometry DDA parameters and global coverage of the metabolome: Spectral molecular networks of momordica cardiospermoides plants. *Metabolomics Off. J. Metabolomic Soc.* **2023**, *19*, 18. [CrossRef]
22. Yu, Z.; Chen, Z.; Li, Q.; Yang, K.; Huang, Z.; Wang, W.; Zhao, S.; Hu, H. What dominates the changeable pharmacokinetics of natural sesquiterpene lactones and diterpene lactones: A review focusing on absorption and metabolism. *Drug Metab. Rev.* **2020**, *53*, 41–44.
23. Shen, N.; Wang, T.; Gan, Q.; Liu, S.; Wang, L.; Jin, B. Plant flavonoids: Classification, distribution, biosynthesis, and antioxidant activity. *Food Chem.* **2022**, *383*, 132531. [PubMed]
24. Yang, J.; Wen, K.; Cheng, K.; Nandakumar, K.; Salem, M.L.; Fang, X.; Yao, Y. Recent Research on Flavonoids and their Biomedical Applications. *Curr. Med. Chem.* **2021**, *28*, 1042–1066.
25. Qiu, X.; Zhang, Y.; Zhou, Y.; Li, G.-H.; Feng, X.-S. Progress in pretreatment and analysis of organic Acids: An update since 2010. *Food Chem.* **2021**, *360*, 129977.
26. Liu, P.; Wang, L.; Li, H.; Tan, L.; Ying, X.; Ju, B. Two new organic acids from *Portulaca oleracea* L. and their anti-inflammatory and anticholinesterase activities. *Nat. Prod. Res.* **2021**, *36*, 4395–4403.

27. Quiroga, P.R.; Nepote, V.; Baumgartner, M.T. Contribution of organic acids to α-terpinene antioxidant activity. *Food Chem.* **2018**, *277*, 267–272. [CrossRef]
28. Zulkifli, N.A.; Hassan, Z.; Mustafa, M.Z.; Azman, W.N.W.; Hadie, S.N.H.; Ghani, N.; Zin, A.A.M. The potential neuroprotective effects of stingless bee honey. *Front. Aging Neurosci.* **2023**, *14*, 1048028. [CrossRef]
29. Liu, T.; Qiao, N.; Ning, F.; Huang, X.; Luo, L. Identification and characterization of plant-derived biomarkers and physicochemical variations in the maturation process of *Triadica cochinchinensis* honey based on UPLC-QTOF-MS metabolomics analysis. *Food Chem.* **2023**, *408*, 135197.
30. Loftus, N.; Miseki, K.; Iida, J.; Gika, H.G.; Theodoridis, G.; Wilson, I.D. Profiling and biomarker identification in plasma from different Zucker rat strains via high mass accuracy multistage mass spectrometric analysis using liquid chromatography/mass spectrometry with a quadrupole ion trap-time of flight mass spectrometer. *Rapid Commun. Mass Spectrom. RCM* **2008**, *22*, 2547–2554.
31. Inada, A.; Somekawa, M.; Murata, H.; Nakanishi, T.; Tokuda, H.; Nishino, H.; Iwashima, A.; Darnaedi, D.; Murata, J. Phytochemical studies on meliaceous plants. VIII: Structures and inhibitory effects on Epstein-Barr virus activation of triterpenoids from leaves of Chisocheton macrophyllus KING. *Chem. Pharm. Bull.* **1993**, *41*, 617–619.
32. Xu, T.; Pan, J.; Zhao, L. Simultaneous determination of four andrographolides in *Andrographis paniculata* Nees by silver ion reversed-phase high-performance liquid chromatography. *J. Chromatogr. Sci.* **2008**, *46*, 747–750. [PubMed]
33. Tajidin, N.E.; Shaari, K.; Maulidiani, M.; Salleh, N.S.; Ketaren, B.R.; Mohamad, M. Metabolite profiling of *Andrographis paniculata* (Burm. f.) Nees. young and mature leaves at different harvest ages using 1H NMR-based metabolomics approach. *Sci. Rep.* **2019**, *9*, 16766.

molecules

MDPI

Review

An Overview of α-Pyrones as Phytotoxins Produced by Plant Pathogen Fungi

Antonio Evidente

Institute of Biomolecular Chemistry, National Research Council (CNR), Via Campi Flegrei 34, 80078 Pozzuoli, Italy; evidente@unina.it

Abstract: Crop diseases negatively affect the quality and quantity of agricultural products, with significant economic and social consequences. These problems become emergencies in a world where the safe production of food for human health is becoming increasingly pressing. Microorganisms, including phytopathogenic fungi, are the main organisms responsible for these diseases, which cause devastating damage. Environmental pollution generated by human activities causes further significant reductions in agricultural production, as well as the expansion of metropolitan areas, and climate change. Phytotoxins produced by pathogenic fungi play a fundamental role in the induction of diseases by directly interfering with the physiological processes of agricultural plants. They are secondary metabolites that can belong to all the different classes of natural compounds, and their structures and biological activities have been extensively studied. These substances have often been shown to possess other interesting biological activities for potential applications both in agriculture and in other fields, such as biotechnology and medicine. This review focuses on phytotoxic α-pyrones produced by plant pathogenic fungi, describing in detail all their chemical and biological properties and, in some cases, the results of studies on their structure-activity relationship and on the potential practical applications in various sectors.

Keywords: crop diseases; phytopathogen fungi; phytotoxins; pyrones; chemical and biological characterization

1. Introduction

Nature is an almost inexhaustible source of a myriad of compounds belonging to several different groups of organic substances, exhibiting specific biological activities [1]. Aromatic heterocycle compounds are about two-thirds of the total organic compounds that define the history, present, and future of modern drugs. Benzene rings in which one carbon (C) is replaced by heteroatoms, such as nitrogen (N), oxygen (O), and sulfur (S), generate different subgroups of heterocyclic compounds [2]. Pyrones are a class of heterocyclic six-membered lactones represented by two isomers, 2-pyrone and 4-pyrone. The number 2/4 is assigned on the basis of the position of the carbonyl group relative to the oxygen atom within the ring system. The 2-pyrone (more commonly known as α-pyrone) structure is found in nature as part of the coumarin ring system. 4-Pyrone (more commonly known as γ-pyrone) is found in some natural chemical compounds such as chromone, maltol, and kojic acid [3]. There is a growing interest in α-pyrones due to their structural diversity and their diverse biological activities, which include anti-inflammatory, cytotoxic, antibacterial, antioxidant, insecticidal, and antifungal activity [4–7]. α-Pyrones are not only produced by fungi, but also, although less frequently, by bacteria, by plants, and by lichens.

Some reviews have previously addressed this topic, but they only report in isolation, either chemical or biological characterization of the α-pyrones, and sometimes also cover a limited time range of publications. Azizian et al. (2024) [8] reported the chemical structures and biological activities of 268 natural α-pyrone derivatives, isolated from January 2016 to October 2023, as fungi (199), bacteria (34), and plant (35) metabolites. Successively, another review describes natural compounds containing a 2-pyrone moiety, emphasizing their role in biological activity, particularly with respect to potential therapeutic or antimicrobial agents [5]. Other authors confirmed the pharmacological properties and potential applicability of the 2-pyrones, focusing attention on their chemotherapeutic activities. The α-pyrones are reported as anti-HIV, anti-TB, and anti-cancer agents, and for their potential role against neurodegeneration, hypercholesterolemia, microbial infections, chronic obstructive lung disease, inflammation, antinociception, and immunomodulation [9]. Some authors reported the relation of the stereochemistry of the α-pyrones with their biological activity [10], while other ones selectively described those produced by fungi and with potential herbicidal activity [11]. Schäberle (2016) [7] specifically reported new insights into additional biosynthetic mechanisms of α-pyrones, while other authors specifically described the chemical and biological properties of natural diterpene pyrones [12].

Thus, the present review is the first one focused on only fungal pyrones with phytotoxic activity. The results discussed in the three different sections were obtained from Sci-Finder and chronologically reported. Furthermore, where reported for some phytotoxic *a*-pyrones, the results of structure–activity, mode-of-action studies, and future perspectives are also discussed.

2. α-Pyrones

2.1. α-Pyrones Produced from Fungi Pathogenic for Agrarian Plants

Some differently substituted α-pyrones were produced in liquid culture by the fungus *Pyrenoclzaeta terrestris*, which is the causal agent of onion pink disease, attracting considerable attention in outbreaks in the land where onion cultivation is widespread. The fungus was also isolated from other plants such as rice and garlic. The first phytotoxins isolated were pyrenocines A and B (**1** and **2**, Figure 1, Table 1) [13]. Toxin **1** was also isolated from *Trichoderma citro-viride* and named citreopyrone [14]. The phytotoxic activity induced by compound **1** on onion root was more strong than that of compound **2** [13]. The first furane-derivative structure, assigned to both phytotoxins, was then revised as that of two α-pyrone derivatives by X-ray analysis of pyrenocine A and that of pyrenocine B by spectroscopic correlation [15]. Successively, from the same culture filtrates, pyrenocine C (**3**, Figure 1, Table 1) was also isolated and showed only a weak phytotoxicity [16]. When *P. terrestris* was grown on solid culture, it also produced three other phytotoxins, named pyrenochaetic acids A-C (**4–6**, Figure 1, Table 1), which are close to pyrenocines. The phytotoxicity of pyrenochaetic acids A-C was tested on the growth of onion and rice seedlings by the germination test using lettuce seed. Pyrenochaetic acid A (**4**) inhibited the root growth of onion and rice seedlings by 100% at 250 and at 5000 ppm, respectively, while its analogue **6** was less toxic. In the germination test on lettuce seeds, the three acids (**4–6**) exhibited equal inhibition at high concentrations, but promoted root elongation at low concentrations [17]. Successively, pyrenocin A (**1**) showed antibiotic activity against plants, fungi, and bacteria. In particular, it showed an effective dose for 50% inhibition (EDSO) of 4 kg/mL for elongation of onion seedlings, and 14, 20, 20, and 25 kg/mL for the germination of asexual spores of *Fusarium oxysporum* f. sp. *cepae*, *Fusarium solani* f. sp. *pisi*, *Mucor hiemalis*, and *Rhizopus stolonifer*, respectively. Compound 1 also inhibited linear mycelial growth of *P. terrestris* and *F. oxysporum* with an EDSO of 77 and 54 kg/mL, respectively. Furthermore, pirenocin A (**1**) showed biostatic rather than biocidal activity against all the bacteria used, with Gram-positive bacteria being more sensitive than Gram-negative bacteria. In fact, the EDOs observed for the growth inhibition of *Bacillus subtilis*,

Staphylococcus aureus, and *Escherichia coli* were 30, 45, and 200 kg/mL, respectively, while *Pseudomonas aeruginosa* appeared to be resistant at the concentrations used. Pirenocins B and C (**2** and **3**) showed weak antibiotic activity in all the tests performed [18].

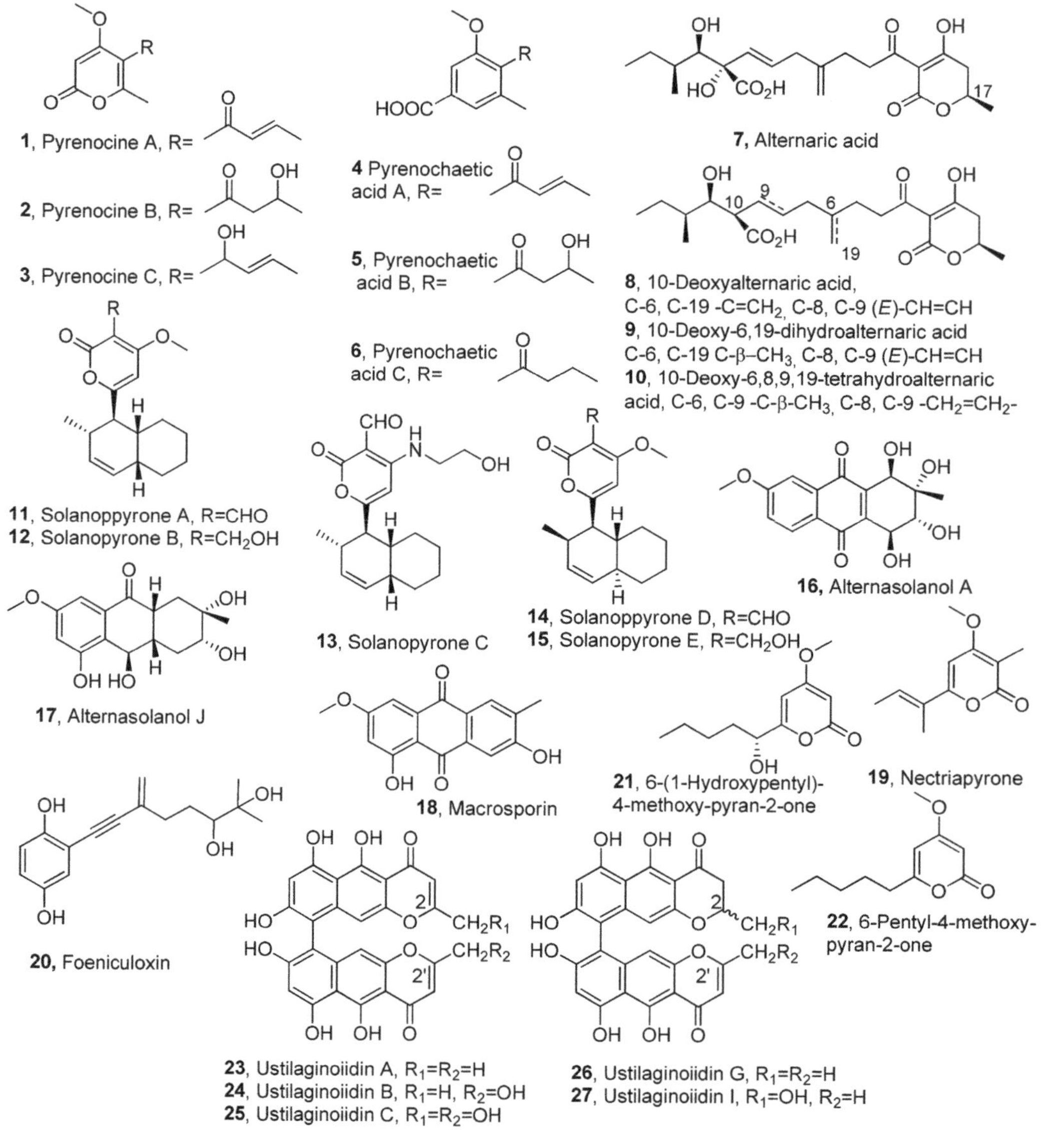

Figure 1. *Cont.*

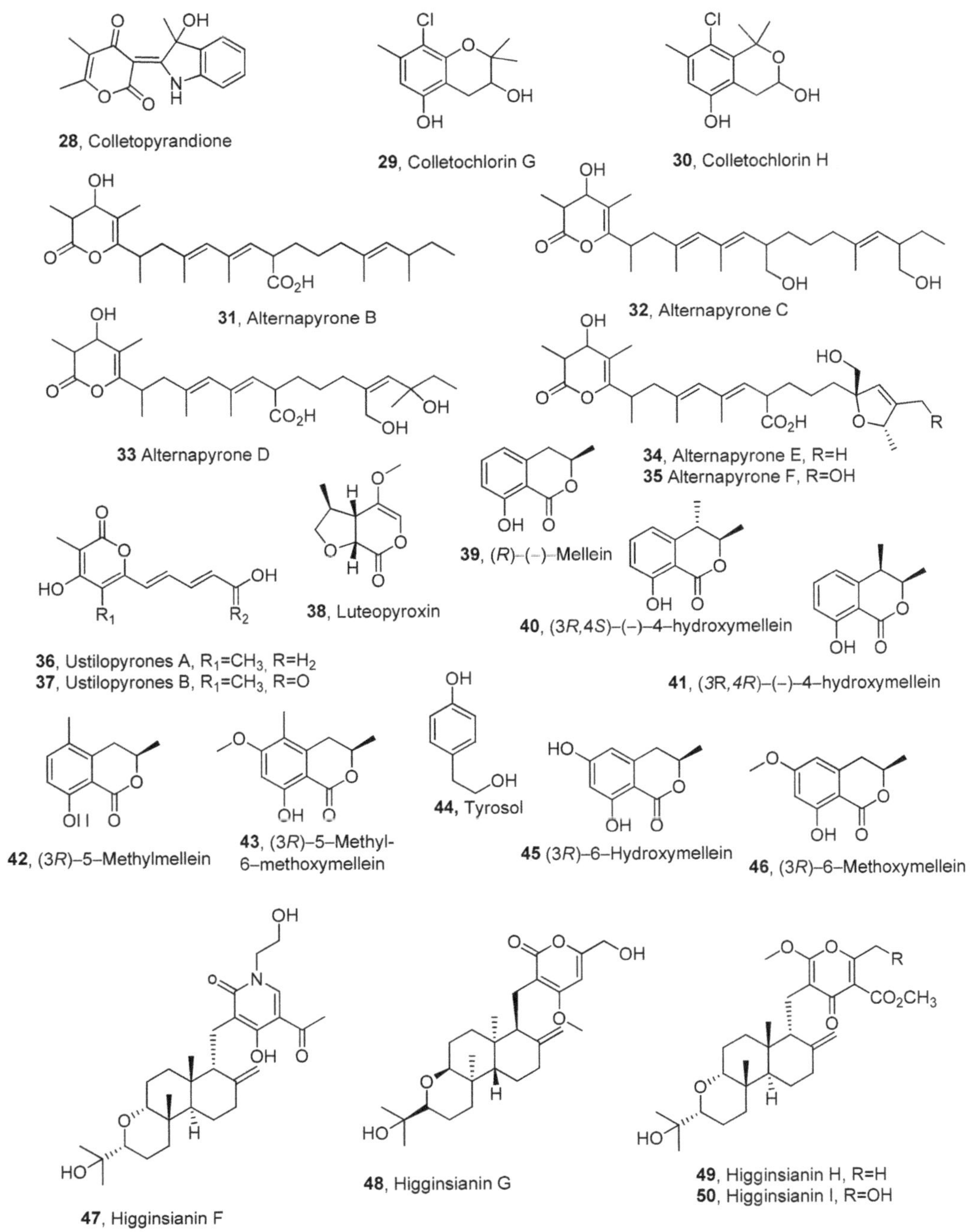

Figure 1. Structures of phytotoxic α-pyrones produced by fungal pathogens for agrarian plants.

Table 1. Phytotoxic α-pyrones produced from fungal pathogens for agrarian plants (″: identical data to the entry immediately above).

Compound	Fungal Producer	Other Biological Activities	Ref.
Pyrenocine A (**1**)	*Pyrenoclzaeta terrestris*	Antibiotic activity	[13,15] [18]
Pyrenocine B (**2**)	″	Weak antibiotic activity	″
Pyrenocine C (**3**)	″	″	″
Pyrenochaetic acid A (**4**)	″	Not reported	[17]
Pyrenochaetic acid B (**5**)	″	″	″
Pyrenochaetic acid C (**6**)	″	″	″
Alternaric acid (**7**)	*Alternaria solani*		[19]
10-Deoxyalternaric acid (**8**)	″	″	[20]
10-Deoxy-6,19-dihydro alternaric acid (**9**)	″	″	″
10-Deoxy-6,8,9,19-tetrahydro alternaric acid (**10**)	″	″	″
Solanapyrones A (**11**)	*A. solani* *Ascochyta rabiei*	″ Antibiotic activity	[21–23] [24]
Solanapyrones B (**12**)	″	Not reported	[21–23]″
Solanapyrones C (**13**)	″	″	″
Solanapyrones D (**14**)	*A. solani*	″	[21,22]
Solanapyrones E (**15**)	″	″	″
Alternasolanol A (**16**)	*Diaporthe angelicae* *Phomopis* sp.	″ Cytotoxic activity	[25] [26]
Alternasolanol J (**17**)	*D. angelica*	Not reported	[25]
Macrosporin (**18**)	″ *Phoma* sp.	″ Antifungal activity	″ [27]
Nectriapyrone (=Pestalopyrone, **19**)	*D. angelica* *Pestalotiopsis oenotherae* *Pestalotiopsis micropspora* *Biscogniauxia rosacearum* *Cosmosporella* sp.	Not Reported ″ ″ ″ Antibiotic	[25] [28] [29] [30] [31]
Foeniculoxin (**20**)	*Diaporthe angelicae*	Not reported	[32]
6-(1-Hydroxypentyl)-4-methoxy-pyran-2-one (**21**)	*Pestalotiopsis guepinii* *Cosmosporella* sp.	″ Antibiotic	[33] [31]
6-Pentyl-4-methoxy-pyran-2-one (**22**)	*P. guepenii* *Cosmosporella* sp.	Not reported″ Antibiotic	[33] [31]
Ustilaginoiidin A, R_1=R_2=H (**23**)	*Villosiclava virens* *Chaetomium* spp.	Not reported Cytotoxic activity	[34] [35]
Ustilaginoiidin B, R_1=H, R_2=OH (**24**)	″ *Villosiclava virens*	Not reported	[34]
Ustilaginoidin C, R_1=R_2=OH (**25**)	″	″	″
Ustilaginoidin G, R_1=R_2=H (**26**)	″	″	″
Ustilaginoidin I, R_1=H, R_2=OH (**27**)	″	″	″

Table 1. *Cont.*

Compound	Fungal Producer	Other Biological Activities	Ref.
Colletopyrandione (**28**)	*Colletotrichum higginsianum*		[36]
Colletochlorin G (**29**)	"	"	"
Colletochlorin H (**30**)	"	"	"
Alternapyrones B (**31**)	*Parastagonospora nodorum*		[37]
Alternapyrones C (**32**)	"	"	"
Alternapyrones D (**33**)	"	"	"
Alternapyrones E (**34**)	"	"	"
Alternapyrones F (**35**)	"	"	"
Ustilopyrones A (**36**)	*Ustilaginoidea virens*	"	[38]
Ustilopyrones B (**37**)	"	"	"
Luteopyroxin (**38**)	*Neofusicoccum luteum*	"	[39]
(*R*)-(−)-Mellein (**39**)	*Neofusicoccum luteum* *Neofusicoccum parvum* *Neofusicoccum australe*	" Antibacterial, insecticidal, and fungicidal activity	[39] [40]
(3*R*,4*S*)-(−)-4-Hydroxymellein (**40**)	*Neofusicoccum luteum* *Neofusicoccum parvum*	Not reported Antibacterial activity	[39] [40]
(3*R*,4*R*)-(−)-4-Hydroxymellein (**41**)	*Neofusicoccum luteum* *Neofusicoccum parvum*	Not reported Antibacterial activity	[39] Antibacterial activity
(3*R*)-5-Methylmellein (**42**)	*Biscogniauxia rosacearum*	Not reported	[41]
(3*R*)-5-Methyl-6-methoxymellein (**43**)	"	" Antibacterial activity	" [40]
Tyrosol (**44**)	"	Not reported Antiatherogenic, cardioprotective, anticancer, neuroprotective, and endocrine effects	[42] [43]
(3*R*)-6-Hydroxymellein (**45**)	"	Not reported	[42]
(3*R*)-6-Methoxymellein (**46**)	"	"	"
Higginsianin F (**47**)	*Colletotrichum higginsianum*		[43]
Higginsianin G (**48**)	"	"	"
Higginsianin H (**48**)	"	"	"
Higginsianin I (**50**)	"	"	"

" It means the species same as above.

Alternaria solani, the causal agent of early blight disease of tomatoes and potatoes [44], produced different non-related toxins as alternaric acids, a5,6-dihydro-α-pyrones and solanapyrones [19]. Alternaric acid (**7**, Figure 1) induced, in the host plant, symptoms similar to those of the so-called host-specific toxins. This phytotoxin (**7**) was also shown to delay the occurrence of hypersensitive death of potato cells infected by an incompatible race of *Phytophthora infestans* [45]. Then the determination of the stereochemistry and the total synthesis of alternaric acid **7** were also reported [46]. Three other alternaric acid-related compounds, 10-deoxyalternaric acid, 10-deoxy-6,19-dihydroalternaric acid, and 10-deoxy-6,8,9,19-tetrahydroalternaric acid (**8–10**, Figure 1, Table 1), were isolated from the same fungus [20]. All the alternaric acids (**7–10**) were tested for their growth inhibition of tomato seedlings and showed a different rate of phytotoxicity on roots and hypocotyls. The results obtained suggested that their phytotoxicity depends on the oxidation levels of the alternaric acids, and that the exo-methylene group at C-6 and the hydroxy group at C-10 in alternaric acid **7** play an important role in the phytotoxic activity. Furthermore, the phytotoxic activity of the degradation and the synthetic segments of alternaric acid suggested that the side-chain moiety and the 3-acyl-4-hydroxy-5,6-dihydro-2-pyrone moiety play different roles in the phytotoxic activity [20]. Solanapyrones A-E (**11–15**, Figure 1, Table 1) were produced from another strain of *A. solani* [21–23]. Both solanapyrones A and D, and B and E were obtained in a diastereomeric ratio of 6:1 [19]. Solanapyrones A and C were also isolated from filtrates of stationary cultures of *Ascochyta rabiei*, the causal fungus of chickpea blight [47], which is the most important disease of chickpea in areas where the growing season coincides with cool and moist weather [48]. The disease caused severe losses around the Mediterranean Basin and in Pakistan, where a loss of up to 50% of the crop was observed. Compounds **11** and **12** showed synergistic activity when tested on potatoes, while on isolated cells of the leaflets of 10-day-old chickpea seedlings, their effect was additive. The solanapyrones share interesting structural similarities to several phytotoxins, such as betaenones A and B isolated from *Phoma betae*, a parasite of sugar beet [49], and stemphyloxin from *Stemphylrum botryosum*, the causal agent of leaf spot on tomatoes [50]. Compounds **11** and **12** could act as siderophores to disturb the non-metabolism of the host. However, solanapyrones probably do not act directly as iron chelators per se, although they may chelate iron or other essential metal ions upon ring opening of the pyrone or upon further biotransformation within the host [47]. Although the phytotoxicity of solanapyrone A has been reported many times, its role in pathogenicity has not been completely clarified. A genetic study was carried out on the *sol5* gene, which encodes Diels-Alderase, which catalyzes the final step of solanapyrone biosynthesis. Silencing of this gene in both *A. rabiei* and *A. solani* leads to the accumulation of prosolanapyrone II-diol, which is the immediate biosynthetic precursor of solanapyrones and is not toxic to plants. Instead, solanapyrone A showed high toxicity against *Arabidopsis thaliana*. Furthermore, pathogenicity tests showed that non-solanapyrone-producing mutants of both fungi retained the virulence of wild-type strains. These results suggested that solanapyrones were not required for the pathogenicity of either fungus [51]. The antibacterial activity of solanapyrones A-C was tested against various human pathogens, such as Gram-positive, *B. subtilis*, *Bacillus megaterium*, *Clostridium perfringens*, *Micrococcus tetragenus*, MRSA (Methicillin-resistant Staphylococcus), and Gram-negative, *E. coli*, using streptomycin, acheomycin, and ampicillin as positive controls. Solanapyrone A (**4**) (MIC (Minimal Inhibitory Concentration) of 12.5 μg/mL) showed the same activity as ampicillin (MIC of 12.5 μg/mL) and better than that of streptomycin (MIC of 100 μg/mL) against *B. subtilis*. Solanapyrone B (**5**) showed better activity than ampicillin (MIC of 50 μg/mL) against *B. megaterium*. None of the tested compounds showed significant inhibition of the growth of *E. coli* and MRSA [24].

Altersolanols A and J, macrosporin (**16–18**, Figure 1, Table 1), three octaketides anthracenones, nectriapyrone (**19**, Figure 1, Table 1), and a pentaketide monoterpenoid, were isolated from *Diaporthe angelicae* (anamorph *Phomopsis foeniculi*), which is the causal agent of a heavy disease in fennel (*Foeniculum vulgare*) in Bulgaria [25]. Nectriapyrone was also named as a pestalopyrone when it was previously produced from an unidentified fungus isolated from the Indo-Pacific sponge *Stylotella* sp. [32,52]. The symptoms induced in the host plant by *D. angelicae* were umbel browning and stem necrosis [25]. The dried fennel seeds are used in phytotherapy and the pharmaceutical [53] and alimentary industries.

When assayed using a leaf puncture bioassay on detached tomato leaves, nectriapyrone and altersolanols A and J showed a modulated phytotoxicity, while macrosporin was not toxic. Altersolanol A was the most phytotoxic compound [52]. The same pathogen fungus, but a strain isolated from diseased fennel near Florence (Italy), produced foeniculoxin (**20**, Figure 1), a phytotoxic geranylhydroquinone [28]. Foeniculoxin (**20**), at 3.6 10^{-3} M, reduced root growth of the germinant seeds of both fennel and tomato while inducing necrosis on tobacco leaves and wilting and/or spots on the leaves of tomato cuttings [28]. Successively, from the same fungal culture filtrates, two phytotoxic exopolysaccharides (EPSs), namely a galactan with the known structure [-->6)-beta-D-Galf-(1-->5)-beta-D-Galf-(1-->5)-beta-D-Galf-(1-->]n and a branched mannan, were isolated too. The branched mannan consists of a backbone of alpha-(1-->6)-linked mannopyranose units. Almost all of these are branched at the 2 position, with arms containing 2- and 3-linked mannopyranose units. The crude polysaccharide and the galactan and mannan showed phytotoxic activity, i.e., chlorosis, necrosis, and/or wilting, on fennel and two non-host plants, tobacco and tomato [54]. Furthermore, altersolanol A (**16**) exhibited in vitro cytotoxicity activity against 34 human cancer cell lines with a mean IC_{50} (IC_{70}) values of 0.005 μg ml^{-1} (0.024 μg ml^{-1}) respectively and inhibited kinase inducing cell death by apoptosis through the cleavage by Caspase-3 and -9 and by decreased anti-apoptotic protein expression [26]. In addition, macrosporin showed antifungal activity against *Colletotrichum musae*, *Colletotrichum gloeosporioides*, *Fusarium graminearum*, *Penicillium italicum*, *Fusarium oxysporum* f. sp. *lycopersici*, and *Rhizoctonia solani* at different levels. Noteworthy activity, compared to that of carbendazim used as a positive control, was shown by compound **18** towards *Fusarium graminearum* [27].

Pestalopyrone (=nectriapyrone, **19**), a pentaketide already known as a minor toxin produced by *Pestalotiopsis oenotherae* [55], was also isolated from *Pestalotiopsis guepinii.* [56]. *P. guepinii* is the fungal causal agent of the so-called 'twig blight', one of the most serious diseases in hazelnuts (*Corylus avellana* L.) in Turkey, which causes severe yield losses [56]. *P. guepinii* was also isolated from walnut (*Juglans* spp.) and gum mastic tree (*Pistacia lentiscus* var. Chia) [56]. When the fungus was grown on a different culture medium besides nectriapyrone, two other phytotoxic pyrones were isolated from *P. guepenii* and identified as 6-(1-hydroxypentyl)-4-methoxy- and 6-pentyl-4-methoxy-pyran-2-one (**21** and **22**, Figure 1, Table 1) [33]. Tested by puncture on leaves of a number of plant species (*Convolvulus arvensis*, *Mercurialis annua*, *Chenopodium album*, and *Ailanthus altissima*), compound **22** showed high phytotoxicity, inducing large necrosis on the leaves of all the species tested, while compound **21** showed a similar toxicity to α-pyrone **22**, although it did not cause necrosis on the leaves of *C. arvensis.* This difference was probably due to a lower sensitivity of the latter plant. These results suggested that the functionalities of the *n*-pentyl side chain are important for the activity. On *Lemna minor* L., compound **22** appeared to be the most toxic compound, causing the complete desiccation of the plantlets, fumonisin B1, which is a powerful phytotoxin used for comparison, while pestalopyrone (**19**) proved to be not toxic [33]. When isolated from *Cosmosporella* sp., an endophytic fungus of *Vinca minor*, pestalopyrone (**19**) showed a selective inhibition of Gram-positive bacteria, such as methicillin-sensitive and methicillin-resistant *S. aureus* with MIC and MBC (Minimum Bactericidal Concentration) values ranging from 125 to 62.5 μg mL^{-1} against MSSA and MRSA strains [31].

Five main bis-naphtho-γ-pyrones, namely ustilaginoidins A, B, C, G, and I (**23–27**, Figure 1, Table 1), were isolated from the rice false smut balls (FSBs) infected by *Villosiclava virens* in rice spikelets on panicles. Rice false smut has become an increasingly serious fungal disease in rice (*Oryza sativa* L.) production worldwide. The contents of five ustilaginoidins (**23–27**) in rice FSBs at early, middle, and late maturation stages were determined by HPLC analysis. The results showed that the highest levels of ustilaginoidins were found in rice FSBs at the late stage, followed by those at the intermediate stage. The contents of ustilaginoidins A (**23**) and G (**25**) were relatively high at the early stage, while the contents of ustilaginoidins B, C, and I (**24, 25,** and **27**), having hydroxymethyl groups at C-2 or C-2′, were relatively high at the late stage [34]. Ustilaginoidin A (**23**) also inhibited ATP synthesis in mitochondria by uncoupling oxidative phosphorylation and depressing state-3 respiration of mitochondria [35].

Colletopyrandione, colletochlorins G and H, a tetrasubstituted chroman, and a tetrasubstituted isocroman-3,5-diol (**28–30**, Figure 1, Table 1), were isolated from the culture filtrates of the fungus *Colletotrichum higginsianum* together with 4-chloroorcinol, colletopyrone, and colletochlorins E and F [36]. *C. higginsiunum*, belonging to the *Colletotrichum destructivum* species complex [57], causes anthracnose leaf spot disease of several Brassicaceae crop species. Previously, from the mycelium of the same fungus were obtained colletochlorins A and B, which showed promising anticancer activity [58]. Assayed in several biological systems, colletopyrandione showed a modest phytotoxic activity, associated with a complete lack of toxicity towards off-target organisms [55]. Alternapyrones B-F (**31–35**, Figure 1, Table 1), which are five new α-pyrone polyketides, were produced by the fungal wheat pathogen *Parastagonospora nodorum*, whose biosynthetic gene cluster, which was significantly upregulated during plant infection, was heterologously reconstructed in *Aspergillus nidulans*. Compounds **34** and **35**, which contain a highly substituted dihydrofuran moiety, showed phytotoxic activity on wheat seed germination. Furthermore, only three enzymes, one highly reducing polyketide synthase and two multifunctional P450 oxygenases, were found to be necessary to synthesize the structurally complex α-pyrone [37].

Ustilopyrones A and B (**35** and **36**, Figure 1, Table 1), two sorbicillinoid-related pyrones, ustisorbicillinols A-F, and six sorbicillinoids were isolated together with nine known cogeners from *Ustilaginoidea virens*, the causal agent of rice false smut [38]. Phytotoxicity assays showed that the major sorbicillinoids bisvertinolone [59], demethyltrichodimerol [30], trichodimerol, and bislongiquinolide (also named trichotetronine) [29,60] showed strong inhibition against the radicle and germ elongation of rice and lettuce seeds, with bisverticolone being the strongest inhibitor. Dihydrotrichodimer ether A [41], and bisvertinolone, demethyltrichodimerol, trichodimerol showed moderate cytotoxicities against the tested cell lines with IC_{50}s of 8.83–74.7 μM, while ustisorbicillinol B, dihydrotrichodimer ether A, oxosorbicillinol [61], bisvertinolone, and demethyltrichodimerol were active against the tested bacteria (MICs (Minimal Inhibitory Concentrations) of 4∼128μg/mL). Furthermore, oxosorbicillinol bisvertinolone, demethyltrichodimerol displayed moderate antifungal activity [41].

Different phytotoxic metabolites were isolated from the organic extract of *Neofusicoccum luteum*, *Neofusicoccum australe*, and *Neofusicoccum parvum*, causal agents of Botryosphaeria dieback in Australia. *N. luteum* produced luteopyroxin (*R*)-(−)-mellein (1), and (3*R*,4*S*)-(−)- and (3*R*,4*R*)-(−)-4-hydroxymellein, (**38–41**, Figure 1, Table 1), a disubstituted furo-α-pyrone, a hexasubstituted anthraquinone, a trisubstituted oxepi-2(7*H*)-one, neoanthraquinone, luteoxepinone, (±)-nigrosporione, and tyrosol. The three melleins (**38–41**) and tyrosol were also produced by *N. parvum*, while *N. australe* produced (*R*)-(−)-mellein (**39**), neoanthraquinone, tyrosol, and *p*-cresol. When assayed on grapevine leaves, neoanthraquinone showed the highest toxic effect, causing severe shriveling and withering. Luteopyroxin (**38**), nigrosporione, and luteoxepinone also showed different degrees of toxicity, while p-cresol displayed low phytotoxicity [39]. Mellein and its two 4-hydroxy analogues (**38–41**) showed other interesting biological activities, including antibacterial activity against MRSA strains, larvicidal activity against *Aedes aegypti*, and antifungal activity towards several pathogens of agrarian plants, as extensively reported by the author of this review [40].

Nectriapyrone (**19**), (3*R*)-5-methylmellein, (3*R*)-5-methyl-6-methoxymellein, and tyrosol (**42–44**, Figure 1, Table 1) were isolated as phytotoxins from *Biscogniauxia rosacearum* isolated from oak trees in Zagros forests of Gilan-e Gharb, Kermanshah Province, Iran. A strain of the same fungus was recognized for the first time as a pathogen involved in grapevine trunk diseases in Paveh (west of Iran) vineyards, and produced meso-2,3-butanediol as the only phytotoxin. When all the metabolites were tested for phytotoxic activity by leaf puncture assays on *Quercus* ilex L. and *Hedera* helix L., and by leaf absorption assays on grapevines (*Vitis vinifera* L.), at a concentration of 5×10^{-3} and 1×10^{-3}, meso-2,3-butanediol and (3*R*)-5-methyl-6-methoxymellein (**42**) were the most toxic compounds. Nectriapyrone (**19**) and tyrosol (**44**) showed severe necrosis at the highest concentration on *Q. ilex*, while none of the compounds were active on *H. helix*. Furthermore, the phytotoxicity of compounds **42** and **43** was also compared with that of some related natural melleins, namely (3*R*)-mellein (**39**), (*3R,4R*)-4-hydroxymellein (**40**), (*3R,4S*)-4-hydroxymellein (**41**), (3*R*)-6-hydroxymellein (**45** Figure 1), and (3*R*)-6-methoxymellein (**46**, Figure 1) with a structure–activity relationship (SAR) study. The results obtained showed that on grapevines *(V. vinifera*, L.*)*, the hydroxy group at C-4 of the pyranone moiety negatively affected the phytotoxicity. Instead, phytotoxicity on the same plant was induced by mellein with the C-6 substitution of the aromatic ring either with a phenolic hydroxy or a methoxy group. Finally, the absence of any substituents on the aromatic ring is an essential feature for the toxicity of *Q. ilex* L., suggesting a different mode of action of the melleins on grapevine and oak leaves [42]. Mellein analogue 42 also showed antibacterial activity [40]. Tyrosol and some of its analogues are well known for their antiatherogenic, cardioprotective, anticancer, neuroprotective, and endocrine effects, as recently extensively reviewed [43]. Higginsianins F-I (**47–50**, Figure 1, Table 1), a diterpenoid α-pyridone consisting of an unreported N-hydroxyethyl-3-(5-acetyl-4-hydroxy)-α-pyridone ring, and three diterpenoid pyrones, were isolated from the mycelium of another strain of *Colletotrichum higginsianum*. Higginsianin F (**47**) could induce the formation of necrotic spots on *Chenopodium album* L. leaves at a concentration of 2 μg/μL. All higginsianin (**47–50**) were also tested on *Amaranthus retroflexus* L. seed germination and applied at four different doses. Higginsianins **47, 49,** and **50** significantly inhibited *A. retroflexus* seed germination, and compound **47** showed the most potent phytotoxicity, indicating that the presence of *N*-hydroxyethyl-3-(5-acetyl-4-hydroxy)-α-pyridone ring could enhance activity. Instead, higginsianin G (**49**) did not exhibit inhibitory activity, suggesting that stereochemistry may influence the activity. In addition, the presence of OH-7′, as in higgisianin I, induced an increase in phytotoxic activity [62].

2.2. α-Pyrones Produced from Fungi Pathogenic for Forest Plants

Pestalopyrone (**19**), hydroxypestalopyrone, and pestaloside (**51** and **52**, Figure 2, Table 2) were isolated from the filamentous fungus *Pestalotiopsis micropspora*, which was found as an endophytic microorganism in the Florida Torreya (*Torreya taxifolia*), whose decline started in the late 1950s and became a rare tree in North America. When assayed at 10 μg using a leaf puncture test on Torreya needles, pestalopyrone, its hydroxy derivative, and pestaloside (**19, 51, 52**) induced chlorosis. Compounds **19** and **51** generated symptoms on *Torreya brevifolia* also at a smaller concentration of 1 μg, showing a modest level of host specificity. Pestaloside (**52**) caused identical phytotoxic symptoms on both *T. taxifolia* and *T. breviflia* [63].

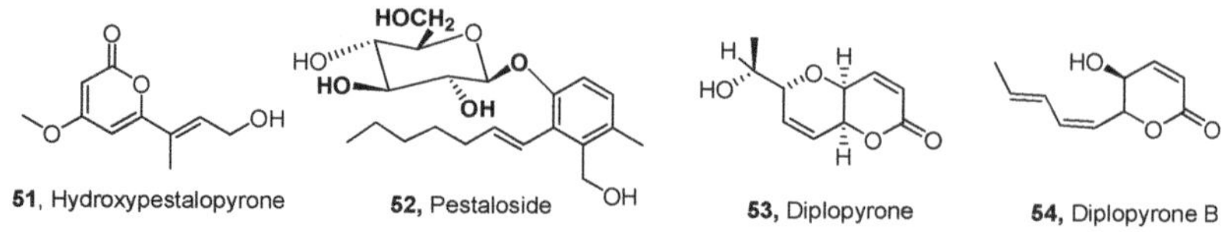

51, Hydroxypestalopyrone **52**, Pestaloside **53**, Diplopyrone **54**, Diplopyrone B

Figure 2. Structures of phytotoxic α-pyrones produced by fungi pathogenic for forest plants.

(+)-Diplopyrone A (**53**, Figure 2, Table 2), a phytotoxic monosubstituted tetrahydropyranpyran-2-one, was isolated as the main phytotoxin from the liquid culture filtrates of *Diplodia mutila*, a fungal pathogen which causes a form of canker disease on cork oak (*Quercus suber*). *D. mutila* is an endophytic fungus, widespread in Sardinian oak forests. When assayed on the host plants, compound **53** induced necrosis and wilting on cork oak cuttings, while brown discoloration or stewing was observed when tested on tomato [64]. The nonempirical assignment of the absolute configuration (AC) of (+)-diplopyrone was approached by two different methods: (a) the exciton analysis of the circular dichroism (CD) spectrum and (b) the ab initio calculation of the optical rotatory power. Both methods indicate that (+)-diplopyrone is 6-[(1*S*)-1-hydroxyethyl]-2,-4a(*S*),6(*R*),8a(*S*)-tetrahydropyrano[3,2-b]pyran-2-one [65]. Successively, this AC was revised, adopting a new experimental-computational strategy based on the combination of diverse experimental spectroscopies with quantum-mechanical simulations. In particular, diplopyrone was chosen. The close match between the new experimental and simulated infrared absorption and vibrational circular dichroism spectra, as well as the AC, as reported in Figure 2, was definitely assigned to compound **53** [66].

Diplopyrone B (**54**, Figure 2, Table 2) was isolated together with other metabolites from *Diplodia corticola*, another pathogen which causes serious and negative impacts on oak ecosystems, limiting both the vitality and the productivity of these trees. From the same fungal culture filtrates, we also isolated three lactones and a fatty acid ester, named sapinofuranones C and D, diplobifuranylone C, sphaeropsidins A and C, diplopyrone, diplobifuranylones A and B, diplofuranone A, and the (*S*,*S*)-enantiomer of sapinofuranone B. All the metabolites isolated were tested at 1 mg/mL on leaves of cork oak, grapevine cv., 'Cannonau', and tomato using the leaf puncture assay. They were also tested on tomato cuttings at 0.2, 0.1, and 0.05 mg/mL. Each compound was tested for zootoxic activity on *Artemia salina* L. larvae. The efficacy of sapinofuranone C and diplopyrone B on three plant pathogens, namely, *Athelia rolfsii*, *Fusarium avenaceum*, and *Phytophthora nicotianae*, was also evaluated. Only diplopyrone B showed strong phytotoxicity inhibition on the vegetative growth of *A. rolfsii* and *P. nicotianae*. All metabolites were inactive in the assay performed for the zootoxic activity, even at the highest concentration used. Diplopyrone B (**54**) also exhibited promising antioomycete activity for the control of *Phytophthora* spp. also considering its lack of zootoxicity [66].

Table 2. Phytotoxic α-pyrones produced from fungi pathogenic for forest plants identical data to the entry immediately above).

Compound	Fungal Producer	Other Biological Activities	Ref.
Hydroxypestalopyrone (**51**)	*Pestalotiopsis micropspora*	Not reported	[63]
Pestaloside (**52**)	"	"	"
Diplopyrone (**53**)	*Diplodia mutila*	"	[64]
Diplopyrone B(**54**)	*Diplodia corticola*	Antifungal	[66]

" It means the species same as above.

2.3. α-Pyrones Produced from Fungi Pathogenic for Weed and Parasitic Plants

The phytotoxic convolvulopyrone, convolvulanic acid, convolvulanic acid B, and convolvulol (**54–57**, Figure 3, Table 3), were isolated together with ergosterol and ergosterol peroxide from *Phornopsis corzvolvulus* [67]. This fungus is a host-specific pathogen which causes leaf spots and anthracnose lesions in the important perennial weed *Corzvolvulus arvensis* (field bindweed). The necrotic lesions surrounded by yellow haloes are characteristic of phytotoxin production. Bindweed is a severe agricultural constraint around the world, with the exception of tropical regions. Field bindweed infestations have been reported along roadsides, in urban gardens, and in new land and cropland throughout much of Canada [68]. This weed has been classified as one of the most damaging weeds worldwide. Herbicides used to control it have been found to be expensive and ineffective [69]. Strong herbicidal activity against *C. arvernsis* was observed with compounds **55** and **57** at concentrations of 3–5 $\times$ 10^{-4} M [67]. The compounds **54–57** were tested for their phytotoxic activity on the aquatic plant *Lemna paucicostata,* which showed high sensitivity. The most phytotoxic compound appeared to be convolvulanic acid B (**56**) which induced total inhibition of growth and 100% chlorosis within 12 h at concentrations of 5.9 $\times$ 10^{-4} M and within 24 h at concentrations of 3.5 $\times$ 10^{-4} M. Metabolites **55** and **57** also inhibited, At concentration of 5.9 $\times$ 10^{-4} M, the growth of the same plant around at 80 and 50%, respectively. Metabolite **54** showed very minor phytotoxicity. Tested by leaf puncture assay on bindweed, similar results of phytotoxic activity were observed for each compound [67].

Gulypyrones A and B (**58** and **59**, Figure 3, Table 3), two a-pyrones, were isolated together with phomentrioloxin, phomentrioloxins B and C, 3-nitropropionic, and 4-methylbenzoic acid from a virulent strain of *Diaporthe gulyae* [70]. The fungus was obtained from stem cankers of sunflower and was also known to be a pathogen to saffron thistle (*Carthamus lanatus* L.). *C. lanatus* is a widespread, winter-growing annual weed of both pastures and crops throughout Australia and is considered the most economically important thistle species in New South Wales [71,72]. When assayed at 5 mM on punctured leaf disks of weedy and crop plants 3,-nitropropionic acid, the main metabolite, caused small, but clear, necrotic spots on a number of plant species (*Papaver rhoes, Ecballium elaterium, Urtica dioica, Hedysarum coronarium, Mercurialis annua, Lactuca serriola, Ailanthus altissima, and Dittrichia viscosa*). Phomentrioloxin B proved to have a weaker toxicity, causing necrosis on *P. rhoeas and U. dioica, M. annua, L. serriola, A. altissima, Picris echioides, D. viscosa, Helianthus coronarium, Helianthus annuus*, and *Aster* sp. Gulypyrone A (**58**), assayed at 5 mM by stem immersion on *Helianthus annuus* plantlets, caused the rapid appearance of clear and very expanded necrosis on leaves, which was associated with the lack of symptoms on the stems. These results suggested that compound **58** can be easily translocated through the vascular system, accumulating in the leaf tissues. 4-Methylbenzoic acid showed a weaker activity, causing small necrosis only to *M. annua, U. dioica, Solanum nigrum*, and *Aster* sp. All the other compounds were either very weakly toxic or non-toxic. Considering the high toxicity of the culture filtrate, an additive or synergistic activity of all the weakly active metabolites could be hypothesized [70].

Acuminatopyrone, chlamydosporol, and isochlamydosporol (**60**, **61**, and **62**, Figure 3, Table 3) were isolated together with blumenol A, isochlamydosporol, ergosterol, and 4-hydroxybenzaldehyde. *Fusarium tricinctum* is one of the several soil fungi, including other *Fusarium* species, pathogens for seeds of the winter annual grass *Bromus tectorum* (cheatgrass). This weed has become highly invasive in semiarid ecosystems of western North America. However, in these areas, a complete cheatgrass stand failure ('die-off'), appearing as a natural phenomenon apparently caused by the above-cited complex soil fungi. Testing 4-hydroxybenzaldehyde against *B. tectorum* in a seedling bioassay exhibited the highest phytotoxicity, significantly reducing the coleoptile and radicle length of cheatgrass seedlings. Compound **60** and blumenol showed moderate activity, while compounds **61** and **62** and ergosterol were not significantly different from the control [73].

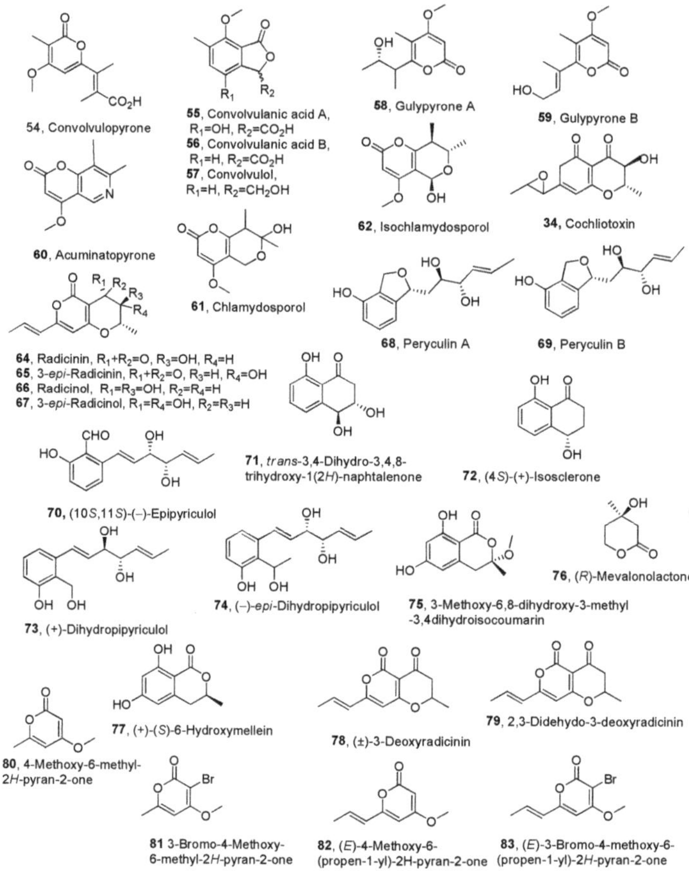

Figure 3. Structures of phytotoxic α-pyrones produced from fungi pathogenic for weeds and parasitic plants.

Cochliotoxin (**63**, Figure 3, Table 3), a dihydropyranpyrone, was isolated together with radicinin, radicinol, and their 3-epimers (**64–67**, Figure 3, Table 3) from *Cochliobolus australiensis*, proposed for the biological control of buffelgrass (*Pennisetum ciliare* or *Cenchrus ciliaris*) [73]. The absolute configuration of cochliotoxin was determined using chiroptical Optical Rotatory Dispersion (ORD), Electronic Circular Dichroism (ECD), Vibrational Circular Dichroism (VCD), and computational methods. The same methods were used to confirm that of radicinin, radicinol, and their 3-epimers, previously determined using chemical, spectroscopic, and ECD methods [74]. Buffelgrass is a perennial grass that has become highly invasive in the Sonoran Desert of southern Arizona. All the compounds were tested by leaf puncture bioassay on buffelgrass at the higher concentration (5×10^{-3} M); cochliotoxin and 3-*epi*-radicinin (**63** and **65**) were strongly and equally phytotoxic, while radicinin (**64**), compared to them, was less toxic. Radicinol and 3-*epi*-radicinol (**66** and **67**) showed lower phytotoxicity. Compounds **63–65** showed high phytotoxicity on tanglehead (*Heteropogon contortus*), but their activity was less than that on buffelgrass, probably as tanglehead is generally less sensitive. Radicinin and 3-*epi*-radicinin (**64** and **65**) were significantly more phytotoxic on Arizona cottontop (*Digitaria californica*) than on buffelgrass and tanglehead, while compounds **66** and **67** were not toxic on tanglehead and Arizona cottontop. Finally, the three most phytotoxic compounds (**63–65**) were assayed at the lower concentration (2.5×10^{-3} M), and cochliotoxin showed lesser toxicity than either radicinin or 3-*epi*-radicinin on all three grass species used [73]. From the point of view of structure−activity relationships, these results showed that the α,β-unsaturated ketone located between C-4 and C-8 in compounds **63–65** should play a significant role in the strong phytotoxic activities of these toxins. The absence of this this moiety in **66** and **67** induced a noteworthy reduction of toxicity. Furthermore, important features involved in modulating phytotoxicity appeared to be the stereochemistry of the chiral C-3 and the presence of the epoxy group in **63–65** and **63**, respectively [73]. Radicinin (**64**), already known as a phytotoxin [75–77], also showed strong antifungal activity against *Magnaporthe grisea* and *Valsa mali* (IC_{50}, the concentration of substance required for 50% inhibition, of 16.3 and 18.2 μg/mL, respectively) [78] as well as strong bacteriocidal activity against *Xylella fastidiosa* [79]. Radicinin (**64**) was isolated as a phytotoxin together with two steroids from the culture filtrates of *Curvularia clavata* when it was obtained by microbiological transformation of progesterone, which was added as substrate when the microorganism reached its exponential growth phase [80].

Successively from the culture filtrate of *Pyricularia grisea*, another pathogen proposed for the biocontrol of buffelgrass, pyriculins A and B (**68** and **69**, Figure 3, Table 3), two mono-substituted hex-4-ene-2,3-diols, together with (10*S*,11*S*)-(−)-epipyriculol, *trans*-3,4-dihydro-3,4,8-trihydroxy-1(2*H*)-napthalenone, and (4*S*)-(+)-isosclerone were isolated (**70–72**, Figure 3, Table 3). All the metabolites were bioassayed in a buffelgrass coleoptile and radicle elongation tests, and (10*S*,11*S*)-(−)-epipyriculol proved to be the most toxic compound. Seed germination was much reduced and slowed, and radicles failed to elongate. All five compounds delayed germination, but only (*10S*,11*S*)-(−)-epipyriculol (**70**) prevented radicle development of buffelgrass seedlings, while it had no effect on coleoptile elongation, and the other four compounds caused significantly increased coleoptile development [81]. Furthermore, from the same fungal culture extract (+)-dihydropyriculol, *epi*-dihydropyriculol, 3-methoxy-6,8-dihydroxy-3-methyl-3,4-dihydroisocoumarin, (*R*)-mevalonolactone, and 6-hydroxymellein (**73–77**, Figure 3, Table 3) were also isolated [82]. When all the metabolites were bioassayed at 5×10^{-3} M on a buffelgrass coleoptile and radicle elongation test, no toxicity was detected. In contrast, (+)-dihydropyriculol and 3-methoxy-6,8-dihydroxy-3-methyl-3,4-dihydroisocoumarin (**73** and **75**) showed a significant stimulation of radical elongation. Moreover, the difference in growth stimulation between compound **73** and its epimer **74** further supported the relationship between absolute configuration and biological activity of these fungal metabolites [82]. Totally, fourteen secondary metabolites were produced by these two pathogens and tested using a leaf puncture assay on the host plant at different concentrations. Radicinin (**64**) and (10*S*, 11*S*)-epipyriculol (**70**) appeared to be the most promising compounds for potential application in agriculture. Thus, their phytotoxicity was also tested on non-host indigenous plants. Radicinin (**64**) showed high target-specific toxicity on buffelgrass, low toxicity to native plants, and no teratogenic, sub-lethal, or lethal effects on zebrafish (*Brachydanio rerio*) embryos. These results prompt the development of a target-specific bioherbicide to be used against buffelgrass in natural systems [83]. These data and the peculiar structural feature of toxin **64** suggested that it be chemically modified to prepare some key hemisynthetic derivatives, and test their phytotoxicity to perform a structure–activity relationship study. In particular, the 3-*O*-*p*-bromobenzoyl, 3-*O*-5-azidopentanoyl, 3-*O*-stearoyl, 3-*O*-mesyl, and 3-*O*-acetyl esters of radicinin were semisynthesized as well as the monoacetyl ester of 3-*epi*-radicinin, the diacetyl esters of radicinol and its 3 epimer, and two diastereomeric hexahydro derivatives in comparison with that of radicinin (**64**). The phytotoxic activity of all derivatives and analogues was assayed by leaf puncture bioassay, and most of the compounds showed phytotoxicity, but none of them had comparable or higher activity than radicinin. Thus, the presence of an α, β-unsaturated carbonyl group at C-4, as well as the presence of a free secondary hydroxyl group at C-3 and the stereochemistry of the same carbon, proved to be the essential feature for activity [84].

Considering these interesting and potential results and a relatively low amount of radicinin produced by fungal fermentation, a novel synthetic strategy to prepare (±)-3-deoxyradicinin (**78**, Figure 3, Table 3) is described. This synthetic method is more efficient than those previously reported in the literature and also shows higher versatility towards the introduction of different side-chains at both C-7 and C-2. Compound **78** showed phytotoxicity against the grass weed buffelgrass comparable to that of the natural phytotoxin radicinin. Therefore, this latter can constitute a more practical synthetic alternative to radicinin as a bioherbicide to biologically control buffelgrass [85].

Radicinin (**64**) and 3-*epi*-radicinol (**64** and **67**) some hemisynthetic radicinin derivative as 3-*O*-acetyl radicinin, 3-*O*-mesyl radicinin, 3-*O*-(5-azidopentanoyl radicinin, 3,4-*O*,*O*′-diacetylradicinol, (±)-3-deoxyradicinin and its synthetic intermediates 2,3-dehydro-3-doxyradicinin 4-methoxy-6-methyl-2*H*-pyran-2-one, 3-bromo-4-methoxy -6-methyl-2*H*-pyran-2-one, (*E*)-4-methoxy-6-(propen-1-yl)-2H-pyran-2-one, and (*E*)-3-bromo-4-methoxy-6-(propen-1-yl)-2*H*-pyran-2 (**79–33**, Figure 3, Table 3) were tested for their in vitro anticancer activity by MTT assays against three cancer cell models harboring various resistance levels to chemotherapeutic drugs. Radicinin (**64**) showed significant anticancer activity in the micromolar range. The results of the SAR study showed that the lack of activity of radicinol and its 3-epimer (**66** and **67**), and the corresponding 3,4-*O*,*O*′-diacetyl derivative, demonstrated that the carbonyl at C-4 is an important structural feature for anticancer activity, because its presence allows a Michael addition of a nucleophile residue. The activities of (±)-3-deoxy- and 2,3-dehydro-3-deoxy-radicinin (**78** and **79**) were slightly less than that of radicinin, showing that the 3-hydroxy group plays a minor role in the activity. Among the four synthetic, intermediate methoxypyrones (**80–83**), only derivative **81** exhibited moderate anticancer activities, while compounds **78**, **82**, and **83** were completely inactive. Interestingly, 4-methoxy-2-pyrone is an important substructural unit of aurovertins B and D, i.e., fungal mycotoxins, showing strong antiproliferative activity against breast cancer cells but with little influence on normal cells [86]. As all four compounds are differently trisubstituted α-pyrones, their difference in activity might be due to the effect of the substituents on the Michael addition of a nucleophilic residue. The presence of the methoxy group at the β-position in all four compounds could reduce their reactivity due to steric hindrance, while the presence of bromine in α-position could instead increase this reactivity; see **81** vs. **80**. The difference between the moderate activity of **81** and the inactivity of **83** may be attributed to the presence of an ethenyl group at the δ-position in the latter, which could strongly reduce its reactivity in the Michael addition. Interestingly, the only active compound (**81**) does not bear a double bond conjugate to the pyrone, which can act as a Michael acceptor. Therefore, it can be hypothesized that its cytotoxicity occurs through a different mechanism with respect to radicinin (**64**) and its derivatives. Not strong variation was observed among the responses of the three different cancer cell lines, suggesting that radicinin (**64**) might exert its anticancer activity through non-apoptotic pathways. Thus, compound **64** could be an interesting candidate to develop further drugs to combat chemoresistant cancers. (±)-3-Deoxyradicinin (**78**), which displays very similar cytotoxicity against the tested tumoral cell lines, may be a more practical alternative to radicinin, as it could be obtained through the novel synthetic strategy, as reported above [87].

Table 3. Phytotoxic α-pyrones produced from fungi pathogenic for weeds and parasitic plants: identical data to the entry immediately above).

Compound	Fungal Producer	Other Biological Activities	Ref.
Convolvulopyrone (**54**)	*Phornopsis corzvolvulus*	Not reported	[67]
Convolvulanic acid A (**55**)	"	"	"
Convolvulanic acid B (**56**)	"	"	"
Convolvulol (**57**)	"	"	"
Gulypyrones A (**58**)	*Diaporthe gulyae*	"	[70]
Gulypyrones B (**59**)	"	"	"
Acuminatopyrone (**60**)	*Fusarium tricinctum*		[73]
Chlamydosporol (**61**)	"	"	"
Isochlamydosporol (**62**)	"	"	"
Cochliotoxin (**63**)	*Cochliobolus australiensis*	"	[88]
Radicinin (**64**)	*Cochliobolus australiensis* " *Curvularia clavata*	"Antifungal Bacteriocide	[78,88] [79] [80]
3-*epi*-Radicinin (**65**)	*Cochliobolus australiensis*	Not reported	[88]
Radicinol (**66**)	"	"	"
3-*epi*-Radicinol (**67**)	"	"	"
Peryculin A (**68**)	*Perycularia grisea*	"	[81]
Peryculin A (**69**)	"	"	"
(10*S*,11*S*)-(-)-Epipyriculol (**70**)	"	"	"
trans-3,4-Dihydro-3,4,8-trihydroxy-1(2*H*)-naphtalenone (**71**)	"	"	"
(4*S*)-(+)-Isosclerone (**72**)	"	"	"
(+)-Dihydropipyriculol (**73**)	"	"	[82]
(-)-*epi*-Dihydropipyriculol (**74**)	"	"	"
3-Methoxy-6,8-dihydroxy-3-methyl -3,4dihydroisocoumarin (**75**)	"	"	"
(*R*)-Mevalonolactone (**76**)	"	"	"
(+)-(*S*)-6-Hydroxymellein (**77**)	"	"	"
(±)-3-Deoxyradicinin (**78**)		Anticancer	[87]
2,3-Dehydro-3-deoxyradicinin (**79**)	"	Not reported	"
4-Methoxy-6-methyl-2*H*-pyran-2-one (**80**)	"	"	"
3-Bromo-4-Methoxy-6-methyl-2*H*-pyran-2-one (**81**)	"	"	"
(*E*)-4-Methoxy-6-(propen-1-yl) -2*H*-pyran-2-one (**82**)	"	"	"
(*E*)-3-Bromo-4-methoxy-6-(propen-1-yl)-2*H*-pyran-2-one (**83**)	"	"	"

" It means the species same as above.

3. Conclusions

In conclusion, this review reports the chemical and biological characterization of phytotoxic α-pyrones, comprising those included in very complex structures, produced by fungal pathogens for agrarian, forest, weedy, and parasitic plants. In some cases, the results of SAR study are described as well as the potential practical application of some of these interesting natural compounds and the synthesis of their key derivatives and phytotoxins, also including the a-pyrones treated in this review, are the secondary metabolites produced athogenic fungi as virulence factors and therefore play a fundamental role in the physiological processes that generate the symptoms of the disease. Their isolation and chemical and biological characterization are the first steps to finding environmentally friendly solutions to save agricultural production. The future directions will provide deeper insights into the chemical ecology of these phytotoxic α-pyrones and their potential roles in the development of plant diseases.

Funding: This research received no external funding.

Institutional Review Board Statement: Not applicable.

Informed Consent Statement: Not applicable.

Data Availability Statement: The data discussed are obtained from the article on the topic trated by SciFinder research.

Conflicts of Interest: The author declares no conflicts of interest.

References

1. Newman, D.J.; Cragg, G.M. Natural products as sources of new drugs over the nearly four decades from 01/1981 to 09/2019. *J. Nat. Prod.* **2020**, *83*, 770–803. [CrossRef] [PubMed]
2. Belennkii, L.I.; Evdokimenkova, Y.B. The literature of heterocyclic chemistry, part XII 2010–2011. *Adv. Heterocycl. Chem.* **2014**, *111*, 147–274.
3. Streitwieser, A.; Heathcock, C.H. *Introduction to Organic Chemistry*, 3rd ed.; Macmillan: New York, NY, USA, 1985; pp. 1038–1040.
4. Dickinson, J.M. Microbial pyran-2-ones and dihydropyran-2-ones. *Nat. Prod. Rep.* **1993**, *10*, 71–98. [CrossRef] [PubMed]
5. McGlacken, G.P.; Fairlamb, I.J. 2-Pyrone natural products and mimetics: Isolation, characterisation and biological activity. *Nat. Prod. Rep.* **2005**, *22*, 369–385. [CrossRef]
6. Lee, J.S. Recent advances in the synthesis of 2-pyrones. *Mar. Drugs* **2015**, *13*, 1581–1620. [CrossRef]
7. Schäberle, T.F. Biosynthesis of α-pyrones. *Beilstein J. Org. Chem.* **2016**, *12*, 571–588. [CrossRef]
8. Azizian, M.; Gheshlaghi, S.; Danesh, A.; Forouzanfar, F.; Shakeri, A. α-Pyrones: Natural occurrence, chemistry, and biological approaches—An Update. *Rev. Bras. Farmacogn.* **2024**, *34*, 1201–1217. [CrossRef]
9. Bhat, Z.S.; Rather, M.A.; Maqbool, M.; Lah, H.U.; Yousuf, S.K.; Ahmad, Z. α-Pyrones: Small molecules with versatile structural diversity reflected in multiple pharmacological activities-an update. *Biomed. Pharmacother.* **2017**, *91*, 265–277. [CrossRef]
10. Evidente, A.; Cimmino, A.; Andolfi, A. The effect of stereochemistry on the biological activity of natural phytotoxins, fungicides, insecticides and herbicides. *Chirality* **2013**, *25*, 59–78. [CrossRef]
11. Cimmino, A.; Masi, M.; Evidente, M.; Superchi, S.; Evidente, A. Fungal phytotoxins with potential herbicidal activity: Chemical and biological characterization. *Nat. Prod. Rep.* **2015**, *32*, 1629–1653. [CrossRef]
12. Al-Khdhairawi, A.A.Q.; Cordell, G.A.; Thomas, N.F.; Nagojappa, N.B.S.; Weber, J.F.F. Natural diterpene pyrones: Chemistry and biology. *Org. Biomol. Chem.* **2019**, *17*, 8943–8957. [CrossRef] [PubMed]
13. Entwistle, A.R. Root diseases. In *Onions and Allied Crops*; Brewster, J.L., Rabinowitch, H.D., Eds.; CRC Press: Boca Rato, FL, USA, 1990; Volume III, p. 284.
14. Niwa, M.; Ogiso, S.; Endo, T.; Furukawa, H.; Yamamura, S. Isolation and structure of citreopyrone, a metabolite of *Penicillium citreo-viride* Biourge. *Tetrahedron Lett.* **1980**, *21*, 4481–4482. [CrossRef]
15. Sato, H.; Konoma, K.; Sakamura, S.; Furusaki, A.; Matsumoto, T.; Matsuzaki, T. X-ray crystal structure of pyrenocine A, a phytotoxin from *Pyrenochaeta terrestris*. *Agric. Biol. Chem.* **1981**, *45*, 795–797. [CrossRef]
16. Sparace, S.A.; Mudd, J.B.; Burke, B.A.; Aasen, A.J. Pyrenocine C, a phytotoxin-related metabolite produced by onion pink root fungus, Pyrenochaeta terrestris. *Phytochemistry* **1984**, *23*, 2693–2694. [CrossRef]

17. Sato, H.; Konoma, K.; Sakamura, S. Three new phytotoxins produced by *Pyrenochaeta terrestris*: Pyrenochaetic acids A, B and C. *Agric. Biol. Chem.* **1981**, *45*, 1675–1679. [CrossRef]
18. Sparace, S.A.; Reeleder, R.D.; Khanizadeh, S. Antibiotic activity of the pyrenocines. *Can. J. Microbiol.* **1987**, *33*, 327–330. [CrossRef]
19. Ichihara, A.; Oikawa, H. Biosynthesis of phytotoxins from *Alternaria solani*. *Biosci. Biotechnol. Biochem.* **1997**, *61*, 12–18. [CrossRef]
20. Tabuchi, H.; Ichihara, A. Structures and stereochemistries of new compounds related to alternaric acid. *J. Chem. Soc. Perkin Trans. 1* **1994**, 125–133. [CrossRef]
21. Ichihara, A.; Tazaki, H.; Sakamura, S. Solanapyrones A, B and C, phytotoxic metabolites from the fungus *Alternaria solani*. *Tetrahedron Lett.* **1983**, *24*, 5373–5376. [CrossRef]
22. Oikawa, H.; Yokota, T.; Ichihara, A.; Sakamura, S. Structure and absolute configuration of solanapyrone D: A new clue to the occurrence of biological Diels–Alder reaction *J. Chem. Soc. Chem. Commun.* **1989**, *17*, 1284–1285. [CrossRef]
23. Oikawa, H.; Yokota, T.; Sakano, C.; Suzuki, Y.; Naya, A.; Ichihara, A. Solanapyrones, phytotoxins produced by *Alternaria solani*: Biosynthesis and isolation of minor components. *Biosci. Biotechnol. Biochem.* **1998**, *62*, 2016–2022. [CrossRef]
24. Wang, X.Z.; Luo, X.H.; Xiao, J.; Zhai, M.M.; Yuan, Y.; Zhu, Y.; Crews, P.; Yuan, C.S.; Wu, Q.X. Pyrone derivatives from the endophytic fungus Alternaria tenuissima SP-07 of Chinese herbal medicine *Salvia przewalskii*. *Fitoterapia* **2014**, *99*, 184–190. [CrossRef] [PubMed]
25. Evidente, A.; Rodeva, R.; Andolfi, A.; Stoyanova, Z.; Perrone, C.; Motta, A. Phytotoxic polyketides produced by *Phomopsis foeniculi*, a strain isolated from diseased Bulgarian fennel *Eur. J. Plant Pathol.* **2011**, *130*, 173–182. [CrossRef]
26. Mishra, P.D.; Verekar, S.A.; Deshmukh, S.K.; Joshi, K.S.; Fiebig, H.H.; Kelter, G. Altersolanol A: A selective cytotoxic anthraquinone from a *Phomopsis* sp. *Lett. Appl. Microbiol.* **2015**, *60*, 387–391. [CrossRef] [PubMed]
27. Huang, S.; Xu, J.; Li, F.; Zhou, D.; Xu, L.; Li, C. Identification and antifungal activity of metabolites from the mangrove fungus *Phoma* sp. L28. *Chem. Nat. Comp.* **2017**, *53*, 237–240. [CrossRef]
28. Evidente, A.; Lanzetta, R.; Abouzeid, M.A.; Corsaro, M.M.; Mugnai, L.; Surico, G. Foeniculoxin, a new phytotoxic geranylhydroquinone from *Phomopsis foeniculi*. *Tetrahedron* **1994**, *50*, 10371–10378. [CrossRef]
29. Shirota, O.; Pathak, V.; Faiz Hossain, C.; Sekita, S.; Takatori, K.; Satake, M. Structural elucidation of trichotetronines: Polyketides possessing a bicyclo [2.2.2]octane skeleton with a tetronic acid moiety isolated from *Trichoderma* sp. *J. Chem. Soc. Perkin Trans. 1* **1997**, 2961–2964. [CrossRef]
30. Abe, N.; Murata, T.; Hirota, A. Novel DPPH radical scavengers, bisorbicillinol and demethyltrichodimerol, from a fungus. *Biosci. Biotechnol. Biochem.* **1998**, *62*, 661–666. [CrossRef]
31. He, T.; Li, X.; del Carmen Flores-Vallejo, R.; Radu, A.M.; van Dijl, J.M.; Haslinger, K. The endophytic fungus *Cosmosporella* sp. VM-42 from *Vinca minor* is a source of bioactive compounds with potent activity against drug-resistant bacteria. *Curr. Res. Microb. Sci.* **2025**, *8*, 100390. [CrossRef]
32. Abrell, L.M.; Cheng, X.C.; Crew, P. New nectriapyrones by salt water cultures of a fungus separated from an indo-pacific sponge. *Tetrahedron Lett.* **1994**, *35*, 9159–9160. [CrossRef]
33. Evidente, A.; Zonno, M.C.; Andolfi, A.; Troise, C.; Cimmino, A.; Vurro, M. Phytotoxic α-pyrones produced by *Pestalotiopsis guepinii*, the causal agent of hazelnut twig blight. *J. Antibiot.* **2012**, *65*, 203–206. [CrossRef] [PubMed]
34. Meng, J.; Sun, W.; Mao, Z.; Xu, D.; Wang, X.; Lu, S.; Daowan, L.; Yang Liu, Y.; Ligang Zhou, L.; Zhang, G. Main ustilaginoidins and their distribution in rice false smut balls. *Toxins* **2015**, *7*, 4023–4034. [CrossRef]
35. Kawai, K.; Hisada, K.; Mori, S.; Nozawa, Y.; Koyama, K.; Natori, S. The impairing effect of chaetochromin A and related mycotoxins on mitochondrial respiration. *Proc. Jpn. Assoc. Mycotoxicol.* **1991**, *33*, 31–35. [CrossRef]
36. Masi, M.; Cimmino, A.; Boari, A.; Zonno, M.C.; Górecki, M.; Pescitelli, G.; Tuzi, A.; Vurro, M.; Evidente, A. Colletopyrandione, a new phytotoxic tetrasubstituted indolylidenepyran-2, 4-dione, and colletochlorins G and H, new tetrasubstituted chroman-and isochroman-3, 5-diols isolated from *Colletotrichum higginsianum*. *Tetrahedron* **2017**, *73*, 6644–6650. [CrossRef]
37. Li, H.; Hu, J.; Wei, H.; Solomon, P.S.; Vuong, D.; Lacey, E.; Stubbs, K.A.; Pigott, A.M.; Chooi, Y.H. Chemical ecogenomics-guided discovery of phytotoxic α-pyrones from the fungal wheat pathogen *Parastagonospora nodorum*. *Org. Lett.* **2018**, *20*, 6148–6152. [CrossRef] [PubMed]
38. Meng, J.; Gu, G.; Dang, P.; Zhang, X.; Wang, W.; Dai, J.; Liu, Y.; Lai, D.; Zhou, L. Sorbicillinoids from the fungus *Ustilaginoidea virens* and their phytotoxic, cytotoxic, and antimicrobial activities. *Front. Chem.* **2019**, *7*, 435. [CrossRef] [PubMed]
39. Masi, M.; Reveglia, P.; Baaijens-Billones, R.; Górecki, M.; Pescitelli, G.; Savocchia, S.; Evidente, A. Phytotoxic metabolites from three *Neofusicoccum* species causal agents of Botryosphaeria dieback in Australia, luteopyroxin, neoanthraquinone, and luteoxepinone, a disubstituted furo-α-pyrone, a hexasubstituted anthraquinone, and a trisubstituted oxepi-2-one from *Neofusicoccum luteum*. *J. Nat. Prod.* **2020**, *83*, 453–460.
40. Reveglia, P.; Masi, M.; Evidente, A. Melleins—Intriguing natural compounds. *Biomolecules* **2020**, *10*, 772. [CrossRef]
41. Zhai, M.-M.; Qi, F.-M.; Li, J.; Jiang, C.-X.; Hou, Y.; Shi, Y.-P.; Di, D.-L.; Zhang, J.-W.; Wu, Q.-X. Isolation of secondary metabolites from the soil-derived fungus *Clonostachys rosea* YRS-06, a biological control agent, and evaluation of antibacterial activity. *J. Agric. Food Chem.* **2016**, *64*, 2298–2306. [CrossRef]

42. Masi, M.; Bashiri, S.; Cimmino, A.; Bahmani, Z.; Abdollahzadeh, J.; Evidente, A. Phytotoxins produced by two *Biscogniauxia rosacearum* strains, causal agents of grapevine trunk diseases, and charcoal canker of oak trees in Iran. *Toxins* **2021**, *13*, 812. [CrossRef]
43. Karković Marković, A.; Torić, J.; Barbarić, M.; Jakobušić Brala, C. Hydroxytyrosol, tyrosol and derivatives and their potential effects on human health. *Molecules* **2019**, *24*, 2001. [CrossRef]
44. Schmey, T.; Tominello-Ramirez, C.S.; Brune, C.; Stam, R. Alternaria diseases on potato and tomato. *Mol. Plant Pathol.* **2024**, *25*, e13435. [CrossRef]
45. Furuichi, N.; Nishimura, S.; Langsdorf, G. Effect of alternaric acid, a toxin of *Alternaria solani*, on the hypersensitive response of potato to *Phytophthora infestans*. *Jpn. J. Phytopathol.* **1992**, *58*, 1–7. [CrossRef]
46. Tabuchi, H.; Hamamoto, T.; Miki, S.; Tejima, T.; Ichihara, A. Total synthesis and stereochemistry of alternaric acid. *J. Org. Chem.* **1994**, *59*, 4749–4759. [CrossRef]
47. Alam, S.S.; Bilton, J.N.; Slawin, A.M.; Williams, D.J.; Sheppard, R.N.; Strange, R.N. Chickpea blight: Production of the phytotoxins solanapyrones A and C by *Ascochyta rabiei*. *Phytochemistry* **1989**, *28*, 2627–2630. [CrossRef]
48. Nene, Y.L. A review of Ascochyta blight of chickpea. *Trop. Pest Manag.* **1982**, *28*, 61–70. [CrossRef]
49. Ichihara, A.; Oikawa, H.; Hayashi, K.; Sakamura, S. Structures of betaenones A and B, novel phytotoxins from *Phoma betae* Fr. *J. Am. Chem Soc.* **1983**, *105*, 2907–290830. [CrossRef]
50. Barash, I.; Manulis, S.; Kashman, Y.; Springer, J.P.; Chen, M.H.; Clardy, J.; Strobel, G.A. Crystallization and X-ray analysis of stemphyloxin I, a phytotoxin from *Stemphylium botryosum*. *Science* **1983**, *220*, 1065–1066. [CrossRef]
51. Kim, W.; Park, C.M.; Park, J.J.; Akamatsu, H.O.; Peever, T.L.; Xian, M.; Gang, D.R.; Wandermark, G.; Chen, W. Functional analyses of the Diels-Alderase gene *sol5* of *Ascochyta rabiei* and *Alternaria solani* indicate that the solanapyrone phytotoxins are not required for pathogenicity. *Mol. Plant-Microbe Interact.* **2015**, *28*, 482–496. [CrossRef]
52. Kimura, Y.; Hamasaki, T.; Nakajima, H. Streochemistry and biological activities of LL-P880g, a pestalotin analogue, produced by *Penicillium citro-viride*. *Agric. Biol. Chem.* **1986**, *50*, 1649–1650.
53. Choi, E.M.; Hwang, J.K. Antiinflammatory, analgesic and antioxidant activities of the fruit of *Foeniculum vulgare*. *Fitoterapia* **2004**, *75*, 557–565. [CrossRef] [PubMed]
54. Corsaro, M.M.; De Castro, C.; Evidente, A.; Lanzetta, R.; Molinaro, A.; Mugnai, L.; Parrilli, M.; Surico, G. Chemical structure of two phytotoxic exopolysaccharides produced by *Phomopsis foeniculi*. *Carbohydr. Res.* **1998**, *308*, 349–357. [CrossRef] [PubMed]
55. Venkatasubbaiah, P.; van Dyke, C.G.; Chilton, W.S. Phytotoxins produced by *Pestalotiopsys oenotherae*, a pathogen of evening primrose. *Phytochemistry* **1991**, *30*, 1471–1474. [CrossRef]
56. Turkann, M. Phytotoxins produced by *Pestalotiopsis guepinii*, the causal agent of halznut twig blight. *Phytopathol. Mediterr.* **2011**, *50*, 154–158.
57. Damm, U.; O'connell, R.J.; Groenewald, J.Z.; Crous, P.W. The *Colletotrichum destructivum* species complex-hemibiotrophic pathogens of forage and field crops. *Stud. Mycol.* **2014**, *79*, 49–84. [CrossRef]
58. Cimmino, A.; Mathieu, V.; Masi, M.; Baroncelli, R.; Boari, A.; Pescitelli, G.; Vurro, M.; Evidente, A. Higginsianins A and B, two diterpenoid α-pyrones produced by *Colletotrichum higginsianum*, with in vitro cytostatic activity. *J. Nat. Prod.* **2016**, *79*, 116–125. [CrossRef]
59. Trifonov, L.S.; Hilpert, H.; Floersheim, P.; Dreiding, A.S.; Rast, D.M.; Skrivanova, R.; Hoesch, L. Bisvertinols: A new group of dimeric vertinoids from *Verticillium intertextum*. *Tetrahedron* **1986**, *42*, 3157–3179. [CrossRef]
60. Andrade, R.; Ayer, W.A.; Trifonov, L.S. The metabolites of *Trichoderma longibrachiatum*. III. Two new tetronic acids: 5-hydroxyvertinolide and bislongiquinolide. *Aust. J. Chem.* **1997**, *50*, 255–258. [CrossRef]
61. Abe, N.; Yamamoto, K.; Hirota, A. Novel fungal metabolites, demethylsorbicillin and oxosorbicillinol, isolated from *Trichoderma* sp. USF2690. *Biosci. Biotechnol. Biochem.* **2000**, *64*, 620–622. [CrossRef]
62. Chen, K.; Song, K.; Hao, X.; Wang, C.; Zhang, L.; Yue, Q.; Xu, Y. Higginsianin F, one skeletal rearrangement diterpenoid α-pyridone with phytotoxic activity isolated from *Colletotrichum higginsianum*. *Phytochemistry* **2025**, *235*, 114475. [CrossRef]
63. Evidente, A.; Maddau, L.; Spanu, E.; Franceschini, A.; Lazzaroni, S.; Motta, A. Diplopyrone, a new phytotoxic tetrahydropyranpyran-2-one produced by *Diplodia mutila*, a fungus pathogen of cork oak. *J. Nat. Prod.* **2003**, *66*, 313–315. [CrossRef] [PubMed]
64. Giorgio, E.; Maddau, L.; Spanu, E.; Evidente, A.; Rosini, C. Assignment of the absolute configuration of (+)-diplopyrone, the main phytotoxin produced by *Diplodia mutila*, the pathogen of the cork oak decline, by a nonempirical analysis of its chiroptical properties. *J. Org. Chem.* **2005**, *70*, 7–13. [CrossRef] [PubMed]
65. Fusè, M.; Mazzeo, G.; Longhi, G.; Abbate, S.; Masi, M.; Evidente, A.; Puzzarini, C.; Barone, V. Unbiased determination of absolute configurations by vis-à-vis comparison of experimental and simulated spectra: The challenging case of diplopyrone. *J. Phys. Chem. B* **2019**, *123*, 9230–9237. [CrossRef] [PubMed]
66. Masi, M.; Maddau, L.; Linaldeddu, B.T.; Cimmino, A.; D'Amico, W.; Scanu, B.; Evidente, M.; Tuzi, A.; Evidente, A. Bioactive secondary metabolites produced by the oak pathogen *Diplodia corticola*. *J. Agric. Food Chem.* **2016**, *64*, 217–225. [CrossRef]

67. Tsantrizos, Y.S.; Ogilvie, K.K.; Watson, A.K. Phytotoxic metabolites of *Phomopsis convolvulus*, a host-specific pathogen of field bindweed. *Can. J. Chem.* **1992**, *70*, 2276–2284. [CrossRef]
68. Alex, J.F. Canada. In *Biology and Ecology of Weeds*, 1st ed.; Holzner, W., Nurnata, M., Junk, W., Eds.; The Hague, Springer Sciences: Dordrecht, The Netherlands, 1982; pp. 309–332.
69. Rosenthal, S.; Andres, L.; Huffaker, C. Field bindweed in California. *Cal. Agric.* **1983**, *37*, 18–22.
70. Andolfi, A.; Boari, A.; Evidente, M.; Cimmino, A.; Vurro, M.; Ash, G.; Evidente, A. Gulypyrones A and B and phomentrioloxins B and C produced by *Diaporthe gulyae*, a potential mycoherbicide for saffron thistle (*Carthamus lanatus*). *J. Nat. Prod.* **2015**, *78*, 623–629. [CrossRef]
71. Briese, D.T. Weed status of twelve thistle species in New South Wales. *Plant Protect. Quaterly* **1988**, *3*, 135–141.
72. Sindel, B. Glyphosate resistance discovered in annual ryegrass. *Resist. Pest Manag.* **1996**, *8*, 5–6.
73. Masi, M.; Meyer, S.; Pescitelli, G.; Cimmino, A.; Clement, S.; Peacock, B.; Evidente, A. Phytotoxic activity against *Bromus tectorum* for secondary metabolites of a seed-pathogenic *Fusarium* strain belonging to the *F. tricinctum* species complex. *Nat. Prod. Res.* **2017**, *31*, 2768–2777. [CrossRef]
74. Santoro, E.; Mazzeo, G.; Marsico, G.; Masi, M.; Longhi, G.; Superchi, S.; Evidente, A.; Abbate, S. Assignment through chiroptical methods of the absolute configuration of fungal dihydropyranpyran-4-5-diones phytotoxins, potential herbicides for buffelgrass (*Cenchrus ciliaris*) biocontrol. *Molecules* **2019**, *24*, 3022. [CrossRef] [PubMed]
75. Nakajima, H.; Ishida, T.; Otsuka, Y.; Hamasaki, T.; Ichinoe, M. Phytotoxins and related metabolites produced by *Bipolaris coicis*, the pathogen of job's tears. *Phytochemistry* **1997**, *45*, 41–45. [CrossRef]
76. Solfrizzo, M.; Vitti, C.; De Girolamo, A.; Visconti, A.; Logrieco, A.; Panizzi, F.P.J. Radicinols and radicinin phytotoxins produced by *Alternaria radicina* on carrots. *J. Agric. Food Chem.* **2004**, *52*, 3655–3660. [CrossRef]
77. Suzuki, M.; Sakuno, E.; Ishihara, A.; Tamura, J.I.; Nakajima, H. Conversions of deoxyradicinin to radicinin and of radicinin to 3-*epi*-radicinin in the phytopathogenic fungus *Bipolaris coicis*. *Phytochemistry* **2012**, *75*, 14–20. [CrossRef] [PubMed]
78. Zhang, Y.L.; Kong, L.C.; Jiang, D.H.; Yin, C.P.; Cai, Q.M.; Chen, Q.; Zheng, J.Y. Phytotoxic and antifungal metabolites from *Curvularia* sp. FH01 isolated from the gut of *Atractomorpha sinensis*. *Bioresour. Technol.* **2011**, *102*, 3575–3577. [CrossRef] [PubMed]
79. Aldrich, T.J.; Rolshausen, P.E.; Roper, M.C.; Reader, J.M.; Steinhaus, M.J.; Rapicavoli, J.; Vosburg, D.A.; Maloney, K.N. Radicinin from *Cochliobolus* sp. inhibits *Xylella fastidiosa*, the causal agent of Pierce's Disease of grapevine. *Phytochemistry* **2015**, *116*, 130–137. [CrossRef]
80. Vujčić, M.; Jankov, R.M. Microbiologic transformation of progesterone by *Curvularia clavata* Jain. *Steroids* **1990**, *55*, 17–21. [CrossRef]
81. Masi, M.; Meyer, S.; Górecki, M.; Mandoli, A.; Di Bari, L.; Pescitelli, G.; Cimmino, A.; Cristofaro, M.; Clement, S.; Evidente, A. Pyriculins A and B, two monosubstituted hex-4-ene-2,3-diols and other phytotoxic metabolites produced by *Pyricularia grisea* isolated from buffelgrass (*Cenchrus ciliaris*). *Chirality* **2017**, *29*, 726–736. [CrossRef]
82. Masi, M.; Santoro, E.; Clement, S.; Meyer, S.; Scafato, P.; Superchi, S.; Evidente, A. Further secondary metabolites produced by the fungus *Pyricularia grisea* isolated from buffelgrass (*Cenchrus ciliaris*). *Chirality* **2020**, *32*, 1234–1242. [CrossRef]
83. Masi, M.; Freda, F.; Sangermano, F.; Calabrò, V.; Cimmino, A.; Cristofaro, M.; Meyer, S.; Evidente, A. Radicinin, a fungal phytotoxin as a target-specific bioherbicide for invasive buffelgrass (*Cenchrus ciliaris*) control. *Molecules* **2019**, *24*, 1086. [CrossRef]
84. Masi, M.; Freda, F.; Clement, S.; Cimmino, A.; Cristofaro, M.; Meyer, S.; Evidente, A. Phytotoxic activity and structure–activity relationships of radicinin derivatives against the invasive weed buffelgrass (*Cenchrus ciliaris*). *Molecules* **2019**, *24*, 2793. [CrossRef] [PubMed]
85. Marsico, G.; Ciccone, M.S.; Masi, M.; Freda, F.; Cristofaro, M.; Evidente, A.; Superchi, S.; Scafato, P. Synthesis and herbicidal activity against buffelgrass (*Cenchrus ciliaris*) of (±)-3-deoxyradicinin. *Molecules* **2019**, *24*, 3193. [CrossRef] [PubMed]
86. Zhong, Y.J.; Cao, F.; Hu, L.S.; Xu, C.X.; Zhu, Y.A.; Chen, X.; Mao, X.M. Complex interplay and catalytic versatility of tailoring enzymes for efficient and selective biosynthesis of fungal mycotoxins. *J. Agric. Food Chem.* **2022**, *71*, 311–319. [CrossRef] [PubMed]
87. Mathieu, V.; Superchi, S.; Masi, M.; Scafato, P.; Kornienko, A.; Evidente, A. In vitro effects of fungal phytotoxins on cancer cell viability: First insight into structure activity relationship of a potent metabolite of *Cochliobolus australiensis* radicinin. *Toxins* **2022**, *14*, 517. [CrossRef]
88. Masi, M.; Meyer, S.; Clement, S.; Cimmino, A.; Cristofaro, M.; Evidente, A. Cochliotoxin, a dihydropyranopyran-4, 5-dione, and its analogues produced by *Cochliobolus australiensis* display phytotoxic activity against buffelgrass (*Cenchrus ciliaris*). *J. Nat. Prod.* **2017**, *80*, 1241–1247. [CrossRef]